Communication Disorders in Multicultural Populations

Second Edition

Dolores E. Battle, Ph.D.

Professor of Speech-Language Pathology,
Buffalo State College, Buffalo, New York

With 18 Contributing Authors

Butterworth–Heinemann
Boston Oxford Johannesburg Melbourne New Delhi Singapore

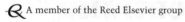

Library of Congress Cataloging-in-Publication Data

Communication disorders in multicultural populations / [edited by]
    Dolores E. Battle. -- 2nd ed.
        p.   cm.
    Includes bibliographical references and index.
    ISBN 0-7506-9825-X
    1. Communicative disorders--United States. 2. Intercultural
communication--United States. 3. Transcultural medical care--United
States.   I. Battle, Dolores E.
RC423.C6425   1997
616.85'5--dc21   97-26065
                                                                                          CIP

British Library Cataloguing-in-Publication Data
A catalogue record for this book is available from the British Library.

Contents

Contributing Authors

Noma Anderson, Ph.D.
Associate Professor and Chair of Communication Sciences and Disorders, Howard University, Washington, DC

Dolores E. Battle, Ph.D.
Professor of Speech-Language Pathology, Buffalo State College, Buffalo, New York

Li-Rong Lilly Cheng, Ph.D.
Assistant Dean of Global Program Development, Office of the President, and Professor of Communicative Disorders, San Diego State University

Eugene B. Cooper, Ed.D.
Professor and Chair Emeritus, Department of Communicative Disorders, University of Alabama, Tuscaloosa; Distinguished Professor, Programs in Communication Sciences and Disorders, Nova Southeastern University, Ft. Lauderdale, Florida

Crystal S. Cooper, M.S.
Adjunct Instructor, Programs in Communication Sciences and Disorders, Nova Southeastern University, Ft. Lauderdale, Florida

Priscilla Nellum Davis, Ph.D.
Professor of Audiology and Speech Pathology, University of Arkansas for Medical Sciences and University of Arkansas at Little Rock

Glenda DeJarnette, Ph.D.
Associate Professor of Communication Disorders, Southern Connecticut State University, New Haven

Betholyn Gentry, Ph.D.
Associate Professor of Audiology and Speech Pathology, University of Arkansas for Medical Sciences and University of Arkansas at Little Rock

Regina B. Grantham, M.Ed.
Assistant Professor, Department of Speech Pathology and Audiology, State University of New York at Cortland

Gail A. Harris, Ph.D.
President, Harris-Fox & Associates, Tucson, Arizona; Adjunct Assistant Professor of Special Education and Rehabilitation, University of Arizona, Tucson

R. Wayne Holland, Ed.D.
Executive Vice President and Chief Operating Officer, Lakeshore Communication Disorders Center, Inc., St. Clair Shores, Michigan

Pamela Hubbard-Wiley, Ph.D.
President, Los Angeles Speech and Language Therapy Center; Executive Director, Wiley Center for Speech and Language Development, Culver City, California

Hortencia Kayser, Ph.D.
Associate Professor of Speech and Language Pathology, New Mexico State University, Las Cruces

Njeri Nuru-Holm, Ph.D.
Vice President for Minority Affairs and Human Relations and Vice Provost for Student Affairs, Cleveland State University

Diane M. Scott, Ph.D.
Former Director of Office of Multicultural Affairs, American Speech-Language-Hearing Association, Rockville, Maryland

Sandra L. Terrell, Ph.D.
Professor of Speech and Hearing Sciences and Associate Dean, Toulouse School of Graduate Studies, University of North Texas, Denton

Gloriajean L. Wallace, Ph.D.
Professor, Department of Communication Sciences and Disorders, University of Cincinnati

W. Freda Wilson, Ph.D.
Speech Manager, Spartanburg Regional Health Care System, Spartanburg, South Carolina; Formerly Executive Director, Jeddah Institute for Speech and Hearing, Saudi Arabia

Toya Wyatt, Ph.D.
Associate Professor, Department of Speech Communication, California State University, Fullerton

Introduction

Change seems to be the only constant in the 1990s. What was new just a few years ago is obsolete today. The IBM 286 computer I used to prepare the first edition of this text is obsolete, having been replaced by a 100+ MHz Pentium PC, which will be out of date by the time this manuscript reaches the bookshelves. Changes in computer technology have overshadowed the changes that have occurred in the demographics of the United States in the last several years.

During the mid-1990s, the demographics of the United States continued to change dramatically as they had in the prior decade. People continued to immigrate to the United States from Europe, Asia, and Central and South America. The 1990s, however, have seen changes in the countries of origin of those coming to the United States. In the 1980s, the leading countries of origin of people immigrating to the United States were the United Kingdom, China, India, Korea, Philippines, Vietnam, and Mexico. In 1993, the Dominican Republic, Poland, and the countries formed from the former Soviet Union were added to the list of leading countries of origin of immigrants into the country (U.S. Bureau of the Census 1995). The number of people admitted to the United States from the African nations, including Ethiopia and Nigeria, in 1993 was nearly double the number admitted in each of the preceding 10 years (U.S. Bureau of the Census 1995). The number of people admitted from Iraq and other countries in the Middle East, including Jordan and Pakistan, in 1993 after the Gulf War was nearly six times the number admitted in each year of the previous decade. By the end of 1995, the U.S. population had grown to nearly 263 million people, of which 12.6% were African American; 10.3% were Hispanic; and 4.4% were American Indian, Aluet, or Pacific islanders (U.S. Bureau of the Census 1996).

The changes in the countries of origin of new arrivals to this country have increased the cultural diversity of the United States. *If the growth rates among those from non-European countries continue at the present rate, the minority groups will become the majority and the majority will become the minority (Cole 1989).* The changes have increased the need for speech-language pathologists to understand the communication and communication disorders of multicultural populations.

In recognition of the changing cultural makeup of the United States, the American Speech-Language-Hearing Association adopted the "Multicultural Action Agenda 2000" (American Speech-Language-Hearing Association 1991). One of its six objectives was "to institutionalize a commitment to sociocultural diversity throughout the Association and professions, particularly in the area of clinical practice, professional education, and research." This objective continues to be important to the professions of speech-language pathology and audiology because of the tremendous increase in cultural diversity in the United States and the greater increase that is projected well into the twenty-first century.

We must not assume that the many cultures coexisting in our society will assimilate into one melting pot. Indeed, it is this country's multicultural character that is one of its great strengths. We are one people under the law, yet we are so diverse in so many ways. As the population becomes increasingly diverse with respect to culture, language, values, and beliefs, speech-language and hearing professions will be increasingly called on to provide services to those from a wide variety of cultures, each with their own normative behaviors, learning styles, social beliefs, and world views. It is important that speech-language pathologists and audiologists be familiar with the cultures of the individuals they serve and that they use the different approaches necessary to assess and treat communication disorders.

This text provides a framework for speech-language pathologists and audiologists to develop an understanding of the many issues related to the provision of clinical services to those from various cultures and of various linguistic backgrounds.

Speech, language, and communication are embedded in culture; therefore, one cannot understand communication by a group without a thorough understanding of the cultural factors related to the group's communication. These factors are linked to the historical, geographic, social, and political histories that bind the group and provide its commonality. Understanding of a culture implies a fully developed sense of the complex web of meanings, perceptions, actions, symbols, and adaptations that make a people who they are. To understand and serve clients from diverse cultural backgrounds, it is important to understand the relationship between culture and communication and communication disorders. Recognizing this relationship will facilitate cross-cultural communication and improve the quality of service to all people in our multicultural society. This is the premise on which this text is built.

The authors in Part I of this text provide an overview of the major cultural groups in the United States, with particular reference to the factors that have had an impact on the assessment and treatment of communication disorders among members of these groups. The authors are leading experts in the study of communication disorders in their particular culture. Each presents a unique survey of the major cultural characteristics of the particular group, speech and language variables for the particular group, and the implications for assessment and intervention related to the group. The text begins with a chapter that stresses that the United States has always been a culturally diverse nation and shows how political and economic factors influenced the nation's development and the perceptions of its peoples. It develops concepts of barriers to assimilation and acculturation in relation to the United States' historical past as well as the present. The remainder of Part I focuses on the major cultural groups in contemporary America and the implications for assessment and intervention for those of the culture. Sandra L. Terrell, Regina B. Grantham, and I provide a comprehensive overview of African American culture. Li-Rong Lilly Cheng provides an extensive survey of Asian and Pacific cultures, their language behaviors, and the issues involved in their acculturation in the United States. She reviews the differences in learning styles of Asian and Pacific children and the impact of these differences on their learning in the United States. New to this edition is information about the cultures and languages of India, which is rapidly becoming one of the major countries of origin of immigrants to this country. Gail A. Harris provides a lesson in cultural diversity and communication disorders among American Indians. Hortencia Kayser discusses the salient cultural and linguistic factors that affect the assessment and treatment of communication disorders among those from Hispanic cultures. New to this edition is information about those from the Caribbean. Also new to this edition is a chapter that discusses the cultures of the Middle East and Northern Africa, areas with significantly increased immigration since the Gulf War. W. Freda Wilson, former director of the Jeddah Institute for Speech and Hearing in Saudi Arabia, provides valuable insights into Middle Eastern cultures and the implication for clinical services for people from this predominantly Muslim area.

Part II focuses on specific communication disorders in culturally and linguistically diverse populations. Noma Anderson and I present the issues related to family and child-rearing practices and the development of language in children of various cultural groups. Eugene B. and Crystal S. Cooper present a unique review of the role of culture in the assessment and treatment of dysfluency. New to this edition is a discussion of the growing body of literature on fluency disorders among bilingual individuals. The current research findings of the assessment and treatment of various cultural groups are presented by Glenda DeJarnette and R. Wayne Holland. Gloriajean L.

Wallace discusses cultural factors related to neurogenic disorders and includes in her chapter current information on communication and speech disorders related to acquired immunodeficiency syndrome, neonatal "crack" cocaine exposure, and traumatic brain injury in various cultural groups.

Part II continues with two chapters that discuss hearing, hearing disorders, and deafness. Diane M. Scott presents a comprehensive review of racial and ethnic diversity in hearing disorders and the implications for auditory assessment. Njeri Nuru-Holm and I present a comprehensive study of the Deaf culture in culturally and linguistically diverse populations. We discuss the interface between the Deaf culture and the cultures of the racially and ethnically diverse. Our treatment of the subculture of the Deaf minority is important reading for all who provide clinical services to hearing-impaired individuals from minority cultures.

The text concludes with two chapters devoted to clinical issues. Toya Wyatt adds her expertise for a new chapter on assessment of communication disorders in diverse cultures. Priscilla Nellum Davis and Betholyn Gentry, who have knowledge and experience with clients in the eastern parts of the United States, have collaborated with Pamela Hubbard-Wiley from culturally diverse California to provide guidelines and resources for successful intervention, including World Wide Web sites that contain cultural and clinical information.

Understanding another culture is a continuous and not a discrete process. This text introduces the reader to the variety of issues related to culture and communication disorders. It is intended to be a catalyst to encourage professionals to learn more about the clients they serve. Because the Unites States is a cultural mosaic, cultural knowledge will greatly facilitate cultural literacy. Cultural literacy requires systematic study to come to a level of cognitive consciousness. Cultural diversity involves far more than an understanding of language form and dialectical considerations. Because culture permeates every dimension of communication, the culturally competent professional must understand that most, if not all, truths are merely perceptions of truth viewed through the prism of culture. Learning to provide clinical services to those from cultures different from one's own involves far more than simply learning culture-specific information, which constitutes, at best, general cultural tendencies and, at worst, cultural stereotypes (e.g., "it is an African American tradition to ...," or "Japanese people are offended by ...," or "Navajo children are required to ..."). Instead, it involves establishing a framework for systematically analyzing cultural similarities as well as differences that can serve as a template to conduct ethnographic inquiries in the clinical setting.

I conclude by proposing several dos and don'ts to consider when treating those from different cultures. The list is not meant to be all inclusive, nor will all items be important for all groups in all circumstances. The items mentioned are meant to challenge the thinking of clinicians as they serve culturally and ethnically diverse clients.

1.   When communicating with individuals from cultural groups other than one's own, learn the name of that culture as assigned by its members, and use it. For example, use *Colombian* to describe a person from Colombia, not *Hispanic*. Use *Japanese* to describe a person from Japan, not *Asian*. Use *Nigerian* to describe a person from Nigeria, not *African*. Adherence to this simple rule will reduce unnecessary cultural conflicts at the outset of interactions. It will also help to reduce the dilemma faced in trying to decide whether to refer to a group as black or African American, Latino or Hispanic, Asian or Oriental, American Indian or Native American, or white or Caucasian.

2.   Do not use generic terms as substitutes or synonyms for more descriptive racial or ethnic terms to avoid using the term *nonwhite*. For example, avoid using *minority* to refer to African Americans, *bilingual* to refer to Hispanics, or *culturally diverse* or *multicultural*. In some areas, such as in Washington, DC, African Americans are not minorities. *Minority* may mean less than 50% to members of the numerical majority, but using the term may be perceived as a way of denigrating the importance of the numerical minority groups. One can be bilingual English-French, or English-Russian, or Spanish–American Sign Language. Remember that because we all are members of several cultural groups, we must all be multicultural. Surely, the term does not mean that only nonwhite non-Europeans have several cultural identities.

3.   Be aware of words, images, and situations that suggest that all or most members of a racial or ethnic group are the same without taking into account intragroup variations related to factors such as gender, age, socioeconomic status, and education. Do not assume that all African Americans speak African American English. Do not assume that standard English is spoken by all white Americans or only by white Americans. Do not assume that all African Americans share the same beliefs and cultural patterns. People with Caribbean roots, for example, have a different social and political history from people whose ancestors were brought to this country in captivity from Africa.

4.   Be aware that some terms have questionable or negative racial, ethnic, or socioeconomic connotations, such as *culturally deprived, at risk, minority,* and *culturally disadvantaged.* Such terms suggest that European Americans are the standard by which all else should be judged and are thus racist and ethnocentric. Do not assume that poverty is the exclusive characteristic of any one cultural group.

5.   Avoid using unnecessary qualifiers, clichés, and color-symbolic language that reinforce racial and ethnic stereotypes, such as the "articulate black student," "Chinese fire drill," "Indian giver," "white lie," "black sheep," and "yellow journalism."

6.   Be aware of the nonverbal sources of miscommunication between people from different cultural groups. These include such factors as the role of touch during conversation, distance between speakers, appropriate topics of conversations, and styles of greeting behavior. I contend that many of the sources of miscommunication between those from different cultural groups are not related to the particular words that are used or the phonologic or syntactic contrasts that exist between two languages, but are more deeply rooted in misunderstandings in role definition, communication style, and a lack of appreciation of the relation between culture and language.

7.   Be aware of verbal sources of miscommunication while communicating when people from other cultures. Such differences go beyond phonologic contrasts and reach to the very roots of the cultures themselves. The importance of the individual in relation to the group, for example, is an important cultural distinction that several authors discuss in this volume.

Every professional must accept the challenges to acquire new attitudes toward cultural diversity and to learn more about cross-cultural communication. If you are ready to commit yourself to an understanding of the issues before you in the changing face of America and you are open to finding new ways to function in a profession that is changing, I applaud you. It is critical to continue to develop the understandings and skills to function as a professional in a world sure to continue to change into the next century. It is through a better understanding of many cultures that we can better understand communication and communication disorders in a world that will never remain the same.

Dolores E. Battle, Ph.D.

References

American Speech Language Hearing Association. (1991). Multicultural Action Agenda 2000. *ASHA, 33(5),* 39–41.

Cole L E. (1989). E pluribus unum: Multicultural imperatives for the 1990's and beyond. *ASHA, 31(9),* 65–70.

U.S. Bureau of the Census. (1995). *Statistical abstract of the United States (115th ed.).* Washington, DC: U.S. Bureau of the Census.

U.S. Bureau of the Census. (1996). *Statistical abstract of the United States (116th ed.).* Washington, DC: U.S. Bureau of the Census.

I

Cultural Diversity: Implications for Speech-Language Pathologists and Audiologists

1

Communication Disorders in a Multicultural Society

Dolores E. Battle

Issues in Multiculturalism

Culture is about the behavior, beliefs, and values of a group of people who are brought together by their commonality. More important, culture is the lens through which one perceives and interprets the world (Vecoli 1995). It is the filter through which all that one does must pass before entering the collective conscious. Religion, language, customs, traditions, and values are but some of the components of culture. Speech, language, and communication are embedded in culture. Edward T. Hall (1959) said, "culture is communication. Communication is culture." Culture can be viewed as a system of competencies shared in broad design and deeper principles and varying among individuals. Its specificities are what an individual knows, feels, and thinks about his or her world. Culture is a theory of what one believes his or her fellows know, believe, and mean. It is more than a collection of symbols fit together by the analyst. It is a system of knowledge sharpened and constrained by the way the human brain acquires, organizes, and creates internal models of reality (Keesling 1974). Culture provides a system of knowledge that allows people of a cultural group to know how to communicate with one another.

The relationship between communication and culture is reciprocal: Culture and communication influence each other (Keesling 1974). Therefore, one cannot understand communication by a group of individuals without a thorough understanding of the ethnographic and cultural factors related to communication in that group. These factors are intricately embedded in the historic, geographic, social, and political history, which binds a group, gives it a sense of peoplehood, and gives it ethnic identity.

Because the roots of communication are embedded in culture, it is logical to assume that one cannot study communication or communication disorders without reference to the cultural, historical, or societal basis for the communication style or language used by the members of the ethnic or cultural group. The social rules of discourse and narratives (e.g., topic selection, who selects the topic, who initiates the conversation, who ends the conversation, distancing, eye gaze, and sense making) are culturally determined. Who speaks to whom, when, where, and about what must be understood in the context of the culture of both partners in the communicative event if the clinician is to determine the presence or absence of a communication disorder.

Communication behavior and the perception of what constitutes a communication disorder within a particular group are the products of cultural values, perceptions, attitudes, and history. These factors must be considered when determining the communication competence of a particular person within a group. For example, reluctance to speak and failure to initiate a conversation or use a particular narrative style can be appropriate to one culture but inappropriate to another. The impact of a voice disorder can be different for speakers of tonal languages than for speakers of nontonal languages. Expectations of the benefits of rehabilitation for the effects of stroke or traumatic brain injury can also differ across cultural groups.

Ethnicity refers to a shared culture that forms the basis for a sense of peoplehood based on the consciousness of a common past. Race, language, and ancestral customs constitute the major expressions of ethnicity in the United States. Ethnicity is not passed genetically from generation to generation. Rather, ethnicity is constructed and reconstructed in response to particular historical circumstances and changes. In its most intimate form, an ethnic group can be based on face-to-face relationships and political realities that mobilize its members into political self-determination. Joined by the aspirations for political self-determination, ethnicity is used to identify groups or communities that are differentiated by religious, racial, or cultural characteristics and that possess a sense of peoplehood.

Ethnography refers to the fully developed sense of the meaning of a culture and the complex manner in which one comes to understand the intricacies of the culture. The ethnographic understanding of a culture implies a fully developed sense of the complex web of meanings, perceptions, actions, symbols, and adaptations that make a people who they are.

Culture should not be confused with race. *Race* refers to the biological and anatomic attributes and functions, such as skin color, facial features, and hair texture. Two people can be of the same race but differ widely in cultural identity, personal history, and their view of the world. For example, a Korean child reared in a Korean family will have Korean cultural values; however, a Korean child adopted at birth by an African American family has the biological and genetic characteristics attributed to his or her genetic ancestors but has the cultural values imparted by the adoptive parents.

Culture is a term that implies the implicit and explicit behavior in a variety of areas. Explicit cultural behaviors are visible to the world and include observable features of dress, language, food preferences, customs, and lifestyle. Explicit behaviors are readily visible and often are used to identify the cultural group to observers. These behaviors are the focus of "culture-of-the-month" activities and programs. Implicit cultural variables are those factors that are not easily depicted and observed. They include such factors as age and gender roles within families, child-rearing practices, religious and spiritual beliefs, educational values, fears and attitudes, values and perceptions, and exposure to and adoption of other cultural norms. Implicit cultural values are beneath the surface, relatively invisible; however, they shape the fiber of those who identify as a member of a cultural group.

Multicultural is used to describe a society characterized by a diversity of cultures with varieties of religions, language, customs, traditions, and values.

Becoming a Multicultural Society in America

History of Immigration in America: 1500–1990

From its beginning, the United States has been a complex ethnic mosaic with a wide variety of communities differentiated by culture, race, religion, and language. From the beginning, the process of peopling this continent has been a story of cultural diversity brought about by immigration. Even the original American Indians walked across a land bridge from Siberia thousands of years ago. Thousands of years later, in 1500, the more than 4.5 million inhabitants of America were divided into hundreds of tribes, each with distinctive cultures, religions, and languages (Vecoli 1995).

Americans are immigrants or the descendants of immigrants. Immigration into America has been a long and continuous process. The early settlers came primarily from the European countries seeking political and religious freedom. They brought with them the ideals and values that formed the foundation of the social, educational, economic, and political systems of the United States. They were held together by shared political beliefs, principles, and practices that were common in Northern Europe. These common beliefs were melded to form the founding principles of the United States.

As the United States grew in economic strength, inexpensive labor became necessary, particularly in the rich farming areas of the Southern colonies and states. By the end of the eighteenth century, some 600,000 Europeans and Africans were recruited or enslaved and transported to the United States, where they contributed to the economic growth of the country.

When the first census was taken in 1790, the United States was already a nation of many cultures. Almost 19% of Americans were of African ancestry; 12% were Scottish and Scotch-Irish; and smaller amounts were German, French, Irish, Welsh, and Sephardic Jews (Vecoli 1995). The census did not include American Indians or Hispanics. Those counted as citizens of the United States comprised only 48% of the total population of the country.

To preserve the national ideals on which the nation was founded, the Naturalization Act of 1790 was passed. It specified that citizenship in the United States was open to "any alien, being a free white person," thus excluding from citizenship of the country those who were not white and those who were enslaved.

The First Wave of Immigration: 1841–1890

After the passing of the Naturalization Act of 1790, population growth in the United States, other than by natural increase, came primarily through three massive waves of immigration. During the first wave of documented immigration to the United States, which included the gold rush period of the 1850s, many Europeans came in search of a better economic opportunity. During this period, almost 15 million immigrants arrived, including 4 million immigrants from Germany after the failure of social reform, 3 million each from Ireland and Britain as a result of the potato famine of 1847, and 1 million from Scandinavia who were seeking land available through the Homestead Act. American capitalism became dependent on the rural workers of Europe, French Canada, Mexico, and Asia to support its factories and mines (Vecoli 1995; Morrison and Zabusky 1980).

By 1882, some Americans became concerned that the newcomers would pose a danger to "American" values and institutions. The slow evolution of a national policy on immigration resulted in a series of laws that progressively restricted immigration or reduced the rights of those who were new to the country (Morrison and Zabusky 1980). For example, The Chinese Exclusion Act of 1882 denied immigration to Chinese laborers and barred Chinese from acquiring citizenship. In addition, immigration laws established qualitative health and moral standards by excluding criminals, prostitutes, "lunatics," "idiots," and paupers from immigrating to the United States.

The Second Wave of Immigration: 1891–1920

The second wave of immigration occurred during the industrial revolution, when Europe was experiencing extreme poverty and political oppression. This wave brought an additional 18 million immigrants to the United States, including more than 4 million from Italy, 3.6 million from Austria-Hungary, and 3 million from Russia (Vecoli 1995).

In addition to the European immigration during this period, a large number of Asians, primarily from China and Japan, also entered the United States. These peoples had language, culture, social institutions, customs, and a collective experience that differed significantly from that of European immigrant groups. The concerns about the differences between Asians and Europeans culminated in the Immigration Acts of 1921 and 1924. These acts denied entry to aliens ineligible for citizenship (i.e., those who were not deemed white) and established national quota systems designed to reduce the number of Southern and Eastern Europeans entering the country and to bar Asians entirely. The laws attempted to freeze the biological and ethnic identity of the American people by reducing the influence from those not like the early immigrants who had gained political and economic power in the country.

The time between 1920 and 1945 marked a hiatus in immigration due to restrictive immigration policies, economic depression, and the effects of two world wars.

The postwar era brought a modest influx of immigrants, followed by a new surge of subsequent changes in laws and immigration policy. As a result, approximately 20,000 Russians and other displaced individuals immigrated to the United States immediately after World War II (Magocsi 1995). Although many Jews leaving Russia after the war were granted permission only to go to Israel, many hoped to go to the United States. By 1985, nearly 300,000 Jews had reached the United States and settled in the major cities of the Northeast (Magocsi 1995). Of the nearly 3 million Americans who identified themselves as wholly or partially Russian in the 1990 Census, nearly 44% resided in the Northeast (Magocsi 1995).

The Third Wave of Immigration: 1965–1990

Abhorring the racism of Nazism and stirred by the valor that the Asian Americans and African Americans showed in the fight to protect the freedom of America during the World War II and Korean War, the nation changed the way it thought about race and equality. A combination of international politics and democratic idealism resulted in the elimination of racial restrictions from American immigration and naturalization policies. The Civil Rights movement in the 1960s and the enactment of the Civil Rights Act of 1964 created a feeling of democratic idealism. The Immigration and Nationality Act of 1965 removed the national origin quotas and opened the United States to immigration from throughout the world by regional quotas. The unexpected consequence of the 1965 act was the beginning of the third wave of immigration. Not only did the total number of immigrants increase steadily to 1 million or more arriving each year, but also the countries of origin changed from being primarily European countries to those of Asia and Latin America (Vecoli 1995). Each year, 170,000 people were allowed to immigrate to the country from the eastern hemisphere, and 120,000 people were allowed to immigrate to the country from the western hemisphere. The Refugee Act of 1980 removed the geographic origin quotas, established an annual general quota of immigration at 270,000 and gave preferences to the family members of American citizens and resident aliens, skilled workers, and refugees.

The third wave of immigration differs from the previous two waves because the major countries of origin of the immigrants have changed. During the first two waves of immigration, almost 90% of the immigrants originated from Europe. During the 1980s, however, only 12% of the 7.3 million immigrants originated from European countries. Nearly 85% of the immigrants in the 1980s came from Asia and Latin America, with Mexico and China being the countries with the largest numbers of immigrants, respectively. More than 1.6 million people came from Mexico; another 4.5 million came from Central and South America and the Caribbean; and more than 2.8 million came from Asia (U.S. Bureau of the Census 1996).

According to the 1990 Census (U.S. Bureau of the Census 1990), immigrants from Asia and the Pacific island nations were well educated, with 70–80% having completed at least a high school education and approximately 50% having advanced degrees. More than 71% of the immigrants from the African countries of Nigeria, Egypt, and Ethiopia had at least a high school education, and 25% had college degrees. Although most of these immigrants are underemployed (i.e., employed in positions of lower income levels than expected based on their education) when they arrive, increased fluency in English and increased immersion into the American culture appear to greatly increase their economic success (U.S. Bureau of the Census 1996).

There was a significant increase of people immigrating to the United States from the Asian countries in the post-Korean war era of the 1970s and the post-Vietnam War era of the early 1980s. Many immigrants from Vietnam and Cambodia who came to the country as impoverished "boat people" had spent many years in refugee camps and did not have viable educations or technological skills before moving to the United States (Galens, et al. 1995).

Immigrants in the late 1980s and the 1990s from Europe, Asia, Central and South America, and the Caribbean came to the United States seeking refuge from political and economic difficulties in their home countries. Between 1980 and 1990, the Hispanic population in the United States grew by 36%, with major countries of origin being Mexico, Haiti, Dominican Republic, and Cuba (U.S. Bureau of the Census 1996).

Immigration in the 1990s

As shown in Table 1-1, immigration into the United States has continued into the 1990s. Between 1991 and 1993, more than 438,000 people from European countries immigrated to the United States, the largest group (159,200) being from the Soviet Union. More than 1 million immigrated from Asian countries, including 192,000 from Vietnam, 182,000 from the Philippines, 137,000 from China, and nearly 122,000 from India (U.S. Bureau of the Census 1996). Nearly 2 million immigrated from North America, including 1.3 million from Mexico and 337,000 from the Caribbean countries (U.S. Bureau of the Census 1996). In 1994, the 10 countries of origin with the largest number of legal immigrants to the United States were the countries of the former Soviet Union, Vietnam, the former Yugoslavia, Laos, Iraq, Somalia, Haiti, Cuba, Sudan, and Iran (U.S. Department of Health and Human Services 1994). Although the largest group continued to be from the Asian and European countries, a significant number of immigrants to the country in 1994 were from the Middle East, Africa, and the Caribbean. When the United States Immigration Services estimates of approximately 3.5–4.0 million undocumented immigrants are added to the actual Census data, it becomes clear why the population projections for nonwhite people in the United States are expected to dramatically increase in this country well into the next century (Fernandez and Robinson 1994).

In addition to the documented legal immigrants to the United States, there are many undocumented or illegal immigrants. A large number of undocumented immigrants who enter the country illegally are from Mexico; however, many undocumented immigrants have origins in El Salvador, Guatemala, Canada, Haiti, Poland, and the Philippines (Fernandez and Robinson 1994). The overwhelming majority of legal immigrants in 1994 settled in California and New York (27,379 and 20,892, respectively). Many also settled in Texas, Washington, Illinois, Florida, Pennsylvania, Massachusetts, Georgia, and Michigan (U.S. Bureau of the Census 1996).

In addition to those illegally crossing the borders, a large number of undocumented immigrants who enter the country as students, tourists, or temporary workers simply stay in the country after their visas have expired. More than 250,000 Chinese intellectuals, scientists, and engineers have come to the United States for advanced degrees and have stayed after their visas expired or have applied for alien resident status. The result of the dramatic increase in immigration shows considerable diversity in the demographic make-up of America, as shown in the demographic data from the 1995 Census reports in Tables 1-1 and 1-2.

Table 1-1   Immigration to the United States by Country of Birth: 1991–1994

Region or country of origin	Number of immigrants (in thousands)
North America	2,168.6
Mexico	1,397.9
Caribbean	441.8
Central America	266.7
Europe	599.8
Soviet Union (former)	222.6
Poland	100.5
United Kingdom	69.0
Asia	1,366.1
Vietnam	234.0
Philippines	241.6
China	191.5
India	156.8
South America	236.6
Colombia	56.5
Peru	45.8
Guyana	36.8
Africa	117.7
Nigeria	20.9
Ethiopia	18.9
Egypt	16.1

Source: Adapted with permission from the U.S. Bureau of the Census. (1996). *Statistical abstract of the United States: 1996 (116th ed.). No. 8: Immigrants, by country of birth: 1971 to 1994*. Washington, DC: U.S. Bureau of the Census.

Population Projections

National estimates of population growth provide a compelling glimpse of the face of the new America. It is estimated that the increase in immigration will continue well into the twenty-first century. If middle population estimates of population changes between 1995 and 2020 are used, the United States population will increase by 8.5% from 1995 to 2020 (U.S. Bureau of the Census 1996). It is projected that by 2020, the white popula-

Table 1-2   Population of the United States by Race: 1995 (Estimated)

Race	Number of residents (in thousands)
White	218,085
African American	33,141
American Indian, Eskimo, Aleut	2,242
Asian/Pacific islander	9,287
Hispanic origin	26,994
Total	263,034

Source: Adapted with permission from the U.S. Bureau of the Census. (1996). *Statistical abstract of the United States: 1996 (116th ed). No. 12: Resident population-selected characteristics: 1970–1995, and No. 2 population: 1950–1995* (pp. 8). Washington, DC: U.S. Bureau of the Census.

tion will increase by 2.4%; however, the African American population will increase by 11.9%, the American Indian population by 13.1%, Asian and Pacific islander population by 26.4%, and Hispanic/Latino population by 26.4% by 2020 (U.S. Bureau of the Census 1996).

First- and second-generation immigrant children are the fastest-growing segment of the United States population younger than age 15 years (Fix and Zimmerman 1993). In 1990, the United States Census counted 2.1 million foreign-born children in the United States (Fix and Passel 1994). Adding second-generation immigrants to that total boosts the number of immigrant children and children of immigrants to more than 5 million. The total school-age population is expected to grow by more than 20%, from 34 million in 1990 to 42 million in 2010 (Fix and Passel 1994). It is estimated that the children of new immigrants will account for more than half of this growth. The number of children of immigrants is expected to rise to 9 million in 2010, representing 22% of the school-age population (Fix and Passel 1994).

Acculturation and Assimilation

Models of Assimilation

Tens of millions of immigrants with differing cultures have been incorporated into American society by the processes of acculturation and assimilation. Acculturation is the process by which newcomers assume American cultural attributes, such as the English language, cultural norms, behaviors, and values. Assimilation is the process of their incorporation into the social and cultural networks of the host society, including work, place of residence, leisure activities, and family. It refers to the process of giving up one's culture and taking on the characteristics of another. Primarily three models of assimilation and acculturation have been used to explain cultural diversity in America.

Anglo-Conformity Model

The Anglo-conformity model of acculturation and assimilation has been favored through much of the history of this country. Convinced of their cultural and biological superiority, early Americans passed laws restricting immigration and citizenship to those from Western Europe. Nonwhite people were expected to abandon their distinctive cultural, religious, and linguistic values and practices and conform to the American model. The "American way" was considered the "only" way. Immigrants strove to adopt as much of the American culture as possible so that they could gain the economic and political benefits of being "American." The immigrants believed that the sooner they assimilated into the American culture, the sooner and easier they could share the riches of America. In their eagerness to become Americans, they either rejected or altered family names and the languages and customs of the "old country" (Morrison and Zabusky 1980).

Melting Pot Model

A competing model of acculturation and assimilation, the melting pot model, is a process whereby, in as much as possible, the elements of culture brought by the immigrants are transmuted into a new American culture that embodies cultural variants. The result is an amalgam of the varied cultures and peoples in which no single culture is dominant and all blend into a rich whole. The melting pot ideology provided a rationale for the more liberal immigration policies in the late 1960s. The policy came under attack, however, as the determination of the ethnic groups to retain their individual identity, traditions, and customs increased.

Cultural-Pluralism Model

The cultural-pluralism model has been offered as an alternative to the meltingpot model in the 1990s. It has been viewed as an internal attitude that predisposes, but does not make compulsory, the display of ethnic identification in interactions. In the cultural-pluralism model, it is valued and accepted to maintain ethnic identity. Although sharing a common American citizenship and loyalty, ethnic groups maintain and foster their particular languages, customs, and cultural values. Cultural pluralism recognizes diversity within the nation.

Levels of Adaptation and Assimilation

The independent variable in the process of acculturation and assimilation is the determination or willingness of the immigrants to assume the culture of America. The degree of adaptation and assimilation varies with each individual and with each group of immigrants. For example, the early immigrants in the first two waves of immigration, influenced by the immigration and naturalization policies of the time, made great efforts to acculturate and assimilate into the fabric of America. The level of assimilation is an important factor to consider in understanding clients and their families. Cheng and Butler (1993) describe six levels of adaptation and assimilation that affect culturally and linguistically diverse immigrants.

At the first level, reaffirmation, the people reject the new culture and attempt to maintain or revive native cultural traditions. Chain migrations and preferences in immigration policies allow relatives and friends to group for mutual assistance. They maintain their customary ways by establishing churches, societies, and newspapers and build institutions and communities that reflect and retain their cultural values and language.

At the second level, people attempt to synthesize a selective combination of cultural aspects of both cultures. For example, they may accept the dress and food of the new culture but retain the native view of health care and education. Through selective assimilation and adaptation, immigrants take from the American culture what they need to survive and keep traditional cultural beliefs and practices that they value. Although many may gradually adapt the parts of the American culture they chose, many hold dear the culture and language of their ancestors. Rather than shed old-country customs, the new immigrants may enroll their children in "cultural schools." Cultural schools ensure that children do not forget the customs of the past. Such schools allow children to adopt ancestral names and to continue speaking their native language in the home, thus ensuring that America remains a culturally pluralistic country.

At the third level, withdrawal, people may reject and withdraw from their native culture or the new culture because of cultural conflict. People who reject their native culture become isolated from their cultural peers and do not maintain relationships with individuals other than immediate family members. People who withdraw from the new culture do not learn the language or culture of the new country. Depending on the level of assimilation, these people may experience loneliness and fear when attempts are made to engage in activities and associations to increase adaptation to the new culture.

People at the constructive-marginality level tentatively accept the two cultures but do not fully integrate into either one. They may feel that they do not belong in either culture and may not be sure of which cultural rule or language to use in a situation.

The biculturalism level refers to the full involvement of both cultures. Bicultural individuals retain fluency in the native language and obtain fluency in the new language. They are equally comfortable functioning in either culture and can switch between the cultures with relative ease.

At the compensatory-adaptation level, people become thoroughly mainstreamed into the new culture, rejecting and avoiding identification with the native culture and language. Young adolescents and young adults at this level reject any knowledge of the native country and try to be as American as possible. They are anxious to learn the new language and cultural expectations as quickly and as thoroughly as possible. They may enroll in accent-reduction programs to remove any trace of their native language in their newly adopted language.

Barriers to Assimilation and Acculturation

There are several barriers to assimilation and acculturation, even for those who intend to be fully assimilated into the American mainstream. Many immigrants experience only limited acculturation and practically no assimilation in their lifetimes. Among the factors that affect the process of acculturation and assimilation are circumstances of immigration, race and ethnicity, class, gender, and the character of community.

Voluntary immigrants, involuntary immigrants, and refugees differ in their circumstances of immigration. Voluntary immigrants are usually prepared for the move, psychologically motivated, and willing to accept the linguistic and cultural changes required to succeed in the new country. Involuntary immigrants, such as those brought to this country in slavery, were resistant to their new circumstances and suffered social and political isolation from the political mainstream that hampered their attempts at assimilation. Refugees, on the other hand, are forced to leave their country because of adverse domestic, social, or political conditions. Preparation for the move is limited, and many enter the country without knowledge of the language or culture of the receiving country. Like involuntary immigrants, they may have been separated from their families and may have spent days or years in unpleasant circumstances before having access to the benefits of the receiving country. As a result, the effects of culture shock are more pervasive on refugees than on voluntary immigrants. Thus, refugees usually achieve low levels of assimilation into the receiving country, do not become proficient in English, and live in ethnic enclaves for longer periods of time (Ima and Keogh 1995).

Race, especially skin color, has been a dominant factor in barriers to assimilation and acculturation for Asians, Hispanics, African Americans, and Native Americans. Among the important factors limiting acculturation and assimilation is the willingness of the dominant culture to accept those perceived as different. Because it is relatively easy to identify those who differ from the mainstream whites by race and skin color, it has been relatively more difficult for African Americans and some Asian Americans to assimilate into the American mainstream.

Other factors also affect acculturation and assimilation. Differences in religious practices, particularly those that require dress codes and religious observances that differ from the Christian mainstream and language, have been construed as barriers to assimilation and acculturation. Social class, dictated largely by economic factors, has also limited interactions among different ethnic groups and has limited assimilation and acculturation along social class and ethnic lines. Traditional roles for women in various ethnic groups have restricted the acculturation and assimilation experience for some women.

The density of the population and the location of the immigrant communities influence the rate and character of incorporation of some immigrants into the mainstream culture. Most immigrants live in densely populated areas of California, Texas, New York, Florida, New Jersey, and Illinois (U.S. Bureau of the Census 1996; Fix and Zimmerman 1993). Seventy-eight percent of all recent immigrant children attend school in just five states—California, Florida, Illinois, New York, and Texas—with 45% attending school in California (Board on Children and Families 1995). Concentration of immigrants in communities in urban cities of the Northeast and in isolated communities of the South and Midwest limits contact between immigrants and mainstream Americans and tends to inhibit the processes of acculturation and assimilation. It can be assumed that adults who remain at home or are employed within the community are more likely to hold customs, language, values, and beliefs of the country of origin than children who attend school or adults who are employed outside the community.

The children and grandchildren of immigrants retain fewer of the ancestral cultural values than their ancestors. This is largely due to attendance in public schools and the interaction with children from other cultures. The language of the home is often lost or does not keep pace with the growing language skills necessary for academic achievement. Although some second- and third-generation immigrants choose to abandon their ancestral customs and traditions, many retain a sense of identity and affiliation with their ethnic group through family and community ties.

The models for assimilation and acculturation have come into question in recent years. As the United States approaches the twenty-first century, its future as an ethnically plural society is questioned. There is need for a new paradigm that encompasses the faith of all Americans by embracing them in their many diversities.

Cultural Diversity in a New America

The three waves of immigration, the adoption of the cultural-pluralism model, and the barriers to acculturation and assimilation have resulted in an America that is culturally and linguistically diverse. The 1990 United States Census report on ancestry identified more than 215 ancestral groups in response to the question "What is your ancestry of ethnic origin?" (Vecoli 1995; U.S. Bureau of the Census 1990). The largest ancestral groups reported were, in order of magnitude, German, Irish, English, and African American. Each of these groups contained more than 20 million people (Vecoli 1995). Groups reporting more than 6 million people were Italian, Mexican, French, Polish, Native American, Dutch, and Scotch-Irish groups; another 28 groups reported more than 1 million each. The rich complexity of diversity in America is marked by the plethora of groups that reported fewer than 1 million members each, including Hmong, Maltese, Honduran, Carpatho-Rusyns, Nigerian, and Egyptian groups (U.S. Bureau of the Census 1990).

Religious Diversity

The importance of religious diversity to the founding of the United States is shown in the guarantee of religious freedom in the First Amendment to the Constitution. Many early settlers came to the country in search of religious freedom. They were primarily Protestants of many denom-inations and sects. Groups who came for religious freedom were Irish, German, Italian, Eastern European, and, more recently, Hispanic Roman Catholics. The Slavic Christian and Jewish immigrants from Central and Eastern Europe established Judaism and orthodoxy as major religious bodies. As a result of Near East and African immigration, as well as the conversion of many African Americans, there are currently nearly 3 million Muslims in the United States. Smaller numbers of Buddhists, Hindus, and followers of other religions have contributed to religious pluralism. Each religion has its own beliefs and practices that affect the identification of communication disorders and the delivery of services to those with communication disorders.

All cultural or ethnic groups have definable implicit characteristics in universal categories of behavior, including views toward education and health care. Many of these beliefs are embedded in religion. Health care in Western or European cultures is based on germ theory (i.e., the theory that a disease or disorder is caused by a germ or a physical malady within the body). To restore health, one must destroy the germ or repair malfunction of the body. For example, by the study of genetics, European medicine hopes to identify the gene related to certain disorders, and, by controlling or altering the genetic structure, control the emergence of the disorder. Also, by attempting to identify a specific virus that causes a disease, scientists hope to develop vaccines to control, or a medicine to cure, the disease. If one can identify the germs or viruses causing or related to the disease, one can control the disease or effect a cure. Those who hold this view of medicine are more likely to seek medical care through medicine or rehabilitation.

Non-European, and often Eastern, views of health care see a connection between illness and internal forces. People who have this point of view believe that health is the result of physical or spiritual harmony with nature and that illness and disease are the result of spiritual or internal disharmony. Eastern medicine and health care is intended to restore harmony. Those with this belief are more likely to seek relief through prayer, incantations, or religious ceremony than through medicine, rehabilitation, or therapy.

Other cultural groups see disease as the result of a specific punishment for an ill deed or religious failing. People with these beliefs are more likely to accept a disorder or illness as a burden that they are obligated to bear. These people do not usually seek assistance from a person who does not share their cultural beliefs (Cole 1989).

Linguistic Diversity

As shown in Table 1-3, according to data from the 1990 Census, there are 26 languages other than English spoken at home by nearly 32 million people 5 years of age and older in the United States (U.S. Bureau of the Census 1996). Although Spanish is the most commonly spoken language other than English, other languages spoken by more than 1 million residents include French, German, Italian, and Chinese. Many other languages are spoken by fewer than 1 million residents. For example, there are more than 100 languages spoken in the school systems of New York, Chicago, Los Angeles, and Fairfax County, VA (Fix and Zimmerman 1993).

The U.S. Census Bureau (1990) estimated that 1.8 million school-age children live in households in which no one older than age 14 speaks English well. Although these figures are not restricted to immigrant children, they contribute to the number of children who are identified as limited English proficient (LEP).

Table 1-3   Languages Spoken at Home by People 5 Years of Age and Older

Language	Number of speakers (in thousands)
Speak only English	198,601
Spanish	17,339
French	1,702
German	1,547
Italian	1,309
Chinese	1,249
Tagalog	843
Polish	723
Korean	626
Vietnamese	507
Portuguese	430
Japanese	428
Greek	388
Arabic	355
Hindi (Urdu)	331
Russian	242
Yiddish	213
Thai (Laotian)	206
Persian	202
French Creole	188
Armenian	150
Navaho	149
Hungarian	148
Hebrew	144
Dutch	143
Mon-Khmer (Cambodian)	127
Gujarathi	102

Source: Adapted with permission from the U.S. Bureau of the Census. (1995). *Statistical abstract of the United States: 1995 (115th ed). No. 57: Persons speaking a language other than English at home by age and language: 1990* (pp. 5). Washington, DC: U.S. Bureau of the Census.

As shown in Table 1-4, the number of people who speak English "less than well" increases with age from 37.8% of school-age children to 47.2% for those older than 65 years of age (U.S. Bureau of the Census 1996). The same pattern is shown for those who speak Asian languages at home. This has implications for the assessment and intervention of older Americans, who are at greater risk for neurologic disease and hearing impairment.

Communication Disorders in a Multicultural Society

The need for speech-language pathologists and audiologists to understand communication disorders in a multicultural society was recognized soon after the passing of the Civil Rights Act in 1964. There was a growing concern that African American children who spoke African American English were being inappropriately classified as having speech-language disorders. Speech-language pathologists and sociolinguists began the study of communication disorders in multicultural populations in response to the need for understanding the linguistic skills of African American children in schools. In recognition of the growing concern, the American Speech-Language-Hearing Association (ASHA) adopted a position paper on social dialects (American Speech-Language-Hearing Association 1983) that recognized that any dialect of English was a legitimate form of the language and that dialect was not to be considered a pathologic form of English.

Although initially the concern was for African Americans, the need to study cultural diversity in communication disorders grew in direct relationship to the third wave of U.S. immigration, the non-European cultural origins of the new immigrants, and the changes in acculturation and assimilation patterns of the new immigrants.

Not only did the increase in immigration population that began in the 1970s continue into the 1980s and 1990s, the new immigrants were also more diverse than before, arriving from a broad spectrum of countries encompassing a range of linguistic variables and increasingly non-European cultural backgrounds. Concerns about cultural and linguistic diversity that once were directed at African American children were related to other ethnic minority groups. In 1985, ASHA published the *Clinical Management of Communicatively Handicapped Minority Language Populations* in recognition of the need to address the needs of those from various cultural and linguistic backgrounds in speech-language and hearing programs (American Speech-Language-Hearing Association 1985).

Table 1-4   People 5 Years of Age and Older Who Speak a Language Other Than English at Home, and Those Who Speak English Less Than "Very Well" by Age and Language: 1990

Age group and language spoken at home	People who speak the language (in thousands)	Percent who speak English less than "very well"
People 5 years old and older	**230,446**	X
Speak only English	198,601	X
Speak other language	31,845	43.9
Speak Spanish or Creole	17,345	47.9
Speak Asian/Pacific island	4,472	54.1
Speak a language other than Asian, Pacific island, Spanish, or English	10,028	32.4
People 5–17 years old	**45,344**	X
Speak only English	39,020	X
Speak other language	6,324	37.8
Speak Spanish or Spanish Creole	4,168	39.3
Speak Asian or Pacific island	816	44.2
Speak a language other than Asian, Pacific island, Spanish, or English	1,340	29.2
People 18–64 years and over	**153,908**	X
Speak English only	132,200	X
Speak other language	21,708	45.1
Speak Spanish or Spanish Creole	12,121	49.6
Speak Asian/Pacific island	3,301	54.7
Speak a language other than Asian, Pacific island, or Spanish	6,286	31.4
People 65 years old and older	**31,195**	X
Speak English only	27,381	X
Speak other language	3,814	47.2
Speak Spanish or Spanish Creole	1,057	62.3
Speak Asian or Pacific island	355	72.0
Speak a language other than Asian, Pacific island, Spanish, or English	2,402	36.9

X = Not applicable.

Source: Adapted with permission from U.S. Bureau of the Census. (1990). *Statistical abstract of the United States: 1995 (115th ed.). No. 57: Persons speaking a language other than English at home, by age and language: 1990* (pp. 53). Washington, DC: U.S. Bureau of the Census.

Communication Disorders in Culturally Diverse Populations

There are little reliable data on the general prevalence or incidence of communication disorders among culturally and linguistically diverse populations in the United States. Estimates are based on projections from data based on the mainstream population. The National Health Interview Survey indicates that there is a greater prevalence of communication disorders among racial and ethnic minorities than among whites (Benson and Marano 1994). ASHA estimates that 10% of the United States population has a disorder of speech, hearing, or language unrelated to the ability to speak English as a native language (Cole 1989). If the prevalence of communication disorders among racial and ethnic minorities is consistent with that of the general population, it is estimated that 6.2 million culturally and linguistically diverse Americans have a communication disorder.

Diversity Among Children in Special Education

According to the U.S. Office of Special Education Programs (1994), 23% of the children served under the Individuals with Disabilities Education Act (IDEA) have speech or language impairments as their primary disability, with significantly more children having speech or language impairment secondary to learning disability, mental retardation, emotional disturbance, or other disability.

One of the more controversial aspects of providing services to culturally and linguistically diverse students is the disproportionate placement of culturally and linguistically diverse students in the various categories of disability. A comparison of ethnic representation in four categories of disabilities based on a 1990 survey by the Office of Civil Rights (Table 1-5) shows that the classification of disability among the African American population is considerably greater than that expected for the American school-age population (U.S. Office of Special Education Programs 1994). Although only 16% of the school population in the United States is African American, 21% of all children classified as seriously emotionally disturbed are African American. African Americans also make up 17% of children classified as learning disabled and 35% of children classified as mildly mentally retarded (Reschly 1996).

Hispanic children are less likely than expected to be identified as learning disabled. Although 12% of the school population is Hispanic, only 11% of those students classified as learning disabled are Hispanic, 6% of those classified as seriously emotionally disturbed are Hispanic, and 8% of those classified as mildly retarded are Hispanic (see Table 1-5) (Reschly 1996).

Table 1-5   Percent of Students by Race/Ethnicity Receiving Special Education Under Selected Categories of Disability

	Asian	Native American	Hispanic	African American	White
Percent of all students (disabled and nondisabled)	3	1	12	16	68
Of students with mild mental retardation, percentage from each ethnic group	<1	<1	8	35	56
Of students with speech impairment, percentage from each ethnic group	1	2	9	16	72
Of students seriously emotionally disturbed, percentage from each ethnic group	<1	<1	6	21	71
Of students who are learning disabled, percentage from each ethnic group	1	1	11	17	70

Sources: Adapted from the Office of Civil Rights. (1992). *The national and state summaries of data from the 1990 Elementary and Secondary School Civil Rights Survey.* Washington, DC: Office of Civil Rights; and Office of Special Education Programs. (1994). *Implementation of the Individuals with Disabilities Education Act: Sixteenth annual report to Congress.* (pp. 198, 201). Washington, DC: U.S. Department of Education.

However, the National Association of State Directors of Special Education (1992) reports that Hispanics were the only ethnic minority group to show an increase in enrollment in special education programs. Enrollment increased from 10% in 1986 to 12% in 1990. The Hispanic population in special education is projected to increase 38% by the year 2000.

Common causes given for the disproportionate representation of African Americans and Hispanics in special education include (1) poverty, (2) cultural bias in referral and assessment, and (3) unique factors related to race and ethnicity. Reschly (1996) and Wagner and Blackorg (1996) implicate poverty and the lack of access to health care caused by poverty with resulting low birth weight as factors that affect a population's representation in special education programs. According to the U.S. Department of Health and Human Services (1985), economically disadvantaged children are more predisposed to disorders related to environmental, teratogenic, nutritional, and traumatic factors than other groups. For example, exposure to carbon monoxide and other chemicals and pesticides found in the air, paint, soil, and plumbing of older homes often located in poverty areas has teratogenic effects on the neurologic functions of young children.

The incidence of neurologic impairment, some of which lead to communication disorders, due to the absorption of lead has been found to be higher in nonwhite children than in white children (National Center for Health Statistics 1994). In addition, although some people from ethnic minority communities have the same type of communication disorders as those in the dominant population, incidences, causes, and effects can be different, indicating different approaches to treatment. For example, African Americans succumb to stroke 306 times more often than whites, and strokes occur in blacks at an earlier age (Singletary 1993). Although 11% of the deaths among white Americans are from stroke, 13% of the deaths among African Americans are from stroke (U.S. Department of Health and Human Services 1985). Death rates from hemorrhage, thrombosis, and embolism (the major types of strokes) are higher for blacks than for whites (Singletary 1993). This is thought to be related to increases in hypertension, differences in diet, and lack of access to health care.

Access to Health Care

Access to health care and health insurance is a critical issue for the immigrant population in the United States. This issue affects the physical and mental well-being of families, as well as the ability to adapt to the culture of the United States. For many immigrants, especially children, the immigration process itself is an event of extraordinary stress. Immigrants are often torn by conflicting social and cultural demands while trying to adapt to an unfamiliar and sometimes hostile and discriminatory environment with limited or no use of the English language. In addition, undocumented immigrants deal with the stress or fear of deportation and separation from family members.

For some immigrants, health worsens in the United States. A study of aggregate data across all immigrant groups found that on virtually every measure of health status, immigrants who had lived in the United States 5 years or less were healthier than those who had lived in the United States more than 10 years (Rumbaut 1995). The findings were explained by a number of factors, including (1) existing physical conditions that were masked during the early years after immigration, (2) deterioration of health due to limited access to health care, and (3) socioeconomic factors. The data point to the importance of identifying conditions under which immigrants do well and those that produce negative health outcomes. Among the factors to consider are family networks and social supports, relationships within families, the effect of mobility on children's lives, segmented assimilation into different kinds of contexts, and cultural medical practices from the country of origin.

Rumbaut (1995) found that generation effects and length-of-residence effects have confirmed associations between these variables and health. For example, difficult pregnancies, low birth weight, and infant mortality increased among Hispanic populations with subsequent immigrant generations in the United States. In contrast, Indo-Chinese immigrants in San Diego County, who appeared to be at risk for poor infant health due to high levels of unemployment, poverty, welfare dependence, and depression, were found to have much lower infant mortality rates than the average resident in San Diego County. This was explained by the nearly universal absence of tobacco, alcohol, and drug abuse among Indo-Chinese women, even though they had less access to prenatal care.

Becoming a Clinician in a Multicultural Society and Understanding Cultural Variables

Understanding another culture is a continuous, not a discrete, process. Identifying the sources of cultural conflict while providing clinical services to those from cultures different from one's own involves far more than learning about the implicit and explicit variables of a culture. It is important for speech-language pathologists and audiologists to understand the importance of potential sources of cultural conflict in the clinic.

Monocultural assumptions in providing clinical services are not relevant for the 1990s and will not be relevant in the coming century. Most literature on communication disorders, intervention, and treatment in multicultural populations assumes that the clinician is a member of the majority culture and that the client is a member of a minority culture. This is a logical conclusion, because less than 5% of the members of the American Speech-Language-Hearing Association identify themselves as nonwhite. It is more accurate to take a broad view of the use of the term multicultural or cross-cultural clinical services. The clinician and the client may differ by culture, racial and ethnic group, sex, age, socioeconomic class, gender, or religion, to name but a few cultural variables that can affect the clinical interaction. The clinician must look to the various parameters of differences, as well as those of similarity, and construct the clinical management program accordingly. Clinicians understand that they must understand their own culture and their own cultural assumptions, as well as those of the client. Whether there is a cultural conflict must be considered in the interaction. The culturally competent clinician seeks continuous self-assessment regarding cultural differences. The clinician needs knowledge and resources to be competent to provide clinical services in an increasingly culturally diverse world.

In becoming a culturally competent clinician, it is important to consider both culture-bound variables and language-communication bound variables. Culture-bound conceptualizations have many variables. Among the most important in studying communication disorders in multicultural society are the importance of individuals and groups in the culture, power and distance, time orientation, and several dimensions of verbal and nonverbal communication.

Individualism and Collectivism

Individualism emphasizes the individual. In collectivism, on the other hand, group goals have precedence over individual goals. Individuals from individualistic cultures are supposed to look after themselves and their immediate family. Individuals from cultures of collectivism look after the needs of the entire group in their social network. Although individualism and collectivism exist in every culture in varying degrees, cultures in which individualism tends to predominate include, but are not limited to, the European countries. Cultures in which collectivism tends to predominate include, but are not limited to, Arab, African, Asian, and Hispanic cultures (Brislin 1994). Individualism and collectivism play an important role in clinical encounters. These factors affect both the client's willingness to establish individual goals and expectations for the individual or the family or group.

The Power-Distance Variable

The power-distance variable focuses on the social relationships between people of different statuses (i.e., superiors and subordinates). This can extend to relationships between men and women. People from high power-distance cultures do not question the orders or suggestions of superiors. On the other hand, people in low power-distance cultures do not necessarily accept superiors' orders. When the clinician and the client are from two different systems, misunderstanding in making and following clinical recommendations is possible.

Time Orientation

Time orientation differs across cultures. When the culture is long term and future oriented, the establishing of long-term goals and priorities is highly valued. When the focus of the culture is on the past, the establishment of long-term goals is not as relevant as preserving the present and the establishment of short-term, more readily attainable, goals. Western cultures are more often oriented toward the future. Many non-Western cultures are focused on the past, as shown by their respect for elders and ancestors.

Nonverbal and Verbal Communication Styles

Language and communication style are highly correlated with race, culture, and ethnicity. All ethnic groups have communication styles that have major implications for clinical services. These language differences have both verbal and nonverbal dimensions.

Nonverbal Communication Styles

In nonverbal communication, information is transmitted by means other than words. This can involve many behaviors, including proxemics, kinesics, eye contact, paralanguage, silence, and directness. Proxemics, or the use of personal space and conversational distance in communication, differs across cultures. Kinesics, or the use of body movements, including facial expressions, smiling, head positioning and nodding, hand shaking, and eye contact, has also been shown to differ across cultures (Battle 1997). In addition, paralanguage variables, such as silence, loudness, inflection, and stress, vary across cultures and can affect the clinical relationship.

Verbal Communication Styles

Verbal communication can also vary across cultures. In addition to the barriers created by differences in the linguistic contrasts between the languages of the client and the clinician, differences in word meanings can affect the clinical encounter. The meanings of words such as *bad* or *normal* can vary across cultures. Pragmatics, or the way language is used in greeting, taking compliments, and more ritualized social rules, can affect the clinical encounter. Social distance can also affect the role that the individuals play in the communication process. In Western cultures, conversation tends to be horizontal, with each person in the communication event having equal responsibility and freedom within the conversation. In non-Western cultures, patterns of communication tend to be vertical, with conversation flowing from those of higher prestige to those of lower prestige (Battle 1997; Sue and Sue 1990).

Conclusion

In becoming a culturally competent clinician, it is important to develop an awareness of the beliefs and attitudes held by the clinician and by the clients. Multicultural awareness is not an end in itself. It is, rather, a means of increasing a clinician's power, energy, and freedom of choice in a multicultural world (Pedersen 1988; Lynch and Hanson 1992). Clinicians need to become culturally aware of their own values and beliefs before they can adjust to the value system of others. Clinicians should understand and value the differences that exist among clients and should develop an awareness of the cultural, verbal, and nonverbal factors that influence the clinical situation. In developing a cultural awareness, the clinician should ask, "What can I do to serve this client in a culturally appropriate manner?" and "How can I best serve this client according to his or her cultural, as well as clinical, needs?"

Clinicians must develop an understanding of the sociopolitical systems operating in the United States and an understanding of the sociopolitical history faced by the client. This knowledge helps the clinician understand the institutional and historical barriers that affect the client as a member of a particular group. This knowledge can also help the clinician understand the client's response to treatment and interaction in the clinical situation.

Finally, clinicians in a multicultural society must develop skill in interacting with clients from a variety of cultures with a myriad of cultural and linguistic variables, none of which are the same for different clients (Lynch and Hanson 1992). Clinicians should be able to both send and receive verbal and nonverbal messages appropriately in each culturally different context.

References

American Speech-Language-Hearing Association. (1985). Clinical management of communicatively handicapped minority language populations. *ASHA, 26(1)*, 55–57.

American Speech-Language-Hearing Association. (1983). Social dialects: A position paper. *ASHA, 25(1)*, 23–24.

Battle, D. (1997). Multicultural considerations in counseling communicatively disordered persons and their families. In T. Crowe (Ed.), *Applications of counseling in speech-language pathology and audiology* (pp. 118–144). Baltimore: Williams & Wilkins.

Benson, C.A., & Marano, A. (1994). Current estimates from the national health interview survey. Washington, DC: National Center for Health Statistics (United States Vital Health Statistics Series 16 No. 173).

Board on Children and Families. (1995). Immigrant children and their families: Issues for research and policy. In *The future of children: Critical issues for children and youths (Vol 5)* (pp. 72–89). Los Angeles: The Center for the Future of Children, The David and Lucille Packard Foundation.

Brislin, R.W. (1994). *Intercultural training: An introduction.* Thousand Oaks, CA: Sage.

Cheng, L., & Butler, K. (1993, March). *Difficult discourse: Designing connections to deflect language impairment.* Paper presented at the annual meeting of the California Speech-Language-Hearing Association, Palm Springs, CA.

Cole, L. (1989). E pluribus unum: Multicultural imperatives for the 1990's and beyond. *ASHA, 31,* 2, 65–70.

Fernandez, E.W., & Robinson, J.G. (1994). *Illustrative ranges of the distribution of undocumented immigrants by state. Technical working paper #8 in U.S. Bureau of the Census. Statistical yearbook annual.* Washington DC: U.S. Immigration and Naturalization Service.

Fix, M., & Passel, J. (1994). *Immigration and immigrants: Setting the record straight.* Washington, DC: Urban Institute.

Fix, M., & Zimmerman, W. (1993). *Educating immigrant children.* Washington, DC: Urban Institute, 1993.

Galens, S., Sheets, A., & Young, R.V. (1995). *Gale encyclopedia of multicultural America.* New York: Gale Research, Inc.

Hall, E.T. (1959). *The silent language.* New York: Doubleday.

Ima, K., & Keogh, P-E. (1995). "The crying father" and "My father doesn't love me": Selected observations and reflections on Southeast Asians and special education. In L.L. Cheng (Ed.), *Integrating language and learning for inclusion: An Asian-Pacific focus* (pp. 149–177). San Diego: Singular Publishing.

Keesling, R. (1974). Theories of culture. *Annual review of anthropology, 3,* 73–97.

Lynch, E.W., & Hanson, M.J. (1992). *Developing cross-cultural competence: A guide for working with young children and their families.* Baltimore: Brookes.

Magocsi, P.R. (1995). Russian Americans. In J. Galens, A. Sheets, & R.V. Young (Eds.), *Gale encyclopedia of multicultural America* (pp. 1159–1170). New York: Gale Research, Inc.

Morrison, J., & Zabusky, C.F. (1980). *American Mosaic: The immigrant experience in the words of those who lived it.* New York: E. P. Dutton.

National Association of State Directors of Special Education. (1992, October). *Winners all: A call for inclusive schools. The report of the NASBE Study Group on Special Education.* Alexandria, VA: NASBE.

National Center for Health Statistics. (1994). *Healthy, United States, 1993.* Hyattsville, MD: Public Health Service.

Office of Civil Rights. (1992). *National and state summaries of data from the 1990 Elementary and Secondary School Civil Rights Survey.* Washington, DC: Office of Civil Rights.

Pedersen, P. (1988). *A handbook for developing multicultural awareness.* Alexandria, VA: American Association for Counseling and Development.

Reschly, D.J. (1996). Identification and assessment of students with disabilities. In *The future of children: Special education for children with disabilities (Vol 6)* (pp. 40–53). Los Angeles: The Center for the Future of Children, The David and Lucille Packard Foundation.

Rumbaut, R.G. (1995). A legacy of war: Refugees from Vietnam, Laos, and Cambodia. In S. Pedraza, & R.G. Rumbault (Eds.), *Origins and destinies: Immigration, race, and ethnicity in America* (pp. 583–621). Belmont, CA: Wadsworth.

Singletary, J. (1993). *The Black health guide to stroke.* New York: Holt.

Sue, D.W., & Sue, D. (1990). *Counseling the culturally different.* New York: Wiley.

U.S. Bureau of the Census. (1990). *Statistical abstract of the United States (110th ed.).* Washington, DC: U.S. Bureau of the Census.

U.S. Bureau of the Census. (1996). *Statistical abstract of the United States (116th ed.).* Washington, DC: U.S. Bureau of the Census.

U.S. Department of Health and Human Services. (1994). *Report from the Congress: FY 1994 Refugee Resettlement Program.* Washington, DC: U.S. Department of Health and Human Services.

U.S. Department of Health and Human Services. (1985). *Report of the Secretary's Task Force on Black and Minority Health (Vol 1). Executive Summary (Pub. No. 491-313/44706).* Washington, DC: U.S. Department of Health and Human Services.

U.S. Office of Special Education Programs. (1994). *Implementation of the Individuals with Disabilities Education Act. Sixteenth annual report to Congress.* Washington, DC: U.S. Department of Education.

Vecoli, R.J. (1995). Introduction. In J. Galens, A. Sheets, & R.V. Young (Eds.), *Gale encyclopedia of multicultural America* (pp. xxi–xxvii). New York: Gale Research.

Wagner, M., & Blackorg, J. (1996). Transition from high school to work or college: How special education students fare. In *The future of children: Special education for children with disabilities (Vol 6)* (pp. 103–120). Los Angeles: The Center for the Future of Children, The David and Lucille Packard Foundation.

Additional Resources

Cheng L. (1995). *Integrating language and learning for inclusion: An Asian-Pacific focus.* San Diego: Singular.

Lynch, E.W., & Hanson, M.J. (1992). *Developing cross-cultural competence: A guide for working with young children and their families.* Baltimore: Brookes.

2

□ □ □
□ □ □
□ □ □

African American Cultures

Sandra L. Terrell, Dolores E. Battle, and Regina B. Grantham

A Brief History of Africans in the Americas

The history of people of African descent in America can be traced to the largest involuntary migration movement in modern times. From the sixteenth to the nineteenth centuries, nearly 40 million people from the countries of West Africa were forced to leave their homelands and sold into slavery. The slaves were transported throughout the world as inexpensive labor to provide for the riches of the British and Spanish empires. More than 20 million Africans were brought to the New World so that Europeans could reap the benefits of the fertile land in the countries of Central and South America, the Caribbean, and North America.

The slave trade in Brazil was used to develop the goods for the Portuguese explorers and settlers. Six percent of the current population of Brazil is of African descent. Great Britain used slaves to develop the products found in the tropical Caribbean. As many of 80% of the inhabitants of the Caribbean countries of Jamaica, Haiti, Dominican Republic, the Bahamas, and Barbados descended from Africa. Although they share the common history of slavery, they have taken on the cultural roots of the British Empire, which controlled the area during the period of slavery. The British influence remains in the area and can be seen in the customs, models of education, and language and dialects used in the countries once dominated by the British Empire. Many of the Caribbean countries speak a dialect of English. Some speak Spanish, German, and French. In Haiti, because of the control of the island by the French, the people speak a dialect of French and English.

Those of African descent in South America and the Caribbean share a heritage of life in the Americas different from that of those in North America (Willis 1992). They rebelled long before the slaves in the United States and gained control of their countries, although they were often subjected to control and corruption from within. They are usually identified as black (not Hispanic) in Census data to distinguish them from the inhabitants of the Caribbean, who share a common connection to Spain and the Spanish conquest of the area.

Many Caribbean people of African descent have made a second migration to North America in search of educational and economic opportunities and freedom from political oppression. In 1990 there were nearly 4 million people from the Caribbean areas of Cuba, Dominican Republic, Jamaica, Puerto Rico, and Trinidad and Tobago living in the United States (U.S. Bureau of the Census 1996). Between 1991 and 1993, an additional 337,000 people immigrated to the United States from Caribbean nations (U.S. Bureau of the Census 1996).

In addition to the Caribbeans with African roots, there are 364,000 people in the United States who were born in the countries of Africa (U.S. Bureau of the Census 1996). Nearly 90% of the Africans in the United States have at least a high school education, and nearly half (47.1%) are college graduates (U.S. Bureau of the Census 1996). The Caribbean descendants of Africa and new African immigrants share a common genealogical root with African Americans, but the history of the Africans who were brought to the United States is different. This distinction is necessary as speech-language pathologists and audiologists come to understand the cultural parameters associated with service delivery to African Americans. It is important to understand that the material that follows cannot be applied uniformly to those in America who appear to have an African heritage. It is important that the speech-language pathologist and audiologist identify the ancestral root of the client to determine the specific psychological, cultural, and linguistic variables that impact service delivery for that client.

African Americans are currently the largest minority population in the United States (U.S. Bureau of the Census 1996). The more than 32 million blacks in the United States are largely descended from West Africa. The 4 million Africans who were brought to North America are the genesis of the African Americans (Willis 1992). The history of African Americans in the United States has been not only a struggle for survival in a period of prolonged slavery but also a struggle for equality in a nation that developed its strength on the backs of those it did not respect. The struggle has not only involved economic conditions but also sociocultural and psychological factors that influence speech and language. These factors overlap to affect the clinical interaction in the delivery of speech-language and audiology services. Although the psychological variables that affect the delivery of speech-language and audiology services to African Americans are many, only four are discussed in this chapter because of their importance in clinical assessment and intervention.

The cultural characteristics of African Americans came into existence based on many different variables, such as racism, African traditions, genetic characteristics, politics, and religion. Although African Americans are a heterogeneous group, many descended from Africans who experienced the involuntary emigration from their homeland to the United States. In spite of economic and political enslavement, they survived and overcame racism and discrimination. The various ways in which African Americans have reacted and responded to these factors largely define the African American culture. This chapter provides information on a variety of elements of African American culture and some common cultural patterns that affect the delivery of effective speech-language and audiology services. This chapter is not definitive or all inclusive; the information should not be applied in a stereotypical manner. It should be viewed as a window into African American culture, describing who African Americans are and how clinical services can be enhanced to serve them.

Cultural Variables Among African Americans

Psychological Variables

Self-Esteem and Attitudes Toward African American English and Its Speakers

Self-esteem refers to the regard or value a person places on oneself (Terrell and Terrell 1996). Early in their history in the Americas, African Americans were led to believe that they were inferior to whites. During slavery, slave owners and other whites adopted the attitude that the slaves were ignorant, substandard, and subservient. This attitude was associated with the slaves' speaking styles. The speaking style used by the slave owners and other upper-class whites was associated with success, wealth, and education. In this way, language style became a means by which whites could show social, economic, and racial dominance over the slaves. Such attitudes toward those who spoke African American English (AAE) continued well into the twentieth century. As a result, many African Americans experience low self-esteem, particularly concerning their use of language.

Anger and Hostility

Research, based on the analysis of case studies, led Grier and Cobbs (1968) to conclude that, because of historical racial injustices, some

African Americans harbor feelings of anger and hostility. Grier and Cobbs argue that African Americans unconsciously act out their anger in symbolic ways and that much of their behavior represents the internal frustration of being dehumanized in a predominantly white society. They suggest that some behaviors of African Americans are latent manifestations of anger. For example, giving incorrect answers, refusing to answer questions, and responding impulsively are behaviors that allow them to subtly vent their anger toward white society. The anger is not only directed toward whites but also toward members of their own culture who have "forgotten where they came from" and who have internalized the white values and traditions and excluded their African heritage. This reaction can have implications for assessing and treating language disorders in African Americans—that is, if an African American client perceives the African American examiner as one who has adopted white values and beliefs, the client may show his or her anger by giving incorrect responses, not responding, or ending the sessions (Terrell and Terrell 1996).

Jealousy

An area that has not been discussed extensively, if at all, in the literature is jealousy among African Americans. *Jealousy* can be defined as the thoughts and feelings that occur when an actual or desired relationship is perceived to be threatened (Salovey and Rodin 1986).

The origin of jealousy among African Americans is unclear. One possibility is that it began in the days of slavery with the house slave–field slave dichotomy. During that period, house slaves were usually treated better than field laborers. They were often given better food and clothing and usually were not required to work as hard as the slaves assigned to the field. House servants were selected because of lighter skin color. They were preferred for house duties because lighter skin color was usually associated with a higher level of mental ability. It was not uncommon for those assigned to domestic duties to be taught to read and write by the slave owners.

This theory has been questioned in recent years with the recognition that the house servants were also often treated with cruelty and severe abuse (Ruffins 1997). Newer research also indicates that there were no clear class distinctions among enslaved African Americans and that some slaves were artisans (e.g., blacksmiths and tanners) and did not work in either the house or the fields. In addition, in Northern and Midwestern cities, where many freed slaves resided, there was no clear evidence that people with lighter skin had better jobs or higher incomes than African Americans with darker skin. More recent studies suggest that light skin is valued more in women than in men, and that such values have more to do with gender than class (Ruffins 1997).

Nevertheless, the phenomenon of jealousy has implications for providing clinical services for African Americans, particularly if the examiner is also an African American. Research consistently indicates that African American examiners do not always get better results than white examiners when testing African American clients (Sattler 1982). In some instances, because of jealousy, African American clients are unmotivated to perform or are uncooperative with an African American examiner (Terrell, et al. 1981). It is possible that, because of jealousy, African American clients may attempt to sabotage the assessment session. Research suggests that both the African American examiner and the white examiner should devote time to establishing rapport with the African American client (Terrell, et al. 1981).

Cultural Mistrust

There is agreement among African Americans across educational, socioeconomic, gender, age, and geographic strata that, in general, African Americans do not trust whites (Terrell and Barrett 1979). Martin Luther King (1958) said that the experiences of slavery, Jim Crow legislation, de facto segregation, institutional racism, and the ongoing economic oppression in America taught African Americans to mistrust whites (i.e., cultural mistrust). He pointed out that too many dreams have been deferred and promissory notes unpaid by the banks of justice for African Americans to be able to trust the white person's words, laws, and institutions (King 1958).

Empirical research seems to show that this mistrust of whites has an effect on the intelligence scores of many African Americans. Terrell, et al. (1981) administered an intelligence test to African Americans with both a high level and a low level of mistrust of whites. They found that individuals with high levels of cultural mistrust obtained lower test scores than individuals with lower levels of mistrust. In another study, similar findings were obtained with elementary school children (Terrell and Terrell 1983). Terrell, et al. (1990) studied the relationship between the academic performance of African American high school students and the level of cultural mistrust they had of whites. Individuals with higher levels of mistrust were found to have lower grades and poorer achievement motivation.

The extent to which African Americans mistrust whites has also been found to affect whether, and the extent to which, African Americans seek treatment. Terrell and Terrell (1984) found that African Americans with high levels of cultural mistrust who visited a mental health center and were seen by a white counselor were more likely to end treatment prematurely than those with low levels of mistrust. These studies exploring trust level, taken collectively, suggest that the mistrust of whites by African Americans is an important variable in the extent to which rapport can be established with the client and the extent to which the client is willing to disclose essential information. Cultural mistrust can also result in limited linguistic production (i.e., restricted word output) in the speech of African American children. This can have a tremendous effect if assessment findings are based on language samples. The low word production may not reflect the child's true capability, but rather, his or her mistrust of the examiner (Terrell and Terrell 1996). It may be useful for examiners working with African American clients to devote additional time to establishing rapport to reduce the level of mistrust at the beginning of the evaluation or intervention process.

African Americans who mistrust whites act in different ways. Among these is the use of a silent code. It is unknown why a communicative code of near silence occurs in formal situations with unfamiliar white speakers, but cultural mistrust may be an explanation. Indeed, the unwritten rule underlying the silent code may be the speaker's intent to reveal as little information about himself or herself as possible because he or she does not know how this information will be used. Regardless of the reason, the implication is that speech-language pathologists, audiologists, and others can misjudge a person's communication abilities on the basis of the person's use of silent code. The use of silent code can result in a restriction of the amount of speech used by the client. Without knowledge of the probable existence of another, more fluent, code, the AAE-speaking child may be judged as shy (at best) or disordered (at worst). Similarly, the AAE-speaking adult may be thought of as having less than adequate communicative abilities.

The psychological and sociocultural variables that influence the communication behavior of African Americans need to be considered in the design and implementation of clinical programs. Procedures that focus solely on the observable communication behavior are likely to result in inappropriate treatment or, worse yet, because the client may withdraw from treatment, no treatment at all.

African American Music

Music has long played a major role in the life of African American people. Music developed by African American people, especially jazz and blues, has achieved the status of a universal language and has been considered America's greatest artistic contribution to world culture. Butcher (1964) identified three types of African American music: Negro folk music, including original work songs; the blues; and jazz, which is a direct descendant of the blues.

The first African immigrants in North America brought with them their native music. The work songs that accompanied work in the fields in Africa became "sorrow songs" in America. They were called sorrow songs because the slaves were working in the fields of the slave holders rather than in their own fields (Jones 1963). Negro spirituals emerged from the earlier work songs. These songs were sung wherever slaves happened to be, whether in the fields or in the kitchen. Spirituals, songs of prayer, generally reflected a topic of looking toward the day when, through death, God would remove the slaves from the life of toil on earth and take them home to heaven. Spirituals expressed such messages as the hell of hard trials and great tribulations; wanderings in some lonesome valley or down some unknown road; and being a long way from home, with a brother, sister, father, mother, wife, husband, or child either sold, dead, or gone. The words often contained cleverly coded messages that had one meaning for slave owners but a different meaning for other slaves. For example, spirituals such as "Steal Away, Steal Away Home: I Ain't Got Long To Stay Here" and "The Old Ship of Zion, Get on Board" were thought by slave owners to be songs of prayer; however, slaves heard underlying messages. Depending on when, where, and by whom the songs were sung, the songs either reflected the intent of a slave to run away to freedom or were a sign to indicate the location of the next station in the Underground Railroad (a secret pathway the slaves followed from South to North). For example, the song "Down by the Riverside" was used to inform those wishing to escape to meet at a specified time by the river.

After the Civil War and the abolition of slavery, African American music adapted to a different set of circumstances. The blues were typically a simple, frank, and honest portrayal of how bad things were at the time. The blues expressed love, family life, or general dissatisfaction with a cold and trouble-filled world.

Jazz, which is derived from the blues, is clearly the most cosmopolitan of Negro music. It stands out as one of the most significant artistic contributions to the history of the United States.

An understanding of African American music is important to the speech-language pathologist providing services to African American clients. African American music was, and continues to be, an important cultural statement. In fact, some African Americans are resentful if spirituals, the blues, or jazz are played or sung by those who are not African American. There is a feeling that the white population has stolen the music of African Americans.

Music used in waiting rooms before clinical sessions relaxes the client. Many professional offices play classical or popular easy-listening music. Not only does this music not relax many African Americans, but it also makes them feel uncomfortable and out of place. Better clinical results may be obtained if music consistent with the African American culture is played while the client waits. Since jazz is universally accepted as a part of American culture, it is appropriate in clinic waiting rooms. In addition, when music is used as a part of an intervention program, it is appropriate to use music consistent with the client's culture.

Religion

Religion has an important role in the lives of many African Americans. Most African American communities have a large number of churches. Indeed, in some communities it is estimated that there is one church for every 400 people. Because the church serves an important function in the lives of African Americans, it is not uncommon to hear African Americans express religious themes in clinical settings. Adult African Americans may share information that seems inappropriate or strange to a speech-language pathologist or audiologist who is unfamiliar with or does not fully appreciate religion in African American culture. In conversations, the client may refer to religious themes, such as getting the spirit and seeing visions or hearing voices. He or she may also use biblical quotes and phrases such as "Yes, Lord" and "Amen."

Some African American clergy have a harsh or hoarse vocal quality because of their loud and emotional manner of delivering sermons. They may sometimes deliver two or three sermons on one Sunday. They may seek help from a physician or speech-language pathologist as a last resort to "God's will" or "God's healing power." The African American preacher is likely to be resistant to any treatment recommendations that call for complete vocal rest for a period of time, as this is in direct conflict with his or her "calling" to preach.

Names

In general, African Americans regard their names as extremely important. According to African tradition, names for children are selected with great care and given in a significant, spiritual ritual. They not only reflect who the child is, but also determine the person who the child will become as he or she matures.

When Africans first experienced the involuntary immigration to America, they were stripped of their given African names and given simple-to-pronounce, one- or two-syllable names. Slaves often took the last names of their owners. Many African Americans still carry these last names. Terrell, for example, was the name of a Georgia plantation owner. Some slaves adopted names, such as Freeman or Newman, that expressed their newly acquired freedom. Others took on the names of important historical figures, such as Washington and Jefferson.

During slavery and long afterward, whites rarely addressed African Americans by their last names. Regardless of status, African Americans were called by their first name or were simply addressed as "boy," "girl," "uncle," "aunt," and so on. The African Americans used a variety of tactics to counteract the methods by which they were addressed. Some gave their children first names of formal address, such as Miss, Princess, Duke, General, and Mister. Whites then had little choice but to use these titles of respect when talking to or calling them.

African American adults frequently report that they resent the use of their first names by professional service providers and consider it a presumptuous practice. This may be surprising to a white practitioner for whom the choice of first name is intended to create informality and friendliness. The resentment of African Americans to this practice must be understood against the historical background of address used by whites toward African Americans. To inappropriately address someone may not be interpreted as a mistake but as an insult.

In the 1960s, Malcolm Little, leader of the Nation of Islam, recognizing that his last name was the name of a slave owner, rejected his last name and became Malcolm X to symbolize the true, rightful, unknown African name that belonged to his ancestors. Also during the 1960s and 1970s, the emergence of the Civil Rights movement motivated many African Americans to search for and embrace elements of their African heritage. Along with wearing African-inspired clothing and hair styles, a number of African Americans rejected their given names and adopted names from an African or Arabic language. This search for and embracing of African heritage continues through the 1990s.

Stemming from African traditions, name giving among African Americans has retained its importance. Like their African ancestors, African American parents take great care in selecting names for their children. Some African American parents give their children either African names or non-European names with unusual pronunciations or spellings, such as LaShawn, Shemeika, Shurtjhana, Latifa, Tanzania, Ivanna Samal, Amani Shama, and Elon Jahdal. Many of these names have important meanings, and as the child grows, the parents share these meanings with the child. Kamau Atu Imarogbe, an African name adopted by the son of an author of this chapter, means quiet warrior (Kamau), born on Saturday (Atu), and of a good family (Imarogbe). Research has shown that African American children who have African names have a higher self-concept than African American children who do not have such names (Terrell, et al. 1988).

It is insulting to an African American child for an adult who is not a member of the child's family or circle of close friends to use a diminutive form of the child's name. For example, Shemeika should never automatically become Mikky, even if this shortened name is what the child's parents and friends call her. Even if an African American child's name is European, it should not be assumed that he or she wants to be called by a nickname. The clinician should always ask the client (or parent) the name of preference and learn how to pronounce and spell the name correctly. To do otherwise is perceived as "calling the person out of his or her name" (an insult) and can negatively affect the clinical service-delivery process.

African American English

As described in "Cultural Variables Among African Americans," there are common elements by which African Americans identify with one another to varying degrees. The language used by African Americans is yet another of these cultural elements. Not only do the language styles of African Americans reflect the history, cultural basis, value systems, customs, and traditions of this population, but these styles also are an integral part of African American cultural identity (Takada and Hamayan, in press). Language systems have been, and continue to be, dynamic forces of the culture, constantly evolving to embrace past communicative styles and to create new ones.

A number of linguistic dialects are spoken among African Americans in the United States. Among these is the Gullah dialect, which is spoken by those living on islands off the coasts of South Carolina and Georgia. There are also various Creole dialects, such as Jamaican Creole English, and dialects spoken by people who immigrated to the United States from the Caribbean or countries in Africa. However, the most prominent linguistic system identified with African Americans is known as AAE.

Definition of African American English

AAE is a dialect of Standard American English (SAE). Its speakers are primarily African American. The highest percentage of users of this dialect are the African American working class (Dillard 1973). Over the years, this dialect has been known by several names, reflecting both the evolving racial name identification and the shifts in focus of the field of linguistics from structuralism during the 1950s and 1960s, to semantics in the 1970s, to pragmatics in the 1980s. The term *nonstandard Negro English* was used during the 1950s and early 1960s. The term *ebonics* was introduced by Williams (1975) during the 1970s to reflect the fusion of ebony and phonics. The term *black English* has been used since the 1980s. In the 1990s, the term *African*

American English has been used most frequently. *Black English vernacular,
African American Language, black English, black dialect,* and *ebonics* are
also in use in the 1990s.

AAE consists of systematic, rule-governed phonologic, grammatical,
syntactic, semantic, and pragmatic characteristics of language. Although
AAE is different from SAE, it maintains enough similarity to SAE that it is
considered a dialect of American English, not a separate language. It includes
not only the verbal spoken word but also nonverbal factors, such as body
language, use of personal space, body movement, eye contact, narrative
sequence, and modes of discourse. AAE patterns are not exclusive to this
dialect, as they contain features that are shared by other social and regional
dialects, such as Southern English.

Although largely identified with African Americans, AAE is not spoken by all African Americans. Additionally, African Americans are not the
only people who speak AAE. Depending on the level and type of socialization with AAE speakers, some whites, Hispanics, and Asians use AAE.
Within the United States, the use of AAE varies from one speaker to the
next. It constitutes a continuum that ranges from African Americans who
do not use the dialect at all to those who use most AAE characteristics in
all communicative contexts (Wyatt 1991). Age, geographic location, occupation, income, and education are a few factors that have been found to
influence the level of usage of AAE among speakers (Wyatt 1991; Labov
1966). Furthermore, the extent to which a person identifies with the culture of the speech community has also been found to influence the use of
the dialect (Terrell and Terrell 1981). Individual speakers can also vary
their use of the dialect along the continuum, switching codes depending on
the communicative context.

History and Evolution of
African American English

There is no empirical evidence that links present-day AAE to
West African languages; however, there are several theoretical explanations
that attempt to make this connection. One hypothesis proposes that when
Europeans and Africans first met on the west coast of Africa during the
1600s, there was a need for a means of communication between the two
groups. Europeans and Africans therefore used a reduced, simplified form of
English, called *pidgin,* whenever communication for essential needs was
necessary (Haskins and Butts 1973).

Additionally, since the Africans who were brought to this country came
from various locations in West Africa, it is highly likely that they did not

speak one another's native languages. With no other means by which to communicate in the New World, the slaves began to use pidgin between themselves and when speaking to their masters. With continued use, pidgin developed into an everyday language with rules, inflections, and other systematic linguistic patterns (Burling 1973; Haskins and Butts 1973).

Some of the English patterns the slaves acquired were nonstandard forms learned from their white overseers. Others were standard English forms learned from the more educated slave owners. The formal patterns, however, remained standard for only a relatively short period of time. Several patterns that are considered to be nonstandard today, such as multiple negation, were acceptable standard forms of English during the seventeenth and eighteenth centuries. As English evolved, these patterns became unacceptable or nonstandard. Because of limited contact with their slave owners, the slaves had no way of keeping up with the evolving nature of the language. The slaves' retention of these previously standard English forms therefore resulted in some of the AAE patterns that are considered nonstandard today.

The slaves also incorporated sounds, grammatical markings, and vocabulary from their traditional African languages into their English. For example, many West African languages have a tense, called the *habitual tense*, that implies an activity of a recurring nature. The slaves relegated this habitual tense to the verb *be* when they learned English, because it most closely approximated the habitual tense. The statement "he be going" means "he usually goes" or "he always goes." This linguistic pattern was not only found in the speech of slaves, but is also a feature of current AAE and of dialects spoken by blacks outside the United States (Haskins and Butts 1973).

In addition to grammatical features, slaves infused West African words into their English. Some of these African words are incorporated into English to the extent that they are currently familiar to many SAE speakers. Words with African origins include *goober, tote, cola, jazz, juke* (as in *jukebox*), and *jive*. The word *john*, meaning the customer of a prostitute, is derived from an African word that is translated as "someone who can be easily exploited." Additionally, the word *okay*, and the sounds *uh-uh* for *no* and *uh-huh* for *yes* are also thought to have West African origins (Burling 1973).

Gradually, the nature of the pidgin English spoken by the slaves changed in three main ways. First, pidgin English became a rule-governed system. African and English words and structures were blended by phonologic, grammatical, syntactic, and semantic rules that provided communicative competence for each speaker of that language. Second, this version of English became the primary mode of communication among slaves. Third, as this English variety became the only language used by the members of the slave community, children born into this community acquired this language as their native tongue. When these changes occurred, this English was no longer pidgin but became a type of Creole language.

Long after slavery was legally abolished, racial separation continued in areas such as politics, education, jobs, and housing. This segregation, along with the continued evolution of the language style, resulted in AAE as it is currently spoken.

Linguistic Features of African American English

Language variation has been attributed to several factors, including race and ethnicity, social class, education, occupation, and geographical region (Taylor 1986). There is evidence to suggest that a combination of these factors contributes to language diversity more so than one factor alone (Terrell 1975). For this reason, the normal characteristics of AAE are not exclusive to this dialect and overlap with other American dialectal systems. Various dialects share many linguistic features; however, some of these features occur more readily in one dialect than in another. AAE can be distinguished from other dialects by the frequency with which various phonologic and grammatical patterns occur.

AAE is a linguistic system and, as such, contains form, content, and use components (Bloom and Lahey 1978; Lahey 1988). These language components are discussed in this section. The following phonologic and grammatical features have been adapted from Williams and Wolfram (1976).

Form

Phonologic Features

There are three major phonologic rules of AAE from which most of the sound features emanate. The first phonologic rule is the silencing or substitution of the medial or final consonant in a word. The consonants affected by this rule include voiced and voiceless fricatives. For example, the fricative *th* is affected, and AAE speakers may say "dey" for *they*, "nofin" for *nothing*, "toof" for *tooth*, and "brovah" for *brother*. The semivowels /r/ and /l/ are also affected. AAE speakers may say "foe" for *four*, "sto'y" for *story*, and "p'otect" for *protect*.

Voiced stops /b/, /d/, and /g/ are generally affected in the final positions of single-syllable words, usually a consonant-vowel-consonant (CVC) combination. In these words, the final voiced stop is pronounced similarly to the consonant's voiceless cognate /p/, /t/, and /k/. In addition, the vowel in CVC words is lengthened. Examples of these changes occur when speakers say "cap" plus the lengthened vowel for *cab*, "but" plus lengthened vowel for *bud*, and "pik" plus the lengthened vowel for *pig*.

The nasals /m/ and /n/ are also affected by this first phonologic rule. Several specific characteristics occur with these nasal consonants. One occurs in CVC-unstressed combinations in a word in which the final consonant in the CVC combination is the /m/ or /n/ (e.g., *mailman*). In these words, the final nasal consonant is silenced, but the quality of nasalization is transferred to the vowel. Some examples of this are "ma" plus the nasalized vowel for *man* and "bu" plus the nasalized vowel for *bun*. This feature is also similar to that that occurs in CVC words such as *pin* and *pen*. In these words, the final nasal consonant /n/ remains intact, but the final consonant nasalizes the adjacent vowels, making these words sound identical.

Other nasalization features in AAE affect the grammatical formulations of the present progressive verb tense (*-ing*) and the articles *a* and *an*. The *-ing* suffix becomes *-in*, as in "singin" and "runnin." The difference between *a* and *an* also becomes neutralized. In this situation, *a* precedes words that begin with either a consonant or a vowel, as in "a apple," "a pear," and "a orange," as opposed to "an apple," "a pear," and "an orange."

The second major phonologic rule is the silencing of unstressed initial phonemes and unstressed initial syllables. Examples of this rule are "bout" for *about*, "cause" for *because*, "matoes" for *tomatoes*, "he uz" for *he was*, and "this un" for *this one*.

The third general rule is the silencing of the final consonant in a consonant cluster occurring at the end of a word. Examples of this are "des" for *desk*, "min" for *mind*, and "ol" for *old*. This rule also affects the AAE grammatical feature for past tense, as in "miss" for *missed* and "slep" for *slept*. Another feature related to consonant clusters is the use of *skr-* for *str-* in the initial position in words, as in "skring" for *string* and "skreet" for *street*. Additionally, "aks" may be used for *ask*.

Morphologic and Syntactic Features

Unlike the phonologic characteristics, AAE morphologic and syntactic or grammatical features are more extensive and cannot be simplified into general rules. However, some of the grammatical features of the dialect affect the past tense of regular verbs (e.g., "cash" for *cashed*) and irregular verbs (e.g., "seen" for *saw* and "done" for *did*). Grammatical features can also affect noun-verb agreement, as in "he walk" (versus *he walks*). They also affect the future tense of verbs through the use of "gonna" and various reductions of "gonna" (e.g., "I'nga," "I'mon," and "I'ma"). Future verb tense is also affected by the silencing of the contraction *'ll* for *will*, as in "she miss you" for *she'll miss you*.

Other AAE grammatical features include the use of double modals (e.g., "used to couldn't"), the use of "like ta" for *liked to have*, differences in the use of the possessive *'s* morpheme (e.g., "the boy hat" for *the boy's hat*), and differences in the use of the plural morpheme *-s* as in "fifty cent" for *fifty cents*.

Some AAE grammatical features attempt to provide regularity to irregular SAE structures. For example, SAE allows for only one comparative or superlative descriptor within a single noun or verb phrase. For example, only *most beautiful* or *prettier* would be allowed in a single phrase. Although standard English does not permit the use of *more* and *most* with words ending with an *-er* or *-est* suffix, this combination is valid in AAE, as well as in several other social dialects. The dialectal formulations of comparatives and superlatives can occur in a variety of combinations serving to carry the comparative or superlative through the entire phrase. Some examples of normal dialectal formulations in this area include "stupidest," "most stupidest," "baddest," "mostest," and "worser."

Negative formulations in AAE also regularize SAE rules. The general logic of negatives within a standard English sentence tells us that two negatives cannot be used together because they negate each other and the sentence becomes positive. In AAE, no such philosophical rule exists. Rather, AAE follows the rules for use of negatives that are present in other languages. In Spanish, for example, the negative is carried throughout the sentence. This means that if the sentence is to be negative, every place in the sentence that can be negated is negated. This same rule applies in AAE, resulting in the normal dialectal feature of multiple negation. Some examples of this feature are "He didn't do nothing," "Couldn't nobody do it?" "Nobody didn't do it," and "Ain't no cat can't get in no coop."

Regularization also extends to reflexive pronouns, where the suffix *-self* can be added to all personal pronouns. The rules used to formulate the first and second person reflexive pronouns *myself* and *yourself* can be extended to the third person, as in "hisself" and "theirself."

Some AAE grammatical forms reflect a feature of hypercorrection. This generally means that the speaker has overgeneralized a grammatical morpheme to an irregular word that already reflects the function of that morpheme. In all cases of hypercorrection, the speaker does not have sufficient knowledge of the SAE rule for the use of a morpheme. Hypercorrected forms are mostly used by older adult dialectal speakers who have realized that they need a more standard language system but do not have a consistent standard English model to imitate. Hypercorrected forms occur in the areas of third person subject-verb agreement (e.g., "I walks," "you walks," and "the children walks"), in pluralization (e.g., "two childrens," "five mens," and "three deers"), and in the use of the possessive morpheme *'s* (e.g., "John's Taylor car").

The use of the word *even* as an intensifying adverb is also an AAE grammatical feature. When this word is spoken in a sentence with an intensifying function, it generally stands out from the rest of the sentence context by a more intense loudness level and its prosodic pattern. When used this way, *even* carries a meaning of finality—that is, there is nothing greater or nothing left to be said about the topic of the sentence. For example, consider a scenario in which a husband enters the house and asks his wife where their son is. The wife responds that the boy is outside but that he'll be in soon for dinner. The husband asks again 10 minutes later, and the wife responds as before. After 5 more minutes have elapsed, the husband asks again, but this time the wife has become irritated and does not want to be asked the same question anymore. She tells him, "I done tol' you he be home for dinner. Don' *even* aks me no more." *Even* is a final, definitive statement on a subject. Likewise, schoolchildren may comment, "I didn't *even* know what that teacher be talkin' about."

Other AAE grammatical features occur in the following areas:

- Pronominal apposition (e.g., "*My brother he* bigger than you" for *My brother is bigger than you* or *He is bigger than you*).
- Demonstratives (e.g., "I want some of *them* candies" and "I like *these here* pants better than *them there* ones").
- Pronouns. For example, "*Him* ain't playing," "*Me and her* will go," "James got *him* book," "Don't eat that candy 'cause it *mines*," "He can dress *hisself*," and "I got *me* one of those."
- The use of *have* and *do*. For example, "I been here for hours," "He *don't* go," "He *have* a bike," and "He always *do* silly things."
- Completed aspects with *done*. This construction is used when an action started and was completed at a certain time in the past. For example, "I *done* tried."
- Remote time construction with *been*. This construction is used when an action has taken place in the distant past. For example "I *been* had it there for about three years."
- Indirect questions. Indirect questions follow the same rules as those for formulating direct questions. For example, "I wonder *was he walking*" for *I wonder if he was walking* and "I wonder *where was he going*" for *I wonder where he was going.*
- Use of *do* for *if*. This feature is related to the indirect question feature: A clause beginning with *if* is reformulated into a direct question format. For example, "I ask' Elon *do he want* to play football" for *I asked Elon if he wants to play football.*

The major grammatical feature of AAE involves variations of use of the verb *to be.* These use rules are as follows:

- Silencing of *is*, *are*, or both in contracted forms. For example, "*He* a man" for *He's a man*, "*He* running home" for *He's running home*, and "*You* good" for *You're good*. Dialectal speakers who use this feature use *is* and *are* in other sentence contexts, such as in tag questions such as "*He* not home yet, *is* he?" Also, some dialectal speakers who use a silenced *are* contraction do not use a silenced *is* contraction. Additionally, this feature extends to contractions of *will be* and *would be*, as in "*He be* here" for *He'll be here* and "*She be* happy" for *She'd be happy*.
- Neutralization of subject-verb agreement. This construction occurs in both past and present forms of *to be*, but the use of this rule is more frequent for the past tense. Examples include "*I was* there," "*She was* there," "*You was* there," and "*They was* there." An example of the more infrequently used present tense form is "*They is* here."
- Use of *be* as a main verb for *is*, *are*, or *am*. This rule is a prominent AAE feature. Examples include "I *be* here in the evening" for *I am here in the evening*, "Sometime he *be* busy" for *Sometimes he is busy*, and "They *be* coming" for *They are coming*.
- Use of *be* for habitual tense. In the most prominent feature of AAE, *be* does not specify a tense, but it reflects the African-based habitual tense, which indicates a permanent or consistent quality or condition. For example, the statement "My momma *be* workin' two jobs" means *my mother has been working two jobs for a while*. And the statement, "Don' min' him; he jus' *be* actin' crazy" means *don't pay any attention to him; acting crazy is his normal tendency*.

Content: Semantic or Lexical Features

Semantics involves learning and using words, which are symbols that represent objects and ideas within and about the world. In the United States, people live under different conditions. These conditions include geographic, economic, regional, sociopolitical, familial, generational, religious, or racial conditions. In most cases, people live with various combinations of these conditions. Because of variations of these factors, reactions, perceptions, experiences, and survival activities of one group of people result in lexical items that are unique to that group. These words constitute a cultural vocabulary.

The lexicon of speakers of AAE is influenced by many of these factors. This means that the person's lexicon is likely to contain words that are unique to the factors that affect the individual's life. Geographically, for example, a carbonated soft drink is "tonic" in the Boston area, "pop" in Pittsburgh, "Coke" in Dallas, and "soda water" in Gainesville, FL. A paper container used to hold groceries is a "bag" in Pittsburgh but a "sack" in Dallas. People in Texas who are getting ready to do something say that they are "fixin' to" do something. An African American who uses AAE who lives on the East Coast might say "What's up, brother?," whereas an AAE user on the West Coast might say "What's up, fool?"

The vocabulary of African Americans can have regional influences as well. A child living in a predominantly African American neighborhood in urban Dallas has a lexicon that is different from that of a child who lives in a rural area near the city. In some cases, the same lexical item symbolizes different referents for these two children. For example, to the rural child, the word *hog* is likely to represent a large pig, but to the urban child, *hog* might symbolize a type of large expensive car.

Generation-influenced lexicon plays a large role in the vocabulary used among many African Americans. Each generation appears to have developed its own unique set of words and meanings, often called *slang*. It is unknown why slang is so prominent among African American youth. It may be that the lack of acceptance of African American youth by white youth in social activities has led to the creation of slang words for each generation of young people. Slang, like African American music, may be a means for African American youth to create something that is uniquely theirs—a code with which they can identify themselves as a group, communicate with each other, and feel good about being together. Slang words are always subject to rapid change: New words are added; others become archaic. Again, it is unknown exactly why this occurs. It could be that new slang words are created to replace words that become popular among mainstream groups. Some examples of generation-influenced lexical items (all of which mean good or great) are "crazy" and "real gone" (1950s); "hep," "bad," and "boss" (1970s); and "fresh," "phat," "smokin," "stompin," and "walk on it" (1990s).

Regardless of geographic or regional location, generational influences, or economic status, some words are commonly used and understood by the majority of African Americans but are generally absent from the lexicon of mainstream populations. Some of these words reflect the physical or racial characteristics of African Americans, such as the vocabulary for hair and skin care. Other words reflect activities in African American churches and other African American organizations. A few examples of this cultural vocabulary are "ash" and "ashy" (referring to dry skin); "grease," "to grease," "glycerine," "perm," "relaxer," and "curl" (referring to oil-based preparations for the hair); and "shout" and "get happy" (referring to outward physical and emotional response to overwhelming joy and mercy of God).

Other examples of lexical differences that occur in AAE include "true dat" (in agreement), "change up or flip the script" (to change), "dis" (disrespect), "down" (cool or nice), "jettin" (quickly), "get my groove on" (have a good time, dancing, romancing), "get my swirve on" (go out with the opposite sex, dance, have a good time), "crib" (home or parent), "fly" (good looking), and "chump change" (small change, insignificant). Word usage and definition are not only influenced by geography, region, generation, and economic status but also by the city or neighborhood. The meaning also changes dependent on the user (adult or teen), the context in which it is being used, or both. Even the way a word is pronounced can change its definition (Foster 1990). Although these are AAE terms that are used in AAE neighborhoods and regions, many are incorporated into SAE because of their use in the lyrics of rap and hip-hop and other cross-over music that is being adopted by white youth.

Form and content areas of language can result in communication failures between speakers of different dialects. Some failures can result from differences in pronunciation, grammar, and vocabulary that create intelligibility problems. In the case of different dialects of a language, the actual linguistic differences can be minor but nevertheless implicated in difficulties in communication and in misunderstandings.

Use: Pragmatic Functions

Just as there are normal systematic phonologic, grammatical, and semantic features of AAE, there are also pragmatic characteristics of the dialect. In recent years, as social scientists have begun to focus on the description and analysis of speech as a communication system, it has become clear that social norms (not just phonologic, grammatical, and semantic rules) operate to influence the communication process. When speakers of different dialects converse, they may find that they must listen more carefully to their interlocutor than when they converse with someone of the same dialect. The flow of conversation may be interrupted by requests for clarification of the meanings of words and idioms. Such difficulties in communication can impair the establishment of rapport between service provider and client and may attenuate the free exchange of information.

Some rules for communicative interactions used by many African Americans are code switching, call and response, wit and sarcasm, eye contact, and topic-associative narrative style.

Code Switching

Code switching is a major pragmatic feature of the speech of most, if not all, American-English speakers. Code switching involves the speaker's ability to make judgments on what linguistic style (formal or informal), dialect, or language is most appropriate for communication. These judgments are based on the age, race, gender, or level of authority of the person with whom one is speaking and the location or other context and event factors of the communication. There is little empirical research on the factors that trigger a speaker to move from one code to another among African Americans. The characteristics of code switching among African Americans may be different for those who (1) speak only SAE, (2) speak both SAE and AAE equally well, and (3) speak only AAE (Seymour and Ralabate 1985). Research also indicates that the ability to code switch seems to increase with age (Seymour and Ralabate 1985).

Call and Response

Call and response is characterized by a choral response to an utterance given by a single person. Largely noticeable within the church and in gospel and rhythm and blues music, call and response is also a feature of conversations among African Americans. There are two specific call-and-response patterns: (1) a statement produced by one person followed by a response by one person and (2) a statement produced by one person followed by responses made by people in a group.

The first type of call and response occurs mostly during a conversational dyad. The response is generally a confirmation or acknowledgment of the speaker's statement. In some instances, the response is confirming (e.g., "I know that's right," "Tell me about it," "You got that right," "Girl, I know what you talkin' 'bout," "Ain't it the truth now," and "Amen"). The response can also acknowledge understanding of the statement or, if the speaker's statement is a request, can answer yes or no (e.g., "You got it, man," "I got you covered," or "Can't fly with that"). Additionally, the response can denote some element of surprise regarding the content of the statement. Examples of this type of response include "Get outta here," "Lawd have mercy," "Lawd Jesus!" "Lawd," "Girl" (pronounced with a lengthened semivowel), "Damn!" "Ooohhh, child!" and "Um-Um-Um."

In some instances, the call-and-response patterns in a dyad are echoic or hyperechoic. The echoic response duplicates or repeats some portion of the speaker's statement, as in the following conversation:

Speaker: I fixed me some turkey and dressing...
Respondent: Um-um! Turkey and dressing!
Speaker: And some sweet potato pie.
Respondent: Potato pie, too? I ain't had no good dinner like that since my wife passed.
Speaker: Then you better come on here and let me fix you a plate.

A pragmatic feature not previously recognized in literature is the hyperechoic response. The hyperechoic response is superimposed on top of the first speaker's utterance. It is a confirmation that the listener not only understands the response but also anticipates, predicts, and verbalizes what the speaker's next words will be while the speaker is talking. If the respondent is wrong, the speaker makes the appropriate adjustments. An example of a hyperechoic response pattern follows:

> Speaker: You know I done tried to be fair. But I s'pose you can'
> teach no ol'...
> Respondent: Man nothin' new... [anticipating "old man, new tricks"]
> Speaker: Nothin' new. I know that's right! [echoed and confirmed]

The second type of call-and-response pattern is a statement produced by one person, followed by responses made by people in a group. It is typically found in church services, rallies, and other situations with a main speaker and an audience. Audience verbal responses in church include "Yea," "Speak the truth, now," "Amen," "Well," "Alright," "Uh-huh," "Hallelujah," "Tell it," and "Preach it." Nonverbal responses to a speaker's statements include hand clapping, head shaking and nodding, hand waving and lifting, standing up, dancing, patting the feet, pointing a finger at the speaker, laughing, and crying. In these situations, the speaker not only looks for the responses but, when the audience is too quiet, also encourages the audience to respond by calling statements such as "Hello?" "Ya'll don' hear me," and "Can I get a witness?"

Call-and-response patterns are considered a beneficial communicative feature among those who use and understand them because the respondents are providing the speaker with complimentary, confirming, and positive feedback. However, these patterns are subject to misinterpretation by people who are unfamiliar with this aspect of AAE. AAE speakers using normal call-and-response patterns may be judged to be rude, interruptive, and disruptive by those who are not familiar with call-and-response patterns.

Wit and Sarcasm

Wit and sarcasm assume a variety of forms by African Americans. Some statements are actual sarcasm, such as the wife who tells her significantly late–arriving husband, "You sho' got home early." Other forms of wit involve creative, verbal turn-taking games, such as *playing the dozens*. Playing the dozens is typically played by school-age African American males. The objective is for a player to create verbal insults about the opponent's mother that are better than the insults directed at the player about his own mother. Following is an example of a typical playing the dozens verbal interchange:

Player 1:   Yo' momma so ugly the dog catcher tried to net her.

Player 2:   Oh yea? Yo' momma so ugly, when the dog catcher got yo'
             momma and put her in his truck, even the other dogs
             didn' know the difference.

On the surface, playing the dozens reflects disrespect of the parent. On the contrary, because of the love and respect the players have for their mothers, a young African American male who can learn to withstand insults about his mother is better prepared to withstand negativism and insults that he will face in the future. It is also an excellent way to develop social and verbal interaction skills.

Eye Contact

Some African Americans are taught as children that eye contact with an adult during a verbal interchange is disrespectful. Some African American adults may therefore find it difficult to speak with those of authority on an eye-to-eye basis. Judging children and adults for not looking at an examiner or other professional (as in "Johnny lacks normal eye contact") or establishing goals for the person to do so (as in "Johnny should establish eye contact with the clinician in response to the command 'Look at me.'") may be a violation of the person's cultural rule for eye contact. This is particularly important in the treatment of dysfluency as described in Chapter 8.

According to Taylor (in press), African Americans demonstrate attentiveness and respect by using indirect eye contact when they are listeners and direct eye contact when they are speakers. SAE speakers could easily misinterpret the lack of eye contact during listening as inattentive or noncaring behavior.

Narrative Style

Heath (1986) describes four types of narrative styles: (1) patterns used to recount past experiences, (2) patterns used to cast or describe present or future activities or events, (3) patterns used to give accounts of what has been experienced, and (4) fictionalized accounts of storytelling. Despite the variable nature of AAE and the awareness of different narrative styles and genres, investigations of the narratives of AAE have generally been restricted to recounts or narratives of personal experiences (Hester 1994, 1996). In the 1980s, several investigators studied AAE narratives in terms of oral and literate styles (Collins 1985; Gee 1985; Heath 1982; Michaels and Collins 1984; Nichols 1989). In oral language style meaning is implicit or indirect—that is, it is expressed through the use of idioms, slang, gestures, and changes in voice and pitch in conversations between familiar individuals. In literate language, style meaning is expressed more directly with specific syntactic and morphological structures as in written language (Olson 1977; Tannen 1982; Westby 1985). Many investigators describe AAE speakers as preferring the oral narrative style because of their relation to the oral tradition of the African ancestry (Baugh 1983; Erickson 1984).

Michaels (1981), Nichols (1989), Collins (1985), Gee (1989), and Westby (1985, 1994) are among several investigators who studied the oral-literate distinction in the narratives of young children. By analyzing narratives during sharing-time activities for African American and white kindergarten children, Michaels (1981) found that the narrative style used by the AAE-speaking children differed from that used by speakers of SAE. When a particular topic was discussed, speakers of SAE used patterns that involved a fairly strict adherence to a central topic. For example, when a teacher asks a class to talk about things seen and done at a zoo, each child using SAE contributes something appropriate to that main topic. This reflects a topic-centered narrative style. On the other hand, some speakers of AAE engage in a more topic-associated narrative style. With a topic-associated narrative style, a child's statements are not linked by a central topic but by ideas generated from an immediately preceding statement. For example, when a group of children who use this style of discussion is asked to talk about things seen and done at a zoo, the first child may respond that he saw a lion, the second child comments that she saw a lion on the *Circus of the Stars* television special, and the third child adds that she got scared when the performer almost fell off the high wire. The investigators reported that AAE-speaking children's narrative skills are restricted to a topic-associated oral style (Collins 1985; Michaels 1981; Nichols 1989; Westby 1985).

More recent investigations, however, have found that AAE-speaking children have more flexible narrative styles than was previously thought. Hyon and Sulzby (1992) and Hicks (1991) studied the use of narrative by kindergarten and first-grade AAE-speaking children, respectively. Hyon and Sulzby (1992) reported that kindergarten children used both topic-centered and topic-associating features while telling stories to a familiar adult. Hicks (1991) found that children who use AAE are able to shift their narrative style according to different task demands.

For some professionals, consistently straying from a main topic during a conversation or discussion is symptomatic of a disorder or disability. Professionals should be aware that this behavior may be a normal narrative style used by some African American children. Regardless of the style preferred by the child, African American children can be expected to tell stories and recount events as do other children.

Other Pragmatic Functions

There are several other pragmatic features of AAE. Turn-taking rules are somewhat different among African American speakers. In AAE, it is not necessary to wait until the first speaker has completed his or her turn before the next speaker begins. Interruptions are acceptable, and the conversational floor is given to the most assertive and aggressive speaker. During AAE conversations, approval or agreement is demonstrated nonverbally through touching, such as touching the listener's hand or arm. However, the touching of one's hair might be considered an insult by speakers of AAE (Taylor, in press; Roseberry-McKibbin 1995).

To summarize, it is important to emphasize that social constraints on speech are culturally organized and vary from culture to culture and from subculture to subculture. Competent speakers of a language must observe a wide range of sociocultural norms in verbal interaction. For example, competent speakers must know when it is appropriate to address a person using a title and a last name or a first name; they must make vocabulary choices appropriate for their addressee and the social situation; and they must know how to phrase requests without violating rules of etiquette. In many cases, it is the violation of such norms, rather than grammatical or phonologic norms, that are the sources of communication failures. The clinical setting, as well as other service-delivery settings, is one in which many people can experience what they feel are violations of their privacy. Compound this with cultural differences in beliefs about what is considered private and pragmatically appropriate, and it becomes easy to envision the barriers of self-defense that clients may erect that block the flow of information necessary for optimal service delivery.

Development of African American English

Morphologic and Syntactic Development

Research on the normal acquisition of AAE morphologic and syntactic patterns is scarce. The few data-based studies that have been conducted have largely investigated grammatical features and suggest that, in addition to sharing linguistic features with other dialects, AAE also shares features of normal linguistic development in young children (Blake 1984; Stockman 1984, 1986a, b; Steffenson 1974; Stockman and Vaughn-Cooke 1982; Stockman 1984; Reveron 1978; Cole 1980).

Blake (1984) and Stockman (1986a) have both shown that the morphosyntactic development of young children who speak AAE is similar to that of children who use SAE up to the age of 3 years, including the development of the mean length of utterance (MLU). Children in homes where AAE is spoken have well developed use of one- and two-word utterances by the age of 18 months, as is observed in children in homes where SAE is spoken (Steffensen 1974; Blake 1984). Their MLU increases with age at least to the age of 2.5 years, with increments similar to those of children who speak SAE (Blake 1984; Stockman 1984).

Research investigating the development of morphologic features shows that children in homes where AAE is spoken acquire early morphologic features in the same pattern as children learning SAE, including features to mark the plural, possessive, past tense, and third-person singular (Stockman 1986a; Blake 1984; Steffensen 1974; Reveron 1978; Cole 1980). As with SAE, the morphologic features of AAE involving tense, mood, and aspect markers of the verb phrase, negation, and later-developing morphologic features develop in the later preschool years. At the age of 3 years, children learning AAE have developed the use of well-formed multiword constructions, simple declaratives, and questions, with subject, verb, and object complements and a few complex utterances also appearing (Stockman 1986a). Elaborated sentences with embedded object complements, negative sentences, and the formation of tag questions appear before the age of 4 years. As children develop through the preschool years, a variety of complex sentences and complex semantic relations are used, including coordinated, subordinate, and relative clause sentences and complex wh- question forms (Washington and Craig 1994; Craig and Washington 1995). Thus, through the early preschool years, there is little difference in the development of morphologic and syntactic forms between children learning AAE and SAE. This implies that the linguistic forms of children acquiring SAE and of children acquiring AAE cannot be distinguished until the children reach about 3 years of age (Steffensen 1974).

The features that contrast AAE and SAE generally involve the later-developing forms. At the age of approximately 4 years, the features of the respective dialects that the children are acquiring begin to emerge. Like the continuum of development of standard English forms, it appears that AAE rules are also learned in a developmental sequence and that the frequency with which these rules are used increases with age (Cole 1980; Reveron 1978). Social class differences become most pronounced after the age of 4 years (Kovac 1980; Reveron 1978; Stockman 1986a; Craig and Washington 1994).

Cole (1980) found that, at the age of 3 years, African American children exhibit the AAE rules for regular past tense, third-person singular, present-tense copula, and remote past (*been*). The AAE features of indefinite article regularization and multiple negation were observed in 4-year-old children. When these children were 5 years of age, the features of reflexive and pronominal regularization occurred. Because Cole analyzed only the speech of 3-, 4-, and 5-year-old African American children, it can be assumed that other AAE features do not emerge until after the age of 5 years. If this is the case, it would make identification of language disorders within AAE-speaking children by conventional standardized tests extremely difficult (Stockman 1986b). AAE forms not used until after 5 years of age include the use of *at* in questions (e.g., "Where my coat at?"), the *go* copula (e.g., "There go my coat."), distributive *be*, first-person future, embedded questions, past tense copula, present copula, and second-person pronouns. Features such as the habitual *be* (e.g., "She be working.") and the use of *what* to mark the relative clause ("He the one what broke it.") develop at much later ages than the other forms (Cole 1980). Among the later emerging contractive AAE forms are the use of *had* to mark the simple past (e.g., "We had went to the store."), the use of *steady* to mark an intensified continuative marker (e.g., "He steady be mockin' me."), and the use of *come* to express indignation about an event or action (e.g., "He come hollering at me.").

Variables in the required use of certain linguistic forms can cause difficulty in distinguishing development from disorders or delays in morphologic development in AAE. For example, although speakers of AAE are required to use the form of *be* in statements such as "yes, he is," it is not obligatory in "John a boy" (Seymour 1995). The expression of habitual *be* (e.g., "he be working"), as opposed to a temporary condition (e.g., "he working"), does not appear in SAE. The feature is not likely to be observed by speech-language pathologists assessing the development of morphologic features using SAE standards.

Phonologic Development

Because SAE and AAE are dialects of the same language, several phonologic features are noncontrastive. Like the early development of morphology and syntax, the early phoneme development of children learning AAE is not different from that of children learning SAE (Seymour and Ralabate 1985; Seymour and Seymour 1981; Steffersen 1974). The features that typically distinguish AAE and SAE involve sounds and phonologic features that develop after the age of 4 or 5 years of age. These features include final consonant deletion or weakening, final cluster reduction, unstressed syllable deletion, and interdental fricative substitution involving final /th/ (Haynes and Moran 1989; Moran 1993; Seymour and Seymour 1981; Vaughn-Cooke 1986; Wolfram and Fasold 1974; Stockman 1991, 1995; Stockman and Settle 1991).

Standard articulation tests vary in the number of items related to AAE. They have limited usefulness in determining phonologic performance of children learning AAE (Cole and Taylor 1990; Washington and Craig 1992). Care must be taken to distinguish between those features that are contrastive and those that are not contrastive of AAE and SAE. According to Bleile and Wallach (1992), the following features are not contrastive between AAE and SAE and can thus be useful in distinguishing between normal disordered or delayed phonologic development in children learning AAE:

- The use of more than one or two stop errors
- Initial word position errors (with the exception of /b/ for /v/)
- Glide errors in children older than 4 years of age
- More than a few cluster errors (with the exception of final clusters)
- Fricative errors other than /th/

The primary indicators of whether a child who speaks AAE is having difficulty in phonologic development is the ability of those familiar with the dialect to understand the child at 5 years of age and the determination of whether the child is considerably more difficult to understand than his or her age and dialect peers (see Chapter 13).

Pragmatic Development

Communicative intent and semantic-linguistic functions in children learning AAE develop along the same lines as children learning SAE. Children between the ages of 18 months and 2 years develop the same functions as children learning other languages. These functions include informative, requestive, regulative, imaginative, affective, participative, and attentive functions (Bridgeforth 1984; Blake 1984; Stockman 1986a). According to Vaughn-Cooke and Wright-Harp (1992) and Davis and colleagues (1992–1993), the similarity in the development of linguistic function appears to continue through the preschool years.

Because of the apparent lack of assessment tools that distinguish between normally developing AAE and true disorders, children developing AAE are often assessed using assessment tools that fail to take into account the normal development of the dialect. It is essential that the normal development of features in AAE be considered in the determination of distinction between the least competent child considered to have normal development and development of language in children considered to be delayed-learning AAE (Stockman 1996).

Nonbiased Clinical Management of African Americans

Nonbiased clinical management is the process of establishing a client's native language, dialect, and culture as the basis on which all speech-language and hearing evaluations are administered and interpreted and on which treatment is prescribed. For nonbiased management to occur with an individual client, the speech-language pathologist must seek out and discover the normal language patterns and cultural views of that client. There are no known valid, empirically based, nonbiased assessment tools for the assessment of the speech of speakers of AAE. This is a critical research objective. Because of the complexity of cultural variables that can affect service delivery, nonbiased management must go beyond the administration of specific tests and procedures. Instead, it must be an entire process, a professional way of life emanating from a basic attitude that respects a person's culture, normal linguistic style, family structure, and beliefs. This process seeks to evaluate normalcy from the client's cultural viewpoint instead of from the morals, values, and standards of language normalcy held by the clinician.

The Individuals with Disabilities Education Act of 1990 reinforces the concept of nonbiased clinical management. It mandates that assessment that determines the need for special education services be racially or culturally nondiscriminatory. The Individuals with Disabilities Education Act requires that tests and other assessment tools be provided and administered in the child's native language, such as AAE, or some other mode of communication, unless it is impossible to do so.

Speech-language pathologists should incorporate the following into a nonbiased clinical management process when treating African Americans as well as people of any culture:

1. The clinician should conduct an attitudinal self-examination. Since nonbiased management requires a respect for the client's race, ethnicity, and culture, the clinician's attitudes toward African Americans or speakers of AAE could impede the process.

2. The clinician should conduct nonbiased services, especially assessment, using ethnographic methods—that is, he or she should obtain information from the point of view of that culture. When ethnographic methods are used as the "umbrella" for all clinical services, clinical services are more culturally relevant.

3. The clinician should refrain from making negative assumptions about the client and family members. Like the majority of people, African American parents love their children and want to provide them with the things that aid in healthy development. However, in a society in which a disproportionate number of people living in poverty are African American, meeting basic survival needs of food, clothing, and housing becomes a time-consuming and thought-consuming task. Educational and rehabilitation efforts, such as speech-language and hearing services, may become low-priority items. This can affect the client's perception of the need for service, the length of time the client stays in treatment, and the motivation for full participation in services.

4. Case history questionnaires, permission forms, and documents authorizing the release of information should be given and explained carefully. The number of forms sent can be overwhelming and the content of the forms too complex to be understood or trusted. Case history information forms typically require answers to personal questions on the birth and medical and health circumstances of the client, including employment and educational levels. The need for having this information about the client and the family should be explained. Asking some African Americans to put answers to personal questions in writing, when the use of the information is unknown, can result in feelings of suspicion and mistrust.

5. The clinician should greet family members and clients using their preferred names. He or she should address African American clients in a formal manner using the appropriate surnames and titles (e.g., Mr. Townsen and Mrs. Grantham) until requested to do otherwise. The use of first names by service providers and others who are not family members can be taken as an insult.

6. Assessment and intervention services should be as family-centered as possible. African Americans have a variety of family units, including two-parent, single-parent, and extended-family systems. In certain economic and familial circumstances, the mother may not spend the most time with the child or necessarily know detailed information about the child's speech, language, and cognitive development. In some instances, for example, an alternate caregiver, such as the child's grandmother or older sibling, may know more about the child than the mother.

Family members should be encouraged and welcomed to attend the sessions. This provides an opportunity for the clinician to observe the normal language use and interactions within the family. The clinician can also observe the client interacting with different family members and obtain accurate, naturalistic information on the client's speech and language skills. Existence of code switching can be more readily observed and recorded during these interactions. Additionally, when the testing has been completed, the clinician can use family members to comment on the validity of the evaluation results and recommendations and to determine priorities for therapy, if therapy is warranted. In treatment sessions, family members can learn speech and language facilitation techniques to help the client at home, especially if regular attendance is difficult or services become interrupted.

Family-centered therapy services can also enhance communication between family members as they join forces to help the client. For example, services were provided to an African American family whose members consisted of the deaf mother who could communicate only in sign language, the hearing father who could not and would not use sign language, the 4-year-old client who had severe receptive and expressive delay, and the toddler daughter who was obviously high-risk for language and speech disorder. All family members came to therapy. During this family-centered treatment, the mother began to teach sign language to the father, and the father began to learn both sign language and to speak to his wife so that she could lip-read his words. The parents not only learned how to provide stimulation for their son using both language systems, but they also enhanced communication between each other. An additional benefit was that the daughter's language skills began to improve.

Family involvement not only helps the client's development but also seems to enhance the communication between family members. Additionally, family involvement can help reduce cultural mistrust or suspicion held by any of the family members.

7. The clinician should determine the client's dialect before interpreting assessment data. Because the client is an African American does not mean that he or she uses AAE. Not all African Americans are speakers of AAE. To determine if a child is learning AAE, Terrell, et al. (1992) recommended comparing the child's performance with that of the child's parents or primary caregivers. Although there are some differences between adult AAE and child AAE forms, it supports the use of this procedure as an indicator of whether or not a person is an AAE user.

8. Specific assessment tools should be adapted to reflect the client's linguistic and cultural orientation. There are two general categories of assessment procedures: standardized and nonstandardized. Within these main categories, clinicians have a choice of ways to use these general procedures with African American clients.

Standardized Tests

The majority of standardized measures are biased against many African Americans in overall testing format and in how items are scored (Taylor and Payne 1983; Washington 1996). If a clinician chooses to use standardized tests, however, the following are several suggestions for strengthening the true meaning of the results:

1. Check the validity of the test. Read the validity data in the test manual to determine if sufficient numbers of African Americans were represented in the sampling data. If African Americans are represented, check to see if there are separate norms for AAE speakers. If included at all, the number of African Americans in the standardization sample usually depends on the most recent U.S. Census available to the authors. According to Washington (1996), even though African Americans are included in the sample, the test items can still be in SAE form. In addition, because a test includes African Americans in the standardization sample does not mean that the test is sensitive to AAE. Usually there is no information as to whether those in the sample speak AAE or SAE. Thus, the test may only be appropriate for African Americans who speak SAE.

2. Analyze the dialectal effect on the test. Before administering a test, analyze each item's stimulus and response for possible dialectal effect. For example, if the correct test response for an item is *two dogs*, the clinician should predetermine that a normal AAE response to that item is *two dog*. The clinician should prepare a list of these dialectal responses for a test. The clinician can then choose to score the test with dialectal variations counted in as normal responses or to score the test according to the manual's guidelines and interpret the results according to dialectal variations. In every case, the report should indicate how the test was scored.

3. Obtain local normative data for a standardized test. This involves administering a test to a local target population and determining the mean scores and standard deviations for this group. In other words, the test is restandardized to be more indicative of the normal performance of the local community. Harris (1993) suggested that at least 50 individuals at each age or grade should be randomly selected from the community to establish the local norm. She also suggests that children who fall between one and one half to two standard deviations might be identified as language disordered.

4. Construct a new test. Possibly the most exciting application of standardized tests to African Americans is to construct a new test that is not racially biased. Although the need for culturally unbiased tests is great and immediate, time and cost have delayed the process. Caution should be taken to ensure that any new test is standardized and validated so that it will yield usable and meaningful results for the group being tested.

5. Modify the testing procedure. To accommodate the AAE speaker the following methods can be used: (a) change the instructions, (b) increase the

response time, (c) test the limits (i.e., test beyond the ceiling and probe for student understanding of a task), (d) provide other practice items to make certain the student knows how to take the test, (e) record the client's comments, changes of answers, or explanations to try to understand his or her reasoning, (f) have the client name objects as well as point to them, and (g) ask the child why he or she selected a specific response. Of course, any modification changes the validity and reliability of a test; thus, the original norms are no longer appropriate. Nonetheless, the results may still give a better picture of the client's capabilities. All adaptations should be noted in the evaluation report (Campbell 1996).

Nonstandardized Procedures

There are a variety of nonstandardized clinical procedures; most involve gathering and analyzing a conversational sample. Since African Americans may switch to a silent code in formal testing situations, it is important for clinicians to obtain conversational samples that are truly representative of the client's language skills. The following are several ways that this can be facilitated:

1. Record the client's conversations with family members or with friends. Compare this with the client's conversation with the clinician.
2. Use culturally relevant or familiar objects to stimulate conversation. These items can include pictures of African Americans engaged in culturally relevant activities; photographs of family members; culturally relevant foods, music, clothing, important persons, and significant African American historical figures, such as Martin Luther King or Jackie Robinson.
3. Determine the client's narrative skills. If the client is 4 years old or older, consider reading a short, culturally relevant story to the child and have the child retell the story. This helps to determine the nature of the client's narrative skills bearing in mind the cultural differences in narrative style. The client's story can also be used to analyze AAE features.
4. Obtain a language sample. Conversational sample analysis should always attempt to identify the dialect that the client uses. Use of a traditional or computer-based language sample analysis can result in biased and incorrect results.
5. Consider using criterion-referenced testing. In this type of testing, a client's responses are not compared with the normative data or performance of other clients; rather, they are compared with a set of behaviors determined to be the criteria for acceptable responses. Criterion-referenced measures are most frequently used in therapy to set performance

levels, such as the 95% criterion for correct production of a phoneme. This technique, however, can also be used for nonbiased assessment, if clinicians have a way to establish valid referent criteria. One way to establish these valid criteria is to use parent-child comparative analysis (Terrell, et al. 1992). This method uses the cultural and linguistic patterns of the parent, caregiver, or person who is the primary language model as the referent criteria. The basic procedure of the parent-child comparative analysis is to administer the same speech and language tests to a parent or caregiver and to the client. The client's speech and language patterns are then compared with the patterns of the parent or caregiver. If the client is a child, patterns that do not match with those of the caregiver are further compared with normal speech expectations for the child's chronological age via normal language charts. Any divergent speech patterns that remain following this two-step comparative analysis have a high probability of being true disorders.

Intervention

If the assessment results indicate a communication disorder, intervention may be recommended. The disorder and not the features of the dialect should be the focus of treatment (American Speech-Language-Hearing Association 1983).

The clinician should be cognizant of the client's preferred learning style and make adaptations to accommodate the style. Learning style is the process of acquiring new information through the organization, perceptions, processing, manipulation, and recall of information. African Americans often prefer a field-dependent learning style in which they are influenced by their surroundings, including peers and authority figures. A high value is placed on social and interpersonal environments and on group achievement and cooperation. They prefer auditory and kinesthetic techniques (cues) and charismatic teaching. These characteristics indicate that speakers of AAE may prefer to work in a group service-delivery model with peers. Being isolated to receive individual treatment can further the feelings of low self-esteem. The group activity may also reduce feelings of mistrust (Battle and Grantham 1997; Terrell and Hale 1992).

Franklin (1992) suggests that an affect-oriented, open, and risk-free environment fosters learning in African American students. She also suggests that African American children demonstrate high proficiency levels with varied stimuli, increased verbal interaction, and modified speaking (using rhythm and intonation). Multisensory stimuli (i.e., oral, print, and visual reinforcements), a varied format, and a faster paced, high energy atmosphere were also noted as techniques that increased learning.

The clinician should be culturally competent. A culturally competent clinician (CCC) is sensitive to his or her beliefs and to how these values and beliefs affect others. The CCC recognizes both similarities and differences among people and adapts his or her teaching techniques to the needs of the clients. The CCC sends and receives signals that are appropriate to the culture, both linguistically and socially (Battle and Grantham 1997). CCCs take the time to visit the community and learn about the culture of the client. They also participate in comprehensive, ongoing, multicultural in-service and workshop programming.

Conclusion

Clinicians should be culturally competent. They should view African American clients as they view all clients—as people who differ in age, sex, culture, region, ethnicity, religion, and social economic backgrounds who might or do have a communication disorder. Indeed, clinicians should consider the total person as they formulate creative, innovative, appropriate and often nontraditional assessment and intervention procedures that can make a true and positive difference in a client's quality of life. Cultural learning is an ongoing process and is essential for successful non-biased clinical management.

References

American Speech-Language-Hearing Association. (1983). Position paper on social dialects. *OSHA, 25,* 23–25.

Battle, D.E., & Grantham. R.B. (1997). Serving culturally and linguistically diverse students. In P. O'Connell (Ed.), *Speech, language and hearing programs in schools: A guide for students and practitioners* (pp. 345–371). Gaithersburg, MD: Aspen.

Baugh, J. (1983). *Black street speech.* Austin, TX: University of Texas Press.

Blake, I.K. (1984). *Language development in working-class black children: An examination of form, content, and use.* Dissertation, Columbia University Teachers College.

Bleile, K., & Wallach, H. (1992). A sociological investigation of the speech of African American preschoolers. *American Journal of Speech-Language Pathology, 1(2),* 54–62.

Bloom, L., & Lahey, M. (1978). *Language development and language disorders.* New York: Wiley.

Bridgeforth, C. (1984). *The development of language functions among black children from working class families.* Paper presented at the presession of the 35th annual Georgetown Univeristy Round Table on Language and Linguistics, Georgetown University, Washington, DC.

Burling, R. (1973). *English in black and white.* New York: Holt, Rinehart & Winston.

Butcher, M.J. (1964). *The Negro in American culture.* New York: Knopf.

Campbell, L. (1996). Issues in service delivery to African American children. In A.G. Kamhi, K.E. Pollock, & J.L. Harris (Eds.), *Communication development and disorders in African American children* (pp. 73–94). Baltimore: Brookes.

Cole, L. (1980). *Developmental analysis of social dialect features in the spontaneous language of preschool black children.* Ph.D. dissertation, Northwestern University.

Cole, P., & Taylor, O. (1990). Performance of working-class African American children on three tests of articulation. *Language, Speech, and Hearing Services in Schools, 24,* 171–176.

Collins, J. (1985). Some problems and purposes of narratives in educational research. *Journal of Educational Research, 167,* 57–68.

Craig, H.K., & Washington, J.A. (1994). The complex syntax skills of poor, urban, African American preschoolers at school entry. *Language, Speech, and Hearing Services in Schools, 25,* 181–190.

Craig, H., & Washington, J.A. (1995). African American English and linguistic complexity in preschool discourse: A second look. *Language, Speech, and Hearing Services in Schools, 26(1),* 87–93.

Davis, P., Williams, J., & Vaughn-Cooke, F.B. (1992–1993). A comparison of lexical development in a child with normal language development and in a child with language delay. *Journal of the National Student Speech-Language Hearing Association, 20,* 63–77.

Dillard, J.L. (1973). *Black English: Its history and usage in the United States.* New York: Vintage.

Erickson, F. (1984). Rhetoric, anecdote, and rhapsody: Cohesion strategies in conversations among black American adolescents. In D. Tannen (Ed.), *Cohesion in spoken and written discourse* (pp. 81–154). Norwood, NJ: Ablex.

Foster, H.L. (1990). *Ribbin' jivin' & playin' the dozens: The persistent dilemma in our schools (2nd ed.).* Williamsville, NY: Herbert L. Foster.

Franklin, M.E. (1992). Culturally sensitive instructional practices for African American learners with disabilities. *Exceptional Children, 59,* 115–122.

Gee, J. (1985). The narrativization of experience in the oral style. *Journal of Education, 167,* 9–35.

Gee, J. (1989). Two styles of narrative construction and their literacy and educational implications. *Discourse Processes, 12,* 263–265.

Grier, W., & Cobbs, P. (1968). *Black rage.* New York: Bantam Books.

Harris, G. (1993). American Indian cultures: A lesson in diversity. In D.E. Battle (Ed.), *Communication disorders in multicultural populations* (pp. 78–113). Boston: Butterworth–Heinemann.

Haskins, J., & Butts, H.F. (1973). *The psychology of black language.* New York: Barnes & Noble.

Haynes, W., & Moran, M. (1989). A cross-sectional developmental study of final consonant production in Southern black children from preschool through the third grade. *Language, Speech, and Hearing Services in Schools, 20,* 400–406.

Heath, S.B. (1982). What no bedtime story means: Narrative skills at home, at school. *Language in Society, 11,* 49–76.

Heath, S.B. (1986). Taking a cross-cultural look at narratives. *Topics in Language Disorders, 7,* 84–94.

Hester, E.J. (1994). *The relationship between narrative style, dialect, and reading ability of African American children.* Ph.D. dissertation, University of Maryland.

Hester, E.J. (1996). Narratives of young children. In A. Kamhi, K.E. Pollock, & J. Harris (Eds.), *Communication development and disorders in African American children* (pp. 227–245). Baltimore: Brookes.

Hicks, D. (1991). Kinds of narratives: Genre skills among first graders from two communities. In A. McCabe, & C. Peterson (Eds.), *Developing narrative structure* (pp. 55–87). Hillsdale, NJ: Lawrence Erlbaum Associates.

Hyon, S., & Sulzby, E. (1992, April). *Black kindergartners' spoken narratives: Style, structure, and task.* Presented at the annual meeting of the American Educational Research Association, San Francisco, CA.

Jones, L. (1963). *Blues people.* New York: Morrow.

King, M.L. Jr. (1958). *Stride toward freedom.* New York: Harper & Row.

Kovac, C. (1980). *Children's acquisition of variable features.* Unpublished doctoral dissertation, Georgetown University, Washington, DC.

Labov, W. (1966). *The social stratification of English in New York City.* Washington, DC: Center for Applied Linguistics.

Lahey, M. (1988). *Language disorders and language development.* New York: Macmillan.

Michaels, S. (1981). Sharing time: Children's narrative style and differential access to literacy. *Language in Society, 10,* 423–442.

Michaels, S., & Collins, J. (1984). Oral discourse styles: Classroom interaction and the acquisition of literacy. In D. Tannen (Ed.), *Cohesion in written and spoken discourse* (pp. 219–244). Norwood, NJ: Ablex.

Moran, M. (1993). Final consonant deletion in African American children speaking Black English: A closer look. *Language, Speech, and Hearing Services in Schools, 24,* 161–166.

Nichols, P. (1989). Storytellin' in Carolina: continuities and contrasts. *Anthropology and Education, 20(3),* 232–245.

Olson, D. (1977). From utterance to text: The bias of language in speech and writing. *Harvard Educational Review, 47(3),* 257–282.

Reveron, W.W. (1978). *The acquisition of four Black English morphological rules by black preschool children.* Ph.D. dissertation, Ohio State University.

Roseberry-McKibbin, C. (1995). *Multicultural students with special language needs.* Oceanside, CA: Academic Communication Associates.

Ruffins, P. (1997). Ten myths, half-truths, and misunderstandings about Black history. *Black Issues in Higher Education, 13,* 23–25.

Salovey, P., & Rodin, J. (1986). The differentiation of social-comparison jealousy and romantic jealousy. *Journal of Personality and Social Psychology, 30,* 1100–1112.

Sattler, J.M. (1982). *Assessment of children's intelligence.* Philadelphia: Saunders.

Seymour, H. (1995, December). *Theory and practice in evaluating child African American English.* Paper presented before the annual convention of the American Speech-Language-Hearing Association, Orlando, FL.

Seymour, H., & Seymour, C. (1981). Black English and standard American contrasts in communication development of 4- and 5-year-old children. *Journal of Speech and Hearing Disorders, 46,* 276–280.

Seymour, H., & Ralabate, P. (1985). The acquisition of a phonological feature of Black English. *Journal of Communication Disorders, 18,* 139–148.

Steffensen, M. (1974). *The acquisition of Black English.* Ph.D. dissertation, University of Illinois.

Stockman, I.J. (1984, September). *The development of linguistic norms for nonmainstream populations.* Paper presented at the National Conference for Concerns for Minority Groups in Communication Disorders, Nashville, TN.

Stockman, I.J. (1986a). Language acquisition in culturally diverse populations: The black child as a case study. In O. Taylor (Ed.), *Nature of communication disorders in culturally and linguistically diverse populations* (pp. 117–156). San Diego: College Hill.

Stockman, I.J. (1986b). The development of linguistic norms for nonmainstream populations. In F.H. Bess, B.S. Clark, & H.R. Mitchell (Eds.),

Concerns for minority groups in communication disorders [ASHA reports 16] (pp. 101–110). Rockville, MD: ASHA.

Stockman, I. (1991, November). *Constraints on final consonant deletion in Black English.* Paper presented at the annual convention of the American Speech-Language-Hearing Association, Atlanta.

Stockman, I. (1995, November). *Early morphosyntactic patterns of African American children.* Paper presented at the annual convention of the American Speech-Language-Hearing Association, Orlando, FL.

Stockman, I. (1996). The promises and pitfalls of language sample analysis as an assessment tool for linguistic minority children. *Language, Speech, and Hearing Services in Schools, 27(4),* 355–366.

Stockman, I., & Vaughn-Cooke, F. (1982). A re-examination of research on the language of black children: The need for a new framework. *Journal of Education, 164,* 157–172.

Stockman, I., & Settle, S. (1991, November). *Initial consonants in young black children's conversational speech.* Poster presented at the annual meeting of the American Speech-Language-Hearing Association, Atlanta.

Takada, N., & Hamayan, E. (in press). Japanese-influenced English. In L.C. Cole, & V. Deal (Eds.), *Communication disorders in multicultural populations.* Rockville, MD: American Speech-Language-Hearing Association.

Tannen, D. (1982). The oral-literate continuum in discourse. In D. Tannen (Ed.), *Spoken and written language: Exploring orality and literacy* (pp. 1–16). Norwood, NJ: Ablex.

Taylor, O. (Ed.). (1986). *Nature of communication disorders in culturally and linguistically diverse populations.* San Diego: College Hill.

Taylor, O.L. (in press). Clinical practice as a social occasion. In L. Cole, & V.R. Deal (Eds.), *Communication disorders in multicultural populations.* Rockville, MD: American Speech-Language-Hearing Association.

Taylor, O.L., & Payne, K.T. (1983). Culturally valid testing: A proactive approach. *Topics in Language Disorders, 3,* 8–20.

Terrell, F. (1975). Dialectal differences between middle-class black and white children who do and do not associate with lower-class black children. *Language and Speech Disorders, 18,* 65–73.

Terrell, F., & Barrett, R.K. (1979). Interpersonal trust among college students as a function of race, sex, and socioeconomic class. *Perceptual and Motor Skills, 48,* 1194.

Terrell, F., & Terrell, S. (1981). An inventory to measure cultural mistrust among blacks. *Western Journal of Black Studies, 5,* 180–185.

Terrell, F., & Terrell, S.L. (1983). The relationship between race of examiner, cultural mistrust, and the intelligence test performance of black children. *Psychology in Schools, 20,* 367–369.

Terrell, F., & Terrell, S.L. (1984). Race of counselor, client, sex, cultural mistrust level, and premature termination of counseling among black clients. *Journal of Counseling Psychology, 31,* 371–375.

Terrell, B.T., & Hale, J. (1992). Serving a multicultural population: Different learning styles. *American Journal of Speech-Language Pathology, 1,* 5–8.

Terrell, S.L., & Terrell, F. (1996). The importance of psychological and socio-cultural factors for providing clinical services to African American children. In A.G. Kamhi, K.E. Pollock, & J.L. Harris (Eds.), *Communication development and disorders in African American children* (pp. 55–72). Baltimore: Brookes.

Terrell, F., Terrell, S.L., & Taylor, J. (1981). Effects of race of examiner and cultural mistrust on the WAIS performance of black students. *Journal of Consulting and Clinical Psychology, 49,* 570–571.

Terrell, F., Terrell, S.L., & Taylor, J. (1988). The self concept of black adolescents with and without African names. *Psychology in the School, 25,* 65–70.

Terrell, F., Watkins, E., & Miller, F.D.S. (1990, August). *Mistrust level, self-esteem, achievement, motivation and academic performance of black students.* Presented at the annual meeting of the American Psychological Association, Dallas.

Terrell, S.L., Arensberg, K., & Rosa, M. (1992). Parent-child comparative analysis: A criterion-referenced method for the nondiscriminatory assessment of a child who spoke a relatively uncommon dialect of English. *Language, Speech, and Hearing Services in Schools, 23,* 34–42.

U.S. Bureau of the Census. (1996). *Statistical abstract of the United States 1996 (116th ed.).* Washington, DC: U.S. Bureau of the Census.

Vaughn-Cooke, F. (1986). Lexical diffusion: Evidence from a decreolizing variety of Black English. In M. Montgomery, & R. Bailey (Eds.), *Language variety in the South* (pp. 111–130). Tuscaloosa, AL: University of Alabama Press.

Vaughn-Cooke, F., & Wright-Harp, W. (1992). *Lexical development in working-class black children.* National Institutes of Health Grant #RR08005-23.

Washington, J.A. (1996). Issues in assessing the language abilities of African American children. In A.G. Kamhi, K.E. Pollock, & J.L. Harris (Eds.),

Communication development and disorders in African American chil-dren (pp. 35–54). Baltimore: Brooks.

Washington, J., & Craig, H. (1992). Articulation test performance of low-income African American preschoolers with communication impairment. *Language, Speech and Hearing Services in Schools, 22,* 203–207.

Washington, J., & Craig, H. (1994). Dialectal forms during discourse of urban African American preschoolers living in poverty. *Journal of Speech and Hearing Research, 37,* 816–823.

Westby, C. (1985). Learning to talk—talking to learn: Oral literate language differences. In C. Simon (Ed.), *Communication skills and classroom success* (pp. 181–212). San Diego: College Hill.

Westby, C. (1994). Multicultural issues. In J. Tomblin, H. Morris, & D. Spriestersbach (Eds.), *Diagnosis in speech-language pathology* (pp. 29–52). San Diego: Singular.

Williams, R. (1975). *Ebonics: The true language of black folks.* St. Louis: Institute of Black Studies.

Williams, R., & Wolfram, W. (1976). *Social dialects: Differences versus disorders.* Rockville, MD: American Speech-Language-Hearing Association.

Willis, W. (1992). Families with African American roots. In E. Lynch, & M.J. Hansen (Eds.), *Developing communication competence: A guide for working with young children and their families* (pp. 120–247). Baltimore: Brookes.

Wolfram, W., & Fasold, R. (1974). *The study of social dialects in American English.* Englewood Clifts, NJ: Prentice Hall.

Wyatt, T. (1991). *Linguistic constraints on copula production in Black English child speech.* Ph.D. dissertation, University of Massachusetts.

Additional Resources

American Speech-Language-Hearing Association. (1983). Position paper on social dialects. *ASHA, 25,* 23–27.

Battle, D.E. (1996). Language development and use in African American children. *Topics in Language Development, 16(4),* 9–22.

Fields, C. (1997). Ebonics 101: What we have learned. *Black Issues in Higher Education, 13,* 18–28.

Gee, J., & Michaels, S. (1989). Discourse styles: Variables across speakers, situations, and tasks. *Discourse Processes, 12,* 263–265.

Kamhi, A., Pollock, K.E., & Harris, J. (1996). *Communication disorders and development in African American children.* Baltimore: Brookes.

Leonard, L.B., & Weiss, A.L. (1983). Application of nonstandardized assessment procedures to diverse linguistic populations. *Topics in Language Disorders, 3,* 35–45.

Taylor, O.L. (1990). Language and communication differences. In G.H. Shames, & E.H. Wiig (Eds.), *Human communication disorders: An introduction* (pp. 126–160). Columbus, OH: Merrill.

3

Asian- and Pacific-American Cultures

Li-Rong Lilly Cheng

If the world were a village of 1,000 people, it would include 584 Asians, 124 Africans, 95 Europeans, 84 Latin Americans, 55 former Soviets, 52 North Americans, and 6 Australians and New Zealanders. The people of the village would have difficulty communicating because they speak hundreds of languages (U.S. Bureau of the Census 1995).

Asian and Pacific Americans (APAs) originate from Pacific Asia or are descendants of Asian or Pacific islander immigrants. Numbering 8.8 million in the United States, APAs are the fastest growing segment of the U.S. population, representing 3.3% of the nation and 10% of California (Gardner, et al. 1985). APAs are fast becoming an influential presence socially, politically, and economically. There has been significant growth in the Asian and Pacific islander population in the United States. In 1970, the Asian and Pacific islander population was less than 1% of the total population of the United States (Rueda 1993). By the year 2000, that population is expected to increase to 4%, a projected growth of 400% in 30 years (Gardner, et al. 1985; Rueda 1993). Approximately 40% of immigrants to the United States in 1990 were from Pacific Asian countries (U.S. Bureau of the Census 1995). During the last two decades, the United States has experienced a great influx of migrants, immigrants, and refugees from Latin America and Pacific Asia, especially from Southeast Asia. The greatest increase in immigration has been by Asian and Pacific immigrants. In 1990, the Census Bureau reported that there were 7,273,662 Asians and Pacific islanders (excluding undocumented aliens) in the United States (2.9% of the population), as compared with 3,500,439 in 1980 (1.5% of the population), representing an increase of 107.8% (Jiobu 1996). More than 300,000 Southeast Asian students are in the K–12 programs in this country.

The Asian-American school-age population increased more than sixfold from 212,900 in 1960 to almost 1.3 million in 1990 (U.S. Bureau of the Census 1995). In 1990, 40% of APA children were first-generation immigrants, 44% were second generation, and 15% were third generation (Jiobu 1996). By the year 2020, the number of Asian-American children in U.S. schools is projected to total about 4.4 million (Jiobu 1996). According to the U.S. census of 1990, the largest number of immigrants to the United States are Chinese (Jiobu 1996).

The number of limited English-proficient (LEP) students in California public schools in the spring of 1996 was 1,323,787, an increase of about 5% over the number in the spring of 1995 (University of California Linguistic Minority Research Institute 1996). Other than Spanish, the languages with greatest representation were Vietnamese, Hmong, Filipino, and Khmer (University of California Linguistic Minority Research Institute 1996).

APAs are extremely diverse in all aspects of their ways of life, including language, culture, religion, attitudes toward education, child-rearing practices, and roles within the family. The Asian and Pacific island cultures have interacted with and influenced one another for many generations and therefore share many similarities. The information in this chapter is presented to provide an understanding of APAs and to assist speech-language pathologists and audiologists in providing services to this culturally and linguistically diverse group of people.

Overview of Asian- and Pacific-American People

Asian and Pacific islander groups have been immigrating to the United States for more than two centuries, with the first records of arrival of Chinese dating from 1785. Since that time, more than 17 Asian groups have immigrated to the United States. The most numerous APAs have origins in China (both Taiwan and the People's Republic of China), Hong Kong, Japan, Korea, India, Vietnam, Cambodia (Kampuchea), Laos, Guam, the Philippines, India, Pakistan, Bangladesh, Malaysia, Indonesia, Singapore, and Samoa. Since 1975, more than 1 million refugees from Southeast Asia have settled in the United States (U.S. Bureau of the Census 1995). Many refugees have settled in California, where the weather is similar to their home countries, and in New York, where there is a large immigrant population.

Refugees and immigrants from Asia and the Pacific islands come from a variety of historical, social, educational, and political backgrounds. Some are affluent, well-educated, voluntary immigrants, and some are preliterate refugees. They bring a variety of financial profiles, languages, folk beliefs, world views, religious beliefs, child-rearing practices, and attitudes toward education, all of which have a profound impact on speech-language pathology services.

Perceptions of Disabilities

A cultural definition of what constitutes an impairment depends on the values of each particular cultural group. Differences exist even within a group, and the expected or anticipated reactions to disabilities can vary considerably. The treatment of birth defects and other disabilities is influenced by cultural beliefs and by the socioeconomic status of the individual and the family within society (Cheng 1990a; Chinn 1990; Gollnick and Chinn 1990; Ortiz-Monasterio and Serrano 1971; Strauss 1985). There are broad similarities and differences among Western and non-Western belief systems and practices. In all cultures, attitudes toward disabilities can be traced, in part, to folk beliefs and superstitions. A tendency exists to define the cause of a health-related problem in spiritual terms (Cheng 1990a; Meyerson 1990; Strauss 1985; Tolliver-Weddington 1990).

Most Asian/Pacific people view a disabling condition as the result of wrongdoing of the individual's ancestors, which results in guilt and shame. The cause of disabilities are explained through a variety of spiritual beliefs, cultural beliefs, or both, such as an imbalance of inner forces, bad wind, spoiled foods, gods, demons or spirits, or hot or cold forces. For example, the Chamorro culture views a disability as a gift from God. They believe the individual with a disability belongs to everyone. The person with the disability is thus protected and sheltered by the family. Some cultures believe disability is caused by karma (fate). These cultures view disability as something meant to be. Other cultures view disability as a curse and may ostracize the individual from society (Cheng 1990b). (For more information about APA views on disability, see Cheng 1990a, Chinn 1990, and Akamatsu 1993.)

Languages

The hundreds of different languages and dialects that are spoken in East and Southeast Asia and the Pacific islands can be classified into five major families: (1) Malayo-Polynesian (Austronesian), including Chamorro, Ilocano, and Tagalog; (2) Sino-Tibetan, including Thai, Yao, Mandarin, and Cantonese; (3) Austro-Asiatic, including Khmer, Vietnamese, and Hmong; (4) Papuan, including New Guinean; and (5) Altaic, including Japanese and Korean (Ma 1985). Additionally, there are 15 major languages in India from four language families: (1) Indo-Aryan, (2) Dravidian, (3) Austro-Asiatic, and (4) Tibeto-Burman (Shekar and Hegde 1996).

Folk Beliefs, Religions, and Philosophical Views

The Asian and Pacific populations hold a variety of religious and philosophical beliefs. Major religions and philosophies include Buddhism, Confucianism, Taoism, Shintoism, animism, and Islam. In addition, because of Western influence, Christianity is also practiced. There are many Catholic churches in the Philippines and across the Pacific islands. The Bible is considered a major source of inspiration by many Pacific islanders.

There are many different Asian and Pacific folk beliefs. People from urban and rural areas and those with different levels of education, exposure to Western cultures, and personal experiences vary in their reactions to folk beliefs. Attitudes toward disabilities are a reflection of current and historical beliefs about the nature of handicapping conditions. Illness is usually treated with all available methods, including consulting with the priest, clansmen, and elders, before a licensed physician is consulted. The particular individuals consulted vary from culture to culture and from individual to individual. Among the Hmong, surgical intervention is viewed as harmful. They believe that spirits may leave the body when the body is cut open, causing death.

Treatments also vary a great deal, ranging from surgery, medication, or therapy to acupuncture, massage, cao (coin rubbing), bat gio (pinching), giac (placing a very hot cup on the exposed area), steam inhalation, balm application, herbs, inhaling smoke or ashes from burnt incense, or the ingestion of hot or cold foods (Cheng 1995a). Other methods of healing include exercises such as Qi-Gong, over-the-counter drugs, prescription drugs, or a combination of methods. The use of non-Western methods of healing may be difficult for Western physicians to manage in their overall treatment of patients because they are not always familiar with such methods. The mixture of medication and herbs can be counterproductive.

Education

The prevailing views toward education in most Asian and Pacific cultures present challenges for American educators and speech-language pathologists. The so-called chopstick cultures (China, Korea, Japan, Vietnam) tend to view education as the most important thing one can achieve in life. This is due largely to the influence of the teachings and principles of Confucius (Cheng 1993). The Asian groups often have different approaches to

Table 3-1   Asian Attitudes Toward Learning

Asian cultural themes	*Educational implications*
Education is formal.	Teachers are formal and are expected to lecture.
Teachers are to be highly respected.	Teachers are not to be interrupted. Students are reluctant to ask questions.
Humility is an important virtue.	Students are not to "show off" or volunteer information.
Reading of factual information is studying.	Fiction is not considered serious reading.
It is important to have order and to be obedient.	Students are to sit quietly and listen attentively.
One learns by observation and by memorization.	Rote memory is considered an effective teaching tool.
Pattern practice and rote learning are studying.	Homework in pattern practice is important and expected.

Source: Adapted from L.L. Cheng. (1991). *Assessing Asian language performance: Guidelines for evaluating LEP students (2nd ed.)* (pp. 14). Oceanside, CA: Academic Communication Associates.

learning, and these approaches have implications for the strategies Asian students use to learn. The selected examples in Table 3-1 are representative of some Asian attitudes toward education and their educational implications. The relative importance of each of the attitudes differs from culture to culture. (For more information about attitudes toward education, see Cheng 1995a.)

As shown in Table 3-2, there are incongruities between Asian students' learning styles and American teachers' teaching styles. These differences can lead to teachers' misconceptions of students and students' confusion over the "proper" way of schooling. The implications for speech-language therapy are obvious, particularly with the naturalistic, whole-language approach to treatment, especially of preschool- and early-elementary–school children. Again, the relative importance of each of the concepts varies with cultural group and among individuals within the group. Educators need to be sensitive to cultural tendencies of various APA groups. These tendencies, however, should not be viewed as static cultural rules: Generalizations must be avoided. Predictions should not be made based on a superficial survey of the culture.

**Table 3-2   Incongruities Between Asian Students' Learning Styles
and American Teachers' Teaching Styles**

American teachers' perceptions	Asian parents' expectations and children's learning styles
Students need to participate in classroom activities and discussions.	Students are to be quiet and obedient.
One learns through inquiry and discussion.	One learns through memorization and observation.
Asian students generally do well on their own.	Teachers need to teach; students need to study.
Critical thinking and analytical thinking are important.	It is important to deal with the real world.
Fantasy is encouraged.	Factual information is more important than fantasy.
Students need to ask questions.	The teacher is not to be challenged.
Reading is a way to discovery.	Reading is decoding of information and facts.

Source: Adapted from L.L. Cheng. (1991). *Assessing Asian language performance: Guidelines for evaluating LEP students (2nd ed.)* (pp. 14). Oceanside, CA: Academic Communication Associates.

Cultural Characteristics of Asian and Pacific Peoples

Although there are many similarities among the various groups, APAs have extremely diverse backgrounds. This section provides a brief description of the major APA groups in the United States: the Chinese, Koreans, Japanese, Southeast Asians, Filipinos, Pacific islanders, and Indians. The immigration history, religious beliefs, family structure, attitudes toward education, and characteristics of the language spoken are presented. This information provides a general background against which speech-language pathologists and audiologists should view the cultural factors of the particular family or client served.

All APA groups and the individuals in those groups present some common background as immigrants or descendants of immigrants. Each may have a very different story to tell. Such diverse personal and group experiences must be taken into consideration when working with individuals.

Clearly intra- and intergroup differences exist among the Asian and Pacific islander immigrant and refugee groups. Caution should be taken to avoid overgeneralization of this information in relation to a particular client or family.

These people represent diverse social, cultural, and linguistic backgrounds. They add to the richness of the American profile. They offer opportunities to understand cultures, languages, and peoples. They challenge our views of the world and Pacific Asia. By learning more about them, speech-language pathologists can provide better services that meet the true meaning of equity.

The Chinese

Immigration History

The Chinese first immigrated to the United States two centuries ago. Records document the arrival of Chinese in the United States in 1785. Chinese immigrants, who came in greater numbers beginning in 1848, worked as miners and farmers and provided the major labor force for building the railroads. Since World War II, Chinese have been immigrating to the United States mainly from Taiwan and Hong Kong to study, to join their families, or for business purposes. In recent years, more Chinese from the People's Republic of China have entered the United States. Although the exit policy in China became more restricted after the 1989 Tienanmen Square incident, many Chinese immigrants received political asylum after that time. Immigrants from the People's Republic of China constituted one of the largest groups of immigrants in the 1990s.

Religion and Values

There are more than 55 ethnic groups in China. They practice a variety of religions, including Buddhism, Taoism, Catholicism and other forms of Christianity, and Islam. They also believe in ancestral worship and Confucianism. One of the most important ideals of the Chinese culture is the pursuit and maintenance of harmony. Value is placed on outward calmness and on control of undesirable emotions, such as anger, jealousy, hostility, aggression, and self-pity. Open expression of emotion and confrontation are viewed as undesirable. The new generation of Chinese, however, may be more competitive and assertive as they face the competition of the world market.

The Family

Chinese culture places a heavy emphasis on respect for elders and the strength of the family as a unit. Each member of the family has a role that is clearly defined through an intricate kinship system. Traditionally, the father was responsible for all family members, with the mother having direct responsibility for the children, and the oldest son having responsibility for the care of his younger siblings. Parents taught their children to behave according to strict rules. In recent decades, the changing role of women and

China's zero population-growth policy have altered traditions. The parents and grandparents can no longer depend on their children to provide filial piety because of the lack of children.

Education

The Chinese traditionally believe that education is extremely important. Chinese Americans work hard to remove any linguistic and cultural barriers to obtaining a good education. Most traditional Chinese families expect their children to do well in school. Teachers are highly respected. If a family member is successful, the entire family receives credit. Parents do not praise their children readily, even when they excel, because excellence is generally expected. If a child does poorly in school or needs special attention, the parents often feel ashamed, perceiving the difficulties as a sign of their own failure. Many Chinese-American parents take their children to Chinese schools on weekends and expect them to learn Chinese and maintain the culture.

Chinese students who have emigrated recently from Taiwan have had quite different educational experiences from students who emigrated from the People's Republic of China. The Taiwanese students' motivation for success is also high. Their overall success in U.S. schools is similar to that of students from South Vietnam, where the educational style is not as competitive. Chinese students who have gone to school in the People's Republic of China, however, do reasonably well in U.S. schools because they have had a competitive education similar to that in the United States. The terms *model minority* and *silent minority* have been used to describe the success of Chinese students. Students in need may be overlooked because they are quiet, and this results in poor school performance and even behavioral problems (Chang, et al. 1995).

Language

More than 80 languages and hundreds of dialects are spoken in China. The Chinese dialects are extremely complex. Some are closely related, whereas others are mutually unintelligible, even though their words are graphically represented by the same characters (Cheng 1991). Of the Chinese population, 94% are reported to speak Han (a Sino-Tibetan language) and its dialects Mandarin, Wu, Yue (Cantonese), Xiang, Gan, Kejia, and Min, with more than two-thirds speaking the Mandarin dialect of Han. The two main dialects spoken by the Chinese in the United States are Mandarin (the national language of Taiwan and of the People's Republic of China) and Cantonese.

Chinese is a tonal language. Each character is phonetically represented by a single syllable, with each syllable having a tone mark. In Mandarin Chinese, there are four tones (and a neutral tone): the first tone has a high level, the second tone is rising, the third tone is falling-rising, and the fourth tone is falling. The same spoken syllable has different meanings depending on the tone and the various characters that the syllable represents. Each Han dialect has its own tonal system with differing numbers of tones. Deaf and hearing-impaired individuals find tones an added challenge in their acquisition of oral language (Ching 1990).

A syllable in Mandarin and Cantonese consists of segmental and suprasegmental features. Segmental features include an initial consonant (optional) and a final sound. Suprasegmental features include the distinct tones that are an intrinsic part of the phonologic make-up of a Chinese syllable.

There are several major differences between the phonetic systems of Chinese and English. Chinese characters are each composed of a single syllable. The rules for syllabification and syllabic stress in English can present difficulty for a Mandarin or Cantonese speaker. The speakers may sound telegraphic and may truncate words. It may also be difficult for Chinese speakers to learn English intonation patterns, such as those signaling the difference between questions and statements.

Because there are only two final consonants in Mandarin, /n/ and /ŋ/, and only seven final consonants in Cantonese, /m/, /n/, /ŋ/, /p/, /t/, /k/, and glottal stop /ʔ/, Chinese speakers often omit final consonants when speaking English. There are no consonant blends in Mandarin or Cantonese, making the double and triple consonant blends of English difficult for Chinese speakers. Chinese learners of English may use Chinese sounds when speaking English, if the sounds are phonetically similar in the two languages such as /s/ and /ʃ/. The differing vowel systems can also cause some confusion. Cantonese speakers, for example, may substitute /e/ for /ɛ/ and /æ/, /i/ for /I/, /ou/ for /ɔ/, (e.g., "boat" for *bought*), or /u/ for /ʌ/ (e.g., "roof" for *rough*).

Unlike English, Chinese is noninflectional and does not use plural markers, tense markers, copulas, the verb *has*, the auxiliary *do*, articles, or conjunctions. In addition, the rules for the use of prepositions, pronouns, negation, and other morphologic and syntactic forms vary, causing considerable difficulty for Chinese speakers when they are learning English. The semantic differences between English and Chinese words further compound the difficulty Chinese speakers have in learning English.

The pragmatic rules of the Chinese language, such as turn-taking, greeting, social distance, proximity, and politeness, vary a great deal from those of the English language. Because Chinese generally do not interrupt a speaker to ask questions, students may appear to be passive or nonparticipatory. A socially appropriate Chinese greeting is "Have you eaten?" to which the accepted response is "Yes," which is similar to the English greeting "How are you?" and the answer "Fine." Social distance is determined by such attributes as age, class, and marital status. Chinese may not express emotion in public, and hugging, kissing, and touching are not frequently observed. A giggle can be used as a sign of embarrassment. The Chinese are taught to be humble and when praised are generally embarrassed. When someone says, "Thank you," the correct response is generally, "No need to thank me."

The Koreans

Immigration History

Koreans have one of the oldest surviving civilizations on earth and have maintained a significant number of their cultural traditions. For many centuries, the Koreans refused to compromise with other nations and remained closed to foreign ideas. As a result, they became a "hermit" nation (Kim 1978). Since World War II, South Korea and North Korea have been clearly divided politically.

Korean immigration to the United States began in the early twentieth century, when Korean laborers came to Hawaii to work in the pineapple and sugarcane plantations and later went to the mainland. Before World War II, however, the Korean community in the United States was not visible because of its small population. Between 1961 and 1970, 35,000 Koreans immigrated to the United States. Between 1971 and 1980, 272,000 immigrated from Korea to the United States (U.S. Bureau of the Census 1995). In the decade from 1981 to 1990, the number of Korean immigrants increased to more than 300,000 (U.S. Bureau of the Census 1995).

Approximately 800,000 Koreans were living in the United States in 1990 (U.S. Bureau of the Census 1995). According to Chu (1990), Korean-American children with LEP have historically been underserved and underfinanced in comparison with LEP children from other non–English-speaking groups.

Religion

Korean immigrants are primarily Christian. Many Christian churches in the Korean community provide services in the Korean language. These churches also have been noted to provide social and emotional support and informational help and to serve as acculturation agents (Kim 1981).

The Family

As with other Asian cultures, Koreans are noted for their extended family, which typically includes three generations (Kim 1978). Traditionally, the father is the head of the family and represents the family honor. He is responsible for the family's welfare and is typically the sole provider. The father or other men in the Korean family do not typically help with household chores (Kim 1984). The Korean mother, who centers her work around the home, may represent the family in dealing with the schools. The elderly family members previously received a great deal of respect from younger family members. Immigration to the United States and acculturation have changed this to some extent.

Parent-child conflicts based on language and cultural differences have increased in the United States between immigrant children and parents. Due to economic pressures, the size of the Korean family has decreased in the United States. Children have begun to question the traditional role of the father and to challenge his authority. Teenage immigrants often feel lost and find it difficult to identify with either the Korean or the American culture (Trueba, et al. 1992).

Education

Since 1945, the educational system in South Korea has been patterned after the American educational system of elementary school, junior high, senior high, and 2 years of junior college or 4 years at a university (Kim 1978). Teachers have a great deal of authority. Korean classrooms are orderly; consequently, Korean-American students now attending American schools who have been educated in Korea may be extremely quiet and not ask questions. Asking questions of the teacher is considered to be a sign of disrespect. However, U.S.-born Korean children may come to school with different experiences and expectations and may not be shy or quiet.

Korean children are socialized into an environment in which going to the best schools is highly valued. They are accustomed to working extremely hard to obtain high scores on college entrance examinations to get into the best colleges. They are directed from the very beginning into specific fields such as science, medicine, or engineering and are not typically encouraged to go into literature, fine arts, human services, or business. There is little room for other alternatives or for students who are not capable of high achievement. Because they are highly disciplined, there are very few reported delinquency problems in school.

More than one-third of the Koreans in the United States have completed 4 or more years of college. In spite of this high level of education, many are employed at middle-level or low-level jobs, due to their language difficulties (Kim 1981, Kim 1984). Many are owners of grocery stores, markets, laundries, and restaurants. Underemployment is common among Korean-American families and causes low self-esteem and, consequently, parenting problems.

Language

The Korean language belongs to the Altaic family. Koreans in North and South Korea speak the same language. There are some variations among the various regional dialects, but they are mutually intelligible. Until

1443, the Koreans used the Chinese written system. After that time, the Hangul system was developed. The Korean written language has 19 consonants and 8 vowels. The sound of a letter is pronounced differently depending on its location in a word.

The phonetic systems of English and Korean are quite different and cause difficulty for Koreans learning to speak English. There are no consonant clusters in the initial and final positions of words in Korean; fricatives and affricates do not occur in the final position of words; and final stops are often nasalized when they occur before a nasal sound (e.g., "banman" instead of "batman"). Korean does not have contrasting vowel length; therefore, the following vowels are problematic: /i/, /I/, /u/, /ʌ/, and /au/. Since there are no labiodental, interdental, or palatal fricatives in Korean, speakers may make the following substitutions: /b/ for /v/, /p/ for /v/, /s/ for /ʃ/, /t/ for /tʃ/, and /dʒ/ for /ð/. Because /r/ and /l/ belong to the same phonetic category, they may be used interchangeably.

Since there is no word stress in Korean, Korean speakers can sound monotonous and have difficulty with interrogative intonation, which is typically found in English question forms. In addition, there are several syntactic and morphologic differences between English and Korean that lead to difficulty for Koreans in learning English. Korean has no gender agreement, no articles, no verb inflections for tense and number, and no relative pronouns.

Korean communication behavior has been influenced by the Chinese. Important factors are harmony, filial piety, social order, fairness, reverence for elders, and the maintenance of human relationships. The choice of words and grammar denote the relationship between the communicators and the importance of that relationship (Chu 1990). Nonverbal communication is very important because taciturnity reduces the amount of verbal interchange. Silence is a much more important part of communication for the Korean speaker than for the English speaker (Chu 1990).

The Japanese

Immigration History

Because land in their native island country was limited, large numbers of Japanese began to immigrate to the United States (first to Hawaii and then to California) between 1891 and 1907. Once in the United States, the Japanese worked at the lowest paying jobs in agriculture, mining, fishing, railroad building, and small businesses (Cheng 1991). Since that time, the Japanese have spent considerable energies to educate themselves and to improve their standard of living. Japanese Americans have assimilated well and participate in social, business, civic, political, and religious groups outside Japanese-American communities. They continue to integrate into predominantly white residential neighborhoods.

Religion

Shintoism, a form of Buddhism, is the dominant religion in Japan today, although Christianity has been adopted by a large proportion of its population. In the United States, many Japanese Americans are Christians. The Japanese are the largest ethnic group in Hawaii, and many are practicing Christians.

The Family

The Japanese group is unique in that it is composed of primarily U.S.-born, second-, third-, fourth-, and fifth-generation Japanese Americans. The terms *ni-sei* (second generation) and *san-sei* (third generation) are commonly used to refer to the number of generations the family has been in the United States. Japanese families generally value obedience, dependence on the family, formality in interpersonal relationships, and restraint in the expression of emotions. As in other Asian families, Japanese family members have well-defined roles and positions of power. Japanese children are expected to maintain emotional bonds with and dependence on their parents, and only secondarily develop self-reliance (Ima and Labovitz 1990). Japanese parents, wanting children to be receptive to adult expectations, continually refer to duty and obligation and invoke fear of ridicule and shame to control their children's lives.

Education

The teaching profession is one of the most highly regarded professions to the Japanese. To the Japanese, education is of prime importance. The Japanese student is expected to be attentive, work cooperatively, and be willing to accept the teacher's word as significant (Ima and Labovitz 1990). In the United States, Japanese-American students are often sent to after-school classes or to private tutors to ensure academic success. This contributes significantly to the pressures placed on children.

Language

Japanese, like Korean, is part of the Altaic language family. The Japanese writing system, which was adapted from the Chinese system, uses characters in writing called *Kanji*. The Japanese modified the Chinese symbols for phonetic purposes, organizing a syllabary called *Kana* (Cheng 1991). The Japanese pronunciation of the characters is entirely different from the Chinese pronunciation. Japanese is polysyllabic; every syllable is given equal stress. Japanese is not tonal, but it has an elaborate inflectional system.

Although there are only a few dialects in Japanese, they are mutually unintelligible because of great dialectal variations. Japanese has 5 vowels (/a/, /i/, /u/, /e/, and /o/) and 18 consonants (/k/, /s/, /t/, /n/, /h/, /m/, /y/, /r/, /w/, /g/, /d/, /b/, /z/, /p/, /tʃ/, /ʃ/, /dʒ/, and /j/). Vowels vary in duration as do English vowels. Only the /n/ phoneme occurs as a final consonant. Double consonants such as /kk/ and /pp/ occur. Difficulties encountered by Japanese people learning English are substitutions (e.g., /r/ for /l/, /s/ for /θ/, /z/ for /ð/, /j/ for /ð/, and /b/ for /v/); addition of vowels to words ending in consonants (e.g., "desker" for *desk* and "milku" for *milk*); and approximations of phonemes (e.g., /f/ phoneme is pronounced between /f/ and /h/, so that *food* becomes "hud").

Several grammatical features of Japanese interfere with learning English. For example, all Japanese verbs appear in the final position of the sentence. Personal pronouns are often omitted, since they are inferred from the context. No distinction is made between the singular and plural, so that, for example, *hon* means both book and books, with the meaning inferred from context. Because yes and no questions are marked by a final particle, question markers (e.g., *what* and *where*) are not needed at the initial position of a sentence.

In a study of narrative and pragmatics among the Japanese, Minami and McCabe (1991, 1995) found that Japanese children speak succinctly about collections of experiences rather than elaborating on any one experience in particular. Furthermore, they found that Japanese mothers request proportionally less description from their children, pay more verbal attention to boys than to girls, give less evaluation, and show more verbal attention than their North American counterparts. Japanese adults expect children to anticipate what will be asked of them and to do it; that value is embedded in the larger context of Japanese culture in which there is a notion of rapport and empathy (*omoiyari*).

The Southeast Asians

Southeast Asia is comprised of Vietnam, Thailand, Laos, Cambodia (Kampuchea), and Burma. These countries have similar foods and are similar in geography and climate but differ in culture and religion. Because the Burmese and Thais are few in number in the United States, these groups are not discussed in this chapter.

Southeast Asian Immigration

Before 1975, there were few Southeast Asians in the United States other than university students. Since 1975, however, more than 1 million Southeast Asians have fled their countries because of communist takeover of their governments.

The first wave of Southeast Asian immigrants (refugees), arriving in the United States in 1975, were Vietnamese who had either worked for or been affiliated with the U.S. government during the Vietnam war and had been airlifted out of Vietnam after Saigon fell to the Communists. They left for fear of persecution, many with only a moment's notice, leaving families behind. These first refugees were well educated and had some previous exposure to Western ideology and culture.

The second wave of refugees arrived between 1979 and 1982 after the brutal takeover of the region by the Khmer Rouge in 1975. This group, including Vietnamese, Cambodians, Laotians, Hmong, and ethnic Chinese, had escaped Southeast Asia after considerable hardship. The second wave of refugees was different from the first in that after 1975, there was no education in Vietnam and Cambodia and only limited education in Laos. Thus, the second wave of immigrants tended to be less well educated. In addition, they were less likely to have had contact with Western culture, were less likely to know English, were mainly rural and less likely to have had any urban experience, and were likely to have spent a long period of time in refugee camps before immigrating to this country.

The third wave of refugees came after the Vietnamese government instituted the Orderly Departure Program in 1982. The main purpose of this program was to allow Amerasians, the elderly, and unaccompanied minors to immigrate to the United States. Some of these refugees were preliterate or illiterate.

Many of the refugees have taken advantage of numerous programs established to assist in their resettlement. For these refugees, life is stable and prosperous, with the children being able to finish school and obtain gainful employment. Other refugees have not adjusted well, have not learned English, are underemployed, and feel a sense of loss and isolation. The problems of isolation are particularly serious for women who, because of staying at home to care for the children, have not had opportunities to learn English or adapt to their new surroundings (Ima and Keogh 1995).

The Vietnamese

Immigration History

Vietnam has a recorded history of more than 2,000 years. It is heavily influenced by Confucianism due to 1,000 years of Chinese rule (from 111 B.C. to A.D. 938). The period from A.D. 938 to A.D. 1883, "the era of independence," began when Ngo Quyen defeated the Chinese forces and liberated the country. In 1883, Vietnam was conquered by the French, whose domination lasted until 1954, when the Geneva agreement ended French rule in Indochina. The agreement also divided Vietnam into two separate states with North Vietnam under communist control and South Vietnam under a noncommunist regime (Te 1987). Two years later, a civil war between North and South Vietnam started that lasted nearly two decades. As the war intensified in 1964, the United States became heavily involved. Finally, when U.S. forces were withdrawn, South Vietnam fell into communist hands, resulting in an evacuation of more than 100,000 Vietnamese.

Religion

The Vietnamese practice a variety of religions and have a pluralistic approach to life (having more than one absolute standard for everything). Therefore, they think nothing of praying in a church different from their own religion's (Cheng 1989). The majority practice is Buddhism, but Taoism, Christianity, and Confucianism are also followed. The teachings from these religions form the foundation of all traditions, customs, and manners.

The Vietnamese celebrate many holidays. The greatest national holiday is the Tet festival, or Lunar New Year, which lasts several days. It is a time for family reunions, spring festivals, paying homage to ancestors, correcting faults, pardoning others, and paying debts. During the Tet festival, all birthdays are celebrated, since everyone becomes a year older on the last day of the twelfth lunar month. There are also holidays dedicated to national heroes, but these holidays are for commemoration and patriotism, not entertainment. The Vietnamese also celebrate the death days of their parents and grandparents.

The Family

In the Vietnamese culture, the family is paternally oriented and is the chief source of social identity for the individual. The family lives and works together, and family members look first to one another in times of crisis. The family consists of three generations and includes the husband and wife, their unmarried children, the husband's parents, and their sons' wives and children. A married woman joins her husband's family. Children are taught to be respectful to their parents and to their elders. The parents consider the education of their children an important responsibility. Both share in disciplining the children. Discipline is usually of a soft, verbal type with no corporal punishment and no extensive limits on behavior. Often the responsibility for the children is given to older siblings.

The Vietnamese name usually consists of three parts, which occur in the following order: family or clan name, middle name, and given name. A common middle name for men is *Van* and *Thi* for women. Common family names include *Nguyen*, *Tran*, and *Le* (Chhim, et al. 1987). There are only approximately 300 family names; therefore, using the family name by itself has little meaning. The given name holds the most meaning. Individuals are normally addressed, for example, as "Mr." plus the given name. A married woman retains her own family name but can be referred to as "Mrs." plus the husband's given name. It is important to keep the correct order, as reversing it means addressing a different person. Also, when writing someone's name, the writer should include diacritical markings, which help to distinguish similar-looking names.

Education

Education is also very important to the Vietnamese people. Educated people have an honored place in society. Overall, in Vietnam, education is free and mandatory; most continue to the college level. It is typically formal, although some parents choose to teach their children at home. Children begin their primary education at 6 years of age and go through the fifth grade. They then begin 7 years of secondary school in vocational arts, humanities, or sciences. Education is teacher-oriented and geared toward memorization and repetition. Learning is achieved by observation, rather than by experimentation. Vietnamese-American children are reported to do well in U.S. schools.

Language

Vietnamese is a tonal language that is essentially monosyllabic. There are three dialects: Northern, Southern, and Central. In the early part of the twentieth century, the Vietnamese adopted a modified romanized alphabet system to replace the old writing system that was based on Chinese characters. Diacritical marks are used to signify the tone of each word. Proficient and educated speakers speak two forms of Vietnamese: the high (formal) form and the vernacular (informal) form (Chuong 1990).

When English and Vietnamese phonetic systems are compared, the following differences are found (Te 1987):

- Consonant blends occur in all word positions in English, whereas there are no consonant blends in Vietnamese.
- Syllabic stress is used for contrastive purposes in English (i.e., to differentiate the noun and verb forms of words such as "convict," "record," and "contrast") but is not phonemic in Vietnamese because lexemes in Vietnamese are typically monosyllabic.
- English uses many final consonants, whereas Vietnamese uses only a limited number of final consonants, including /p/, /t/, /k/, /m/, /n/, and /ŋ/.

Vietnamese includes many words derived from other languages, such as English, French, Malay, and Chinese. Vietnamese speakers may mispronounce certain English phonemes by substituting a similar Vietnamese phoneme. Vietnamese learning English may display phonetic interference with distortions (e.g., /c/ + /ʃh/ for /tʃ/), substitutions (e.g., /z/ for /dʒ/), and omission of final consonants.

An important part of the Vietnamese language is the use of pronouns, which must be used appropriately to maintain proper social distance and inter-personal relationships. Different personal pronouns are used when addressing persons of differing age or status (Chuong 1990). The appropriate pronouns are used to show the intensity of respect or disrespect. Another feature of Vietnamese is the use of a number of fixed verbal formulas in daily conversa-tion. These emphasize the importance of family hierarchy and the social order.

The Hmong
Immigration History

Originally from China, the Hmong (also spelled Miao, Mung, Muong, H'mong, Hmoob, and Hmuoung) moved to the mountainous area of Southeast Asia, primarily Laos, centuries ago. After the fall of South Vietnam in 1975, approximately 100,000 Hmong fled to escape retaliation for assisting the South Vietnamese in the struggle against the Communists. Most of them had never been outside their mountain homeland before evacuation. The majority of them were illiterate. Before their uprooting, they had not been exposed to the conveniences (and stresses) of the "modern world." Thus, the Hmong who resettled in the United States faced tremendous problems.

As of 1987, approximately 60,000 Hmong were living in the United States, mostly congregated in the so-called Indochinese communities, the de facto Southeast Asian ghettos (Trueba, et al. 1992). The immense social and psychological upheaval the older Hmong experienced left them physically and financially dependent on their children, physically and psychologically isolated, lacking in self-esteem, and with few of the skills that are necessary for life in American mainstream society.

The elderly Hmong in the United States practice folk medicine and con-tinue to perform indigenous religious rituals. They wear native costumes and eat ethnic foods. An agrarian people, the Hmong prefer to grow their own vegetables. They find it extremely difficult to adjust to an urban lifestyle that makes it impossible to continue their customary way of life (Trueba, et al. 1992). They have difficulty learning to use modern home appliances, such as the refrigerator, washer and dryer, stove, and toilet. Many have combined traditional ways with the newly acquired American customs (Meredith and Cramer 1982).

Education

The Hmong view of education is different from that of other Asian refugee groups, in that they have not had a long tradition of literacy and schooling. The parents' insistence on discipline in education is a part of their Confucian tradition. Currently, Hmong students in the United States appreciate being able to read and use written language as a way to communicate. Hmong students often perform better than Khmer and Laotian students in school because they understand that a good education leads to better employment opportunities. Girls, however, often feel obligated to honor their parents' wishes to marry early and thus do not attend college.

Language

The linguistic characteristics of the Hmong language create difficulties for Hmong people attempting to learn English. The Hmong language, which is a Sino-Tibetan language, has two dialects: White (Hmoob Dawb) and Green (Hmoob Ntsuab). Hmong has 56 initial consonants, seven tones, and one final consonant /ŋ/. There are four series of stopped consonants, voiced and voiceless fricatives, nasals, liquids, and a single voiced glide. Several consonant sounds, such as /p/, /r/, and /t/, have both aspirated and unaspirated forms. The sound /r/, which is a stop rather than a liquid, is produced in the midpalatal area and may sound like either /t/ when aspirated or /d/ when unaspirated. Consonant clusters, which occur only in the initial position of words, include nasals plus stops (e.g., /np/ and /nt/) and nasals plus stops plus /l/ (e.g., /npl/).

Tones and vowels are more important for understanding than the many initial consonants. White Hmong has 13 vowels, whereas Green Hmong has 14 vowels. No vowels are reduced to the schwa. There are six basic vowels (/i/, /ɪ/, /u/, /ey/, /ɔ/, and /ɑ/), two nasalized vowels ("ong" and "eng"), and five diphthongs (/iɑ/, /uɑ/, /ɑi/, /ɑu/, and /ɔɪ/).The sounds of Hmong are represented in the romanized alphabet, developed in the late 1950s by missionary linguists. Tones are indicated by final letters but are never produced as final consonants in Hmong. For more information about the Hmong language, consult Cheng (1991) and Lewis and colleagues (1989).

Hmong speakers may experience difficulty with final consonants, particularly final consonant clusters. On the other hand, pronouncing polysyllabic words with correct primary and secondary stress is fairly easy, once the syllables are thought of as individual words with tones. A Hmong speaker may place too much importance on the vowel sound in unaccented syllables, not understanding that in English these vowels are often schwa sounds.

Hmong words are essentially monosyllabic. Compound words are disyllabic or polysyllabic. Unlike English, Hmong is a noninflectional language. Although many Hmong students have oral English fluency, they may still experience difficulty with tenses, using infinitives and gerunds, stringing several verbs together, and using adjectives after nouns.

The many homonyms, homophones, and synonyms in English cause difficulty for Hmong learners. Hmong, like other Asian languages, uses classifiers with nouns. These reveal the attributes of nouns in ways that English does not. For example, *tus* goes with a living or a long thing; *lub* goes with a bulky thing, a body part, or an abstract concept; *daim* goes with a flat, sheet-like thing; and *cov* indicates plurality (Bliatout, et al. 1988).

Cambodia or Khmer (Kampuchea)

Immigration History

Cambodia, also known as Kampuchea, is located in mainland Southeast Asia. France colonized the region in the mid 1800s, and in 1863 Cambodia became a French protectorate. In 1953, however, Cambodia gained independence, and the country was proclaimed the Khmer Republic in 1970. Although Cambodia was considered a nonaligned neutral country in the war in Southeast Asia, military actions against North Vietnam pushed the Vietnamese Communists into Cambodia. Cambodia fell into the hands of the communist Khmer Rouge in 1975. There was a complete devastation of the economic, social, and educational systems, which had been established by the French.

Many of the 7 million Cambodians tried to escape the communist takeover. Those caught trying to escape faced horrible brutalities, including torture, robbery, and rape. The families that successfully escaped were settled in refugee camps. Many families were separated, some losing contact forever. Many refugees had to spend years in the camps, waiting for permits to enter the United States. A majority of the families who arrived in the United States were headed by single parents (usually mothers), many of whom had mental health problems from the years of brutality and devastation during and after the war.

Because of previous hardships experienced during the war and in the refugee camps, Cambodians in the United States may display considerable distrust. Distrust, which was a method of survival during the war, was carried to refugee camps and into the country of permanent resettlement.

Religion

Approximately 85% of the population in Cambodia adheres to Buddhism, the official religion in Cambodia. The temple was the place of worship and was traditionally located in the center of each rural community. Since the communist takeover, all religious activities in Cambodia have been suppressed (Chhim, et al. 1987).

The Family

Traditionally, the Cambodian woman held a high place in society and was associated with responsible and important positions in the family. She was, and still is, considered the mentor of educational, social, and moral values, as well as the manager of all financial matters. Elderly family members are responsible for making important decisions concerning family issues, especially child care. The father has the role of head of the household (Rumbaut and Ima 1987).

Education

After Cambodia gained independence from France in 1953, interest in education grew tremendously to serve the needs of the people. A reform in education was begun in 1967, which was called the "Khmerization of Education," since the Khmer language was substituted for French as the language of instruction (Ouk, et al. 1988). When the Khmer Rouge took total control of Cambodia in 1975, schools were destroyed, and educated people were executed. Because education was not available after the communist takeover, students born after this time have most likely had no formal education. Recently, a minimal amount of education has been offered, with most children completing elementary school.

Language

Khmer is a language of the Austro-Asiatic family, which consists of more than 100 languages scattered from Eastern India to the South China Sea. Approximately 90% of Cambodians speak Khmer, although many other languages, such as Thai, Lao, and Cham, are also spoken (Ouk, et al. 1988). Khmer is a homogeneous language with very little dialectal variation from one region to the next. Several dialects can still be identified, including the following:

1. Standard Khmer is the form of the national language taught in schools and used for mass communication. Normally, standard Khmer is spoken in the central provinces.
2. Northern dialect is characterized by a change in some vowels and the retention of the final /r/.
3. Southeastern dialect is characterized by a simplification of the vowel system.
4. Phnom Penh dialect is characterized by the loss or change of /r/ to /h/ in initial or second position and an accompanying rising tone.

The Khmer alphabet was derived from Sanskrit and Pali (Ouk, et al. 1988). The written system has two forms, Aksar Mul and Aksar Crieng, which are used for different purposes. Various groups of people must be addressed differently in Cambodia, as in Laos. Therefore, four different forms of Khmer exist: the language of the ordinary people, the formal language, the language of the clergy, and the royal language.

Khmer words are usually monosyllabic or disyllabic, with stress always on the second syllable. The few polysyllabic words are either compound words or derived from other languages. Khmer is a nontonal language. Many lexical terms are derived from the French, particularly technical terms such as *aeroplane*, *café*, and *poste* (stamp).

Many consonant sounds are shared between Khmer and English, but some English consonant sounds do not occur in Khmer. Others that are shared may not be exactly alike. There are 85 different initial consonant clusters in Khmer but no final clusters. Most, but not all, are very different from those in English (e.g., *Mtyul* and *Sdap*). Khmer stops /p/, /t/, /k/, /ʔ/, and /d/ are both aspirated and nonaspirated. There are only two fricatives.

Khmer has approximately 50 different vowels and diphthong sounds, as compared with 14 in English. Even though the vowels are divided into short and long vowels, as in English, the sounds differ. Thus, Khmer speakers have to learn the differences between similar sounds and learn to hear and produce those that are new to them. Khmer speakers learning English often substitute /k/ for /g/, /v/ for /w/, /f/ for /b/, /tʃ/ for /s/, /s/ for /θ/, and /t/ for /θ/. The /r/ is approximated as a trill *r*. Many final consonants, such as /r/, /d/, /g/, /s/, /b/, and /z/, are omitted. The /b/ and /d/ are implosive, and there are possible vowel distortions of /ɛ/, /i/, /u/, and /æ/.

The Khmer often have difficulty with forms of the verb *to be*. Khmer speakers learning English may have difficulty with copula and auxiliary verbs and progressive and future tense markers. In addition, they may experience difficulty with placement of negative markers.

The Laotians

Immigration History

As part of French Indochina, Laos was under French rule between 1893 and 1954. Soon after the fall of South Vietnam and the Vietcong invasion in 1973, many Laotians, fearing for their lives, escaped and resettled in the United States. Major cultural differences have contributed to the adjustment problems of Laotians who have settled in the United States. Parents have had difficulty coping with the changes their children have rapidly undergone; many do not cope well and suffer deep depression. In addition, some Laotians were rural agrarians and were illiterate in their native language. Never having learned to read and write in their native language, they have found it extremely difficult to learn English. Without language skills in English, they have encountered difficulty in obtaining training and employment in the United States.

Religion

The Laotian refugees bring many customs and beliefs. Most Laotians are Theravada Buddhists, and most Laotian men are required to spend 2 or 3 weeks as monks before they marry. Many believe in the practice of folk medicine and the ritual of Baci. In the belief that every human being has 32 souls, many Laotians ask a sorcerer to perform the ritual of Baci to call back the soul outside of one's body of a person who is sick to bring about that person's recovery (Lewis and Luangpraseut 1989).

The Family

The Laotians revere the elderly (as do all Asians). They have large families, and extended families are not uncommon. Their community is not as cohesive as other Asian communities and has different factions based on political positions. They continue to complain about their lack of moral leadership and are constantly accusing each other of immoral leadership. Anyone who becomes a leader is suspect and must face accusations concerning his immorality in the leadership position. It is very difficult to form a cohesive community within this political atmosphere in which members accuse each other of untrustworthiness (Trueba, et al. 1992).

Education

Many Laotian refugees lacked basic literacy skills when they first immigrated to the United States, and so they found it difficult to learn English. The main focus of Laotian education is the Pagoda, which teaches how to read the sacred Buddhist texts. It takes great effort for Laotian parents to convince their children to continue their education beyond high school. Students work for prestige or community recognition, but education in itself is not seen as a requirement.

Teachers working with Laotian children should become familiar with the Laotian way of life to understand the children's behavior. For example, Laotian students generally do not say, "I don't know," believing it is a sign of disrespect to the teacher. Similarly, they rarely say "no," because they think that saying "no" will hurt the teacher's feelings. They generally do not look the teacher in the eye because staring is regarded as a sign of challenge, disrespect, and aggression (Chhim, et al. 1987).

Language

In the Laotian language, most words are monosyllabic, although there are some compound and polysyllabic words borrowed from Indian languages. The Laotian alphabet is based on Sanskrit and Pali of India.

In their system there are more symbols than sounds. Laotian is tonal like Chinese and Vietnamese. There are six tones (Chhim, et al. 1987).

Laotian culture plays an important role in the lexicon. This can be seen in the contrasting sets of lexical items used in conversations with various people of different social status. For example, seven different words may be used by a Laotian to refer to himself or herself, depending on the partner in conversation. Consequently, Laotian speakers must determine the listener's social rank before having a conversation. If the rank is unclear, Laotians are uneasy about responding (Lewis and Luangpraseut 1989).

Six different tones are used to denote syllables in Laotian. Individual words also have tonemes. Laotians sound monotonous because there is no stress in the language. Laotian words usually end in a vowel. Indicating stress and adding final consonants are therefore difficult for Laotian speakers learning English.

The basic word order of a Laotian sentence is similar to that of an English sentence (i.e., subject plus verb plus object); however, there are many syntactic and morphologic differences that interfere when a Laotian is learning English. Subjects are often omitted. Adjectives follow nouns, plurality and possession are expressed with different combinations of words rather than morphologic markers, and there are no tense markers. In addition, there are no articles, the verb form does not change when there is a change in subject (e.g., "I go," "you go," "he go"), and there is no verb *to be* for sentences with predicate adjectives (e.g., "food good," "dress beautiful"). Interrogatives are marked by placing *bo* at the end of the sentence as a marker.

India

Immigration History

India is one of the most populous countries in the world, with a population of nearly 1 billion. The Indian subcontinent includes India, Bangladesh, Nepal, Pakistan, Sri Lanka, and Buttan. Most immigrants to the United States from the area come from India and Pakistan. In the 1980s and 1990s, more Indians have come to the United States than all of the years before combined. According to the 1990 Census, there were 815,447 Indian immigrants in the United States (U.S. Census Bureau 1990).

Religion

India is the birthplace of many religions. The main religions are Hinduism, Jainism, Buddhism, and Sikhism. Others deserving special mention are Christianity, Zoroastrianism, and Islam. Hinduism is the oldest religion in the world and is traced back to 1500 B.C. Under its umbrella, monists, monotheists, polytheists, pantheists, animists, toremists, agnostics, and even atheists are sheltered. All Hindus believe in the doctrine of karma, or predestination. The caste system is another unique feature of Hindu life. The Brahmins have the highest place as the priestly clan, the Kshatriyas are the warrior class, the Vaisyas are the cultivators and merchants, and the Sudras are the menials. Postindependence reform abolished the caste system legally, but in practice it still lingers.

Buddhism was a dominant religion in India and spread to many parts of Asia, including China, Korea, Japan, and Sri Lanka; however, Buddhism has declined in India. The nations of India and Pakistan were divided because of strife based on the difference in religious beliefs. Pakistan's majority religion is Islam.

The Family

Families in India are typically very large and include extended families. All members, including three or four generations, live under the same roof. In contrast, immigrant Indian families in the United States are smaller in size. Although the traditional caste system is no longer promoted, individuals from different castes still do not maintain contact. The "untouchables" are still considered the lowest in the social stratum. Marriage is a necessity for Hindus on religious grounds. A male descendent is required to conduct the funeral rites of his parents. The Hindu joint family is either patrilineal or matrilineal and share a common god. Decision making is based on common opinions. However, the head of the joint family is empowered with all the powers and privileges and his decision is unquestioned and unchallenged (Jha 1995).

Education

The educational system in India is based on the British system, and English is taught in the schools. The educated are bilingual or multilingual. Literacy rates range from below 50% in some areas to more than 75% in other areas. The illiteracy rate is high in India due to the large number of people living in extreme poverty (Shekar and Hegde 1995). Immigrants to the United States, however, have achieved high academic success and are, in general, well educated. Most are college educated and are fluent English speakers. Indian immigrants have the highest educational attainment of all ethnic groups in the United States (U.S. Department Commerce 1993a, b). They tend to hold technical, managerial, professional, and sales positions. They also have higher income than the general U.S. population (Shekar and Hegde, 1995).

Languages

Linguists have listed 845 dialects and 225 distinct languages in India. The constitution of India recognizes 15 major languages, including Sanskrit and English. Hindi, the national language, is spoken or understood by 40% of the population. The Indian branch of the Indo-European language family contains Hindi, Bengali, Marathi, Punjabi, Gujarati, Sindhi, Oriya, and Assamese. These languages are spoken in part of India, Pakistan, and Bangladesh. The Dravidian branch languages include languages such as Kannada, Malayalam, Tamil, and Telugu, which are spoken in South India. India has produced its own dialect of English, known as the *Hobson Jobson*, with a dictionary of its own (Moraes and Howe 1991).

Both Hindi and Kannada have five short vowels /ɑ/,/e/, /i/, /o/ and /u/ and their longer counterparts. The following Hindi and Kannada consonants are not found in English: (1) voiced bilabials and velar aspirated stops, (2) dental and retroflex consonants, (3) voiced and voiceless palatal affricates, and (4) palatal nasal. In English /v/ is a labiodental fricative, whereas in Hindi the /v/ phoneme is a bilabial fricative. The English /w/ is an allophonic variation of the Hindi phoneme /v/. Wells pointed out that labiodental and interdental fricatives (i.e., /f/, /v/, /θ/, and /ð/) do not occur in these languages. Because of this, Hindi and Kannada speakers often substitute /f/ with a voiceless bilabial fricative /ɸ/, /v/ with a labiodental approximate /ʋ/, or /θ,ð/ with dental stops /t/ and /d/ (Wells, 1982). Indian speakers often substitute the alveolar series /t, d, l, r, n, s, z/ with the retroflex /ṭ, ḍ, ḷ, ṇ, ṛ, ṣ, ẓ/ found in Indian languages. Bansal (1978, 1990) pointed out the distinct stress and intonation patterns of Indian English, which can negatively affect intelligibility.

Other Groups from Pacific Asia

The Filipinos

Immigration History

Before 1521, the Philippines was a sovereign state that traded with China and many other Eastern and Middle Eastern nations. In 1521, the Philippines was taken over and ruled by the Spanish until it became a protectorate of the United States after the Spanish-American War in 1898. It was granted independence after World War II. Due to its history of trade and repeated colonization, the Filipino culture is a mosaic, with input from Spanish, American, Chinese, Malay, Indian, and other cultures. The multicultural influences on the Philippines make it difficult to identify Asian, Pacific, or European influences.

Filipino immigration to the United States began after the onset of American rule because of an unstable political climate, poverty, the search for better economic and educational opportunities, and reunion with family members. The Filipinos came to the United States in three major waves.

The first wave, which began in 1903, consisted of a highly select group of young men seeking college educations who gained the reputation of being serious scholars (*pensionado*) (Takaki 1989). These students returned to the Philippines after completion of their education and encouraged other young men and women to seek education in the United States (Melendy 1977). Between 1910 and 1938, almost 14,000 Filipinos were educated in the United States (California State Department of Education 1986).

The second wave of immigration, which began in 1906 and lasted until the 1930s, was directed toward Hawaii and was composed of Filipinos seeking agricultural employment in Hawaiian pineapple and sugarcane plantations. Many Filipinos eventually moved to the mainland of the United States and were employed in agricultural jobs on the West Coast.

The third wave of Filipino immigration, which began in 1965, included many well-educated families with school-age children, many of whom were seeking family reunions. Between 1965 and 1984, Filipino immigration increased by 950%, as more than 200,000 immigrants entered the United States (California State Department of Education 1986). The Filipinos constitute the largest single group of Asian immigrants (Cheng and Ima 1989). By the year 2000, the Filipino population in the United States is projected to reach 2 million (Chinn 1990).

The Family

The Filipino people practice a bilateral system of family responsibility, by which they are obligated to both sides of the family. The extended family is common. Filipino values place importance on specific roles and responsibilities that are hierarchically defined. The specific roles remain in effect even after children reach adulthood. Thus, each family is tied by defined roles. The child is not viewed as an individual but rather as an extension of many family generations. The family is seen as a family unit (R Galang, V Noble, L Halog, unpublished data, 1985). Adherence to traditional values varies among families.

Filipinos from different parts of the Philippines have different traditions, customs, languages, and religious beliefs. Their diversity is reflected in regional loyalties, which are often associated with language.

Education

Public education is compulsory (although this is not enforced by the authorities) through the elementary level in the Philippines. The Filipino people are status conscious and view education as a key measure of status. They believe in education and respect scholars. Many believe the way to succeed in life is through education. As a result, parents are eager for their children to do well in school and to perfect their English language skills (Monzon 1984).

Languages

Authorities disagree on the exact number of Filipino languages. It is estimated that there are 75 mother tongues. All of the languages are from the Malayo-Polynesian group. The major languages are Tagalog (the national language), Ilocano, and Visayan.

Tagalog is a polysyllabic language with its own dialectal variations. The sound system has 27 phonemes. There are sounds that are different from those in English and sounds that do not exist in English. Most words consist of roots and affixes. The combination of the root and its affix or affixes determines the meaning of the word. The usual word order in a sentence in Tagalog is the reverse of that in English (i.e., predicate plus subject, as in "slept the dog").

The Tagalog lexical, syntactic, morphologic, and phonologic features of language also can interfere with learning English. The Tagalog verb system does not make true time distinctions but characterizes something as begun or not begun, and if begun, as completed or not completed. Also, verbs are not inflected for number but are the same form for both singular and plural. Furthermore, Tagalog does not indicate gender in third-person singular pronouns.

The phonetic and syntactic differences between English and Tagalog cause many frustrations for the native Filipino learning English. In the following excerpt, this is expressed by a tenth grade Filipino boy who immigrated to the United States at age 14 (Olsen 1988):

> There is lots of teasing me when I don't pronounce right. Whenever I open my mouth I wonder, I shake and worry, will they laugh? They think if we speak Tagalog that we are saying something bad about them, and sometimes they fight us for speaking our language. I am afraid to speak English, I am afraid to try. And I find myself with fear about speaking Tagalog.

Tagalog has 27 phonemes: 16 consonants, including the significant glottal stop, 5 vowel sounds, and 6 diphthongs. Although many of these phonemes are similar to those used in English, nine English phonemes do not occur in Tagalog: $/v/$, $/z/$, $/\theta/$, $/\eth/$, $/d\mathcurrent{3}/$, $/f/$, $/\int/$, $/t\int/$ and $/\mathcurrent{3}/$. The Philippine speaker substitutes $/p/$, $/b/$, $/s/$, and $/t/$ for $/f/$, $/v/$, $/z/$, and $/\eth/$, respectively, because these sounds closely resemble sounds produced in

Tagalog. Differences in vowel boundaries lead Philippine speakers to have difficulty distinguishing, for example, between "lift" and "left."

In Filipino languages, plurality is marked by the word *onga* placed before the pluralized nominal (e.g., "onga bata" meaning *children*) or by another word carrying the concept of plurality (e.g., "dala wang bata" meaning *two children*). The Filipino speaker learning English has difficulty with the marking of plurality with the morpheme *-s*, particularly when it is redundant to the context (e.g., many friends).

The Pacific Islanders

The Pacific islands are grouped into three clusters: Polynesia, Melanesia, and Micronesia. Most numerous among the islanders are the Hawaiians, Samoans, and Chamorros, in that order. The Pacific islanders have different views and ways of life based on their experiences. The Hawaiian, Tongan, Samoan, Fijian, and other groups may share commonalities. The abundance of food, the mild temperature, the collective nature of their traditions, and the ritualized behavior of a group make it less important for an individual to strive and compete to become the best. Community orientation and group tradition make it difficult for a child to stand up and say, "I know how to do this, but you don't." He or she is more likely to state, "Let's all work on it together. I'll show you, and you show me." The Pacific islanders treasure and value collective behavior—that is, the reliance of existence on the group rather than on the individual. In the school environment children read, chant, and practice in unison. The American tradition of individualism violates the Pacific islander's principles of collective work and community-oriented education.

Religion and Folk Beliefs

Many religions are practiced in the Pacific islands. As a result of contact with Westerners, Pacific islanders have been converted to various forms of Christianity, including Catholicism, Mormonism, and Protestantism. In addition, many islanders have combined Western religions with indigenous folk beliefs. Suruhana and Surahano (practitioners of folk medicine) are often consulted for treatment in case of illness.

The Family

Families in the Pacific islands are usually extended and can include three generations living in the same house. Whether matrilineal or patrilineal, islander families place heavy emphasis on authority and expect children to comply with the wishes of elders and authority figures. The primacy of parents corresponds to the apparent lack of concern over the individual and the focus on the well being of the family.

Education

Formal education was not part of Pacific islander history until the Europeans came. They were essentially a premodern, preliterate society. Much of their educational tradition is still based on oral learning. Learning style is considered to be passive, with rote memorization being preferred (Cheng 1989). The child is taught not to be too individualistic, and emphasis is on conformity. Teaching is authoritarian in style. Teachers are respected, and children go to great lengths to please their teachers. Studies of Hawaiian, Tahitian, and Samoan children have suggested that they are likely to be unaccustomed to interacting with adults on a one-on-one basis, since they are often in situations in which direct communication is with other children and not adults (Jordan and Tharp 1979). In addition, absenteeism is common, reflecting not only the more relaxed style of the islanders but also a different emphasis on academic expectancies, such as being on time and completing projects.

As a result, when Pacific island children come to school in the United States, they are struck by the differences between the two cultures. The culture of the U.S.-based schools emphasizes the individual, individual excellence, and creativity. This contradicts the Pacific islander's learning style, and it basically undermines their sense of well-being, as their identity is tied to the group and is not individualistic. Data from the California State Department of Education (1986) indicate that, as a group, the Pacific islanders perform at much lower levels in school than their Hispanic and African American counterparts (Ima and Labovitz 1990).

Languages

Among the 5 million inhabitants of the Pacific islands, more than 1,200 indigenous languages are spoken. These include Carolinian, Chamorro, Fijian, Hawaiian, Korean, Marshallese, Papua New Guinean, Paluan, Pompean, Samoan, Tahitian, Trukese, and Yapese. The five lingua francas used by the Pacific islanders are French, English, Pidgin, Spanish, and Bahasa Indonesian. Languages are heavily influenced by multicultural sources. Culture also places emphasis on certain groups of words. For example, in Carolinian, there are many words to describe the different stages of the coconut, including *atil, ghurub, ttach, seew, apeel, luu, mwosoow, schoo,* and *faar,* among others (Cheng and Ima 1989).

The People of the Hawaiian Islands

The Hawaiian Islands are multiethnic and multicultural. The main ethnic groups are Japanese, Caucasian, Filipino, Chinese, and Korean. At least 22 languages are spoken by children enrolled in the Honolulu public schools, representing the major languages from Southeast Asia and the

Pacific islands. The most important values are expressed by *aloha*, meaning generosity, graciousness, spirituality, friendliness, and hospitality. The extended family, or *ohana*, is highly valued (Kanahele 1986). For more information about Hawaiian and Pacific families see Mokuau and Tauili'ili 1993.

The Hawaiian language is polysyllabic and alphabetical. It has the shortest alphabet in the world, with five long vowels (a, e, i, o, and u) and eight consonants (h, k, l, m, n, p, w, and ?). The basic phonologic rules are that the stress is placed on the second to last syllable, consonant clusters do not exist, the final phoneme is always a vowel, and the glottal stop is phonemic.

The Samoans

In the beginning of the nineteenth century, Samoa's isolation was broken by missionaries and traders from Germany, Great Britain, and the United States. In 1899, Western Samoa became a German colony, and the United States acquired American Samoa for its naval station. After Germany's defeat in World War I, Western Samoa was given to New Zealand under a League of Nations mandate. In 1962, Western Samoa became an independent nation, whereas American Samoa continues to be a possession of the United States.

During the 1920s, some Samoans left their homeland to provide free labor to build a Mormon temple in Hawaii. It was not until the 1950s, however, that large groups of Samoans left for Hawaii and the U.S. mainland. There are approximately 60,000 Samoans living in the United States (including Hawaii), and only 30,000 remaining in American Samoa. Among the many reasons Samoans give for leaving their homeland are a search for a better life, access to health care, better education, and an escape from the traditional authoritarian system (Cheng 1989).

The Samoans have an extended family system based on a clan culture. The chief *(matai)*, who is elected by the clan members, is responsible for locating resources (e.g., food, fish, land titles, and housing).

The Chamorro of Guam

A territory of the United States, Guam has a population of approximately 116,000 (U.S. Bureau of the Census 1995). Chamorros make up the largest ethnic group, representing approximately 42% of the total population.

The Chamorros are believed to have migrated to Guam from Indonesia and the Philippines as early as 2000 B.C. Guam today is an island society of diverse ethnic elements that draws its strength from Asian, American, and indigenous Chamorro sources. The Chamorro people control the political structure of the government of Guam. Based on the rate of Chamorro immigration and Asian (especially Filipino) immigration to Guam during the past three decades, this will not be the case in the twenty-first century. As many as 40% of all Chamorros now reside outside of Guam and the Northern Marianas (U.S. Bureau of the Census 1995). Forty-nine thousand people from Guam lived in the United States in 1990 (U.S. Bureau of the Census 1995).

Chamorro is one of the official languages of Guam. Chamorro has six vowels and at least 11 vowel allophones. There are 18 consonants and one semiconsonant (/w/). Words are divided into classes, and each class has separate rules it follows. Chamorro speakers are likely to have difficulty learning English because of the characteristics of their native language.

Overview of Assessment and Intervention Principles and Guidelines for Asian and Pacific American Populations

Assessment Strategies

Chapter 13 focuses on assessment. This section offers brief principles and guidelines specific for the APA population.

APA LEP children with speech-language disorders face tremendous problems in school. To provide quality education to students with speech-language and hearing disorders, appropriate assessment is necessary. The purpose of assessment is to identify strengths and weaknesses of the individual, so that appropriate clinical intervention can be provided if necessary.

APA children and adults who are in need of speech, language, and hearing services often are underserved due to the lack of trained bilingual professionals and a lack of understanding of the life history of the clients. The number of speech-language pathologists and audiologists in the United States who speak Vietnamese, Laotian, Khmer, Chamorro, Tagalog, Hmong, Korean, or Yiu-Mienh is minuscule. Only a few bilingual speech-language pathologists speak some of the other more widely used Asian languages, such as Chinese and Japanese. Furthermore, only a few bilingual speech-language pathologists work in settings where they have regular contact with bilingual clients. Consequently, speech-language disorders in APA children and adults are sometimes not identified, or language differences are identified incorrectly as language disorders.

Due to a federal mandate requiring that the abilities of children with limited English proficiency be assessed in their native language (Diana v. California State Board of Education 1970), speech-language pathologists and audiologists need to develop competency in providing appropriate service to APA clients. This may necessitate seeking the assistance of interpreters.

Clients have diverse linguistic, paralinguistic, stylistic, and discourse backgrounds and experiences. It is important that assessment determine the degree to which the problems observed are due to these diversities rather than to an inability to communicate. Not all Asian Americans have the same values and beliefs, so an awareness of the particular cultural and linguistic values of the particular population to which the client belongs is an essential tool for the speech-language pathologist. The traditional mode of assessment may not be appropriate for the assessment of APA clients.

Feasibility of the Traditional Approach to Assessment

Traditional assessment approaches, which use standardized formal tests designed to measure discrete areas of language, are not able to effectively account for cultural diversities. When incongruities between the native culture and the mainstream American culture exist, clients, particularly children, tend to experience confusion. The translation of standardized tests into other languages to accommodate the needs of culturally and linguistically diverse students is inappropriate. There are many words that cannot be translated from one language into another language without losing meaning. Also, words or concepts that may be considered common in English may not be common in the language of the Asian- or Pacific-American being tested. According to Cheng (1991), these include vocabulary related to household objects, clothing, sports, musical instruments, professions, historically related events and holidays, as well as games, values, and stories. Thus, formal assessment instruments, translated tests, and their interpretive scores are inappropriate for the APA population.

Recommended Assessment Procedures

The following are general guidelines for diagnosis, which are often referred to as the *RIOT* procedure (Cheng 1995b). They are adapted here for APA populations:

1. **R**eview all pertinent documents and background information. Many Asian countries do not have cumulative school records. When available, the records may not be in English. The subjects on the records may not match those of the traditional American curriculum. Oral reports are

sometimes unreliable; yet, they may be the only way to find information. Parents may be reluctant to discuss social and family background. An interpreter may be needed to obtain this information because of the lack of English language proficiency of the parents or guardians. Medical records may be difficult to obtain. Pregnancy and delivery records might not have been kept, especially if the birth was a home birth or in a refugee camp. Medical care may have been provided by a family member or other person who would not have kept records. Records, if available, may not be provided in English.

2. Interview teachers, peers, family members, and other informants and work with them to collect data regarding the client and the home environment. The family can provide valuable information about the communicative competence of the client at home and in the community, as well as historical and comparative data on the client's language skills. The clinician needs information regarding whether or not the client is proficient in the home language. The atmosphere of the home environment and cultural differences must also be discovered. The family's home language, their proficiency in different languages, the patterns of language usage, and the ways the family spends time together are some areas for investigation. Often a family and the clinician do not agree on the priorities for the client. It is important to determine the family's concerns and priorities. Mainstream American sociolinguistic patterns, school behaviors, and expectations must be explained to children and their families.

If the client is in school, consult with classroom teachers and aides. Classroom teachers can provide valuable information about a child's behaviors and performance (e.g., rate and style of learning, cognitive style, personal relational style, and behavior in multiple contexts). Resource teachers can provide information about the child's performance in any special program in which he or she is enrolled. Interactional and sociolinguistic patterns are often different across diverse cultures. Comments from school personnel should be examined in relation to what a particular child has experienced and learned from the home environment and culture. This can explain behavior that is different from mainstream American behavior. Rather than stressing the importance of compensating for or tolerating a child's difference, stress enhancement and addition to the student's repertoire of communication behaviors.

Interview questions are available from multiple sources (Cheng 1990a, 1991; Langdon and Saenz 1996). Questions should focus on obtaining information on how the client functions in his or her natural environment in relation to age peers who have had the same or similar exposure to language or to English.

3. *O*bserve the client over time in multiple contexts with multiple communication partners. Observe interactions at school, both in and outside the classroom, and at home. This cognitive-ecological-functional model takes into account the fact that clients often behave differently in different ecological settings. Clinicians determine who the clients like to be with, how they interact with others, how they react to different situations and individuals, and how they adapt to social communication barriers. Successes, as well as difficulties, are recorded. Direct observation of social behavior with multiple participants allows the evaluator to observe the ways members of different cultures view their environment and organize their behavior within it. Experiences depend on how clients interpret their world, given their cultural and experiential categories.

Knapp (1972) suggested that 35% of an utterance's social meaning is transmitted by words, whereas 65% of the social meaning is conveyed through nonverbal channels. Proximity, gestures, and facial expression are some features of nonverbal communication. People from different cultures interpret nonverbal signals in different ways. For example, because of his or her cultural upbringing, an Asian student may nod a "yes" sign when he or she actually means "no," especially in response to negative questions (e.g., "Don't you have your book?"). Sensitivity to and acknowledgment of these diverse communicative mannerisms signals the acceptance of the client's unique traits. Clients need to feel confident about themselves and not feel embarrassed about speaking and communicating. Perhaps speech-language pathologists can be enriched by the client's different modes and ways with words as the client becomes empowered through increased self-esteem (Damico 1990).

Some APA families may find it embarrassing to open their home to visitors and may not be clear on why such a visit is important. Observe family dynamics, with consideration to the family role. Observe the proficiency of the parents in the native language and English. What language do the parents use in addressing the client? Do the parents use the same level of language in addressing the client as they do to his or her age peers?

4. *T*est the client using informal dynamic assessment procedures in both school language and home language. Use the portfolio approach by keeping records of the client's performance over time. Interact with the client, being sensitive to his or her need to create meaning based on what is perceived as important, the client's frame of reference, and his or her experiences. It is necessary to understand the client's perspective. Clients should be allowed to succeed, struggle, or even fail with their interactions without interruptions from the clinician. Describe the client during gen-

uine communication in a naturalistic environment with low anxiety and high motivation. Assessment procedures should be culturally and pragmatically appropriate. Detailed information on the client's background and past experiences is helpful in finding activities that are stimulating and still permit an accurate evaluation of the client's communication skills. Collect narrative samples using wordless books, pictures, or other stimuli. Asking the client to describe experiences, retell stories, predict future events, and solve problems provides rich data for analysis. Literature from the client's background or narratives can be used to assess skill in accounting (description of a present event), recounting (description of a past event), and event casting (description of a future event). Stories translated into English may not be easily adapted to make them culturally appropriate. Thus, clients have the opportunity to have the process of acculturation take place without feeling that they have to give up their culture.

As professionals, clinicians should allow clients the luxury of acculturation and not demand complete assimilation into American society. Clinicians should nurture the growth of cross-cultural communicative competence by critically examining their own world view, values, beliefs, way of life, communicative style, learning style, cognitive style, and personal biases. Clinicians should attempt to explain the communicative patterns observed in their culture and in that of the client. The clinician should then determine if there are difficulties due to possible cultural and social mismatches between the two.

Special Challenges in Treating Asian- and Pacific-American Populations

What clinicians learn from the assessment should be integrated into their intervention strategies. Intervention should be constructed based on what is most productive for promoting communication and should incorporate the client's personal and cultural experiences. Salient and relevant features of the client's culture should be highlighted to enhance and empower the client.

Working with the Family

Sociologic and psychological difficulties arise in the conflict of culture, language, and ideology between Asian students, their parents, and the American educational system. These difficulties can include the background of traditions, religions, and histories of the Asian and Pacific population; problems of acculturation; the understanding of societal rules; contrasting influences from home and the classroom; confusion regarding one's sense of identity relating to culture, society, and family; the definition of disability; and the implications of special education services.

Intervention activities and materials can be selected based on the client's family and cultural background, using activities that are culturally and socially relevant. In addition to traditional intervention techniques of modeling and expansion, the speech-language pathologists can include activities such as those discussed by Cheng (1989) and Heath (1985).

Alternative strategies should be offered when clients or caregivers are reluctant to accept the treatment program recommended by the speech-language pathologist or audiologist. Inviting them to special classes or speech and language sessions is a useful way to provide the needed information. Seeking assistance from community leaders and social-service providers may also be necessary to convince the clients of the importance of therapy or recommended programs. The clients or caregivers may also be asked to talk with other APAs who have experiences with treatment programs. Other individuals can be effective in sharing their personal stories about their experiences with therapy. The clinician should be patient with the clients by letting them think through a problem and waiting for them to make the decision to participate in the treatment program.

The Experiential Approach to Intervention

Activities that provide interesting content and natural opportunities for social interaction can provide a rich environment for language learning to occur (Goodman 1986). The recognition of language as a social activity fosters a learning environment in which children are encouraged to talk and to exchange ideas (Norris and Damico 1990). The principles of experiential learning can be applied to intervention with the APA child, with the understanding that the approach is contrary to the teaching and learning styles of some cultural groups where more direct instruction is the norm.

Johnston and colleagues (1984) provided therapy guidelines useful for pragmatic activities, some of which can be adapted for APA clients. For example, the conversation module includes talking on the telephone, and asking for directions.

The following are specific guiding principles for all educators and specialists to enrich language learning in real-life contexts for APA children (Cheng 1994):

1. Use language in multiple social contexts. Students should be encouraged to participate in high-interest activities that are familiar to them. For example, Japanese students could be encouraged to tell a native folk story, and Chinese students could be asked to demonstrate how to use chopsticks.

2. Facilitate language learning in low-risk and low-anxiety contexts. The teacher should get to know the students better. He or she should approach and talk to the student to ascertain his or her likes and dislikes, to learn about his or her interests and strengths, and to ask the student to present work in which they excel to the class.

3. Use language activities that are experiential and relevant. When a teacher learns more about the students and his or her experiences, students can be asked to tell stories about experiences that are not only relevant but also meaningful to the student. Such activities can be a source of learning and bonding for everyone.

4. Encourage language interactions in comprehensible contexts, starting from the least demanding and proceeding to more cognitively challenging tasks. Art, music, and experiential activities should be used before activities that require high verbal ability or high cultural knowledge.

5. Respect differences between home discourse and school discourse. Teachers need to make the effort to explain explicitly what is expected in school discourse. Games and activities that are common and understood by American children may be unfamiliar to APA children who have recently arrived in the country. The concepts of winning a game may also be new. Concepts in games such as Monopoly may be unfamiliar to clients unfamiliar with the American system of real estate and finance.

6. Seek natural support systems and allow students to have self-selecting cooperative groups. Students should be allowed to select their own groups, seeking out peers with whom they are comfortable. Such an atmosphere provides the support they need to socialize.

7. Provide culturally familiar activities and unfamiliar activities. Most Asian newcomers do not know much about the Cub Scouts, the YMCAs, YWCAs, the PTA, Boys and Girls Clubs, and the numerous programs that the schools and community offer to the students and their families. They should be guided to participate in some of these programs. The schools, on the other hand, can invite family or community members to come into the schools and provide information on ethnic cultural activities from the various ethnic groups, thus providing the youngsters the opportunity to show their peers the activi-

ties that they are familiar with and value. This exchange is mutually empowering and provides the school-home-child connection.

8. Use a "talk story" approach. Au and Jordan (1981) propose establishing contact with students first by chatting with them without any set agenda, capitalizing on the preexisting cognitive and linguistic experiences of the children. The approach allows the students to "talk story" (a major speech event in Hawaiian culture).

Special Clinical Considerations: Accent, Stress, Voice, and Tones

Accent identifies a person as a member or nonmember of a particular linguistic community (Ainsfeld, et al. 1962). Everyone speaks with an accent, ranging from a New York accent to a Southern accent to a Cantonese accent. For tonal languages, tones are phonemic, and each syllable is assigned a specific tone. In English, intonation patterns are suprasegmental, and a variation of tones does not result in a completely different meaning. Individuals from tonal languages may apply their tonal patterns in their delivery of English, which makes their speech patterns distinct; hence, there are many versions of the English language, including French-influenced English, Hindi-influenced English, Tagalog-influenced English, Singaporean English, and so on. These distinct patterns and thick accents are not easy to change and can interfere with communication. Voice patterns also differ from culture to culture. A deep, soft voice indicates authority in Japan, but the same voice pattern may not be viewed the same way in the United States. The esthetics of voice also differ from culture to culture. For example, Chinese opera singers can use falsetto for performance, which sounds very pleasant to the audience; however, to the Western ear, Chinese opera may sound piercing and unpleasant. An easy way to understand this is to compare Chinese opera or Japanese No opera with Western opera.

Conclusion

Providing speech-language and hearing services to APA individuals is challenging. Preassessment information on the language, culture, and personal life history of the individual lays a solid foundation to further explore the client's strengths and weaknesses. Assessment procedures need to be guided by the general principles of being fair to the culture and nonbiased. Results of assessment should take into consideration the cultural and pragmatic variables of the individual. Intervention can be extremely rewarding when culturally relevant and appropriate approaches are used. The goals of intervention must include the enhancement of appropriate language and communication behaviors, home language, and literacy. Clinicians need to be creative and sensitive in their intervention to provide comfortable, productive, and enriching services for all clients.

References

Ainsfeld, M., Bogo, N., & Lambert, W. (1962). Evaluational reactions to accented English speech. *Journal of Abnormal Psychology, 65,* 223–231.

Akamatsu, C.T. (1993). Teaching deaf Asian- and Pacific Island–American children. In K.M. Christensen, & G.L. Delgado (Eds.), *Multicultural issues in deafness* (pp. 127–142). White Plains, NY: Longman Publishing.

Au, K., & Jordan, K. (1981). Teaching reading to Hawaiian children: Finding a culturally appropriate solution. In H. Trueba, G.P. Guthrie, & K. Au (Eds.), *Culture and the bilingual classroom* (pp. 139–152). Rowley, MA: Newbury.

Bansal, R.K. (1978). The phonology of Indian English. In R. Mohan (Ed.), *Indian writing in English* (pp. 101–114). Bombay, India: Orient Longman.

Bansal, R.K. (1990). The pronunciation of English in India. In S. Ramsaran (Ed.), *Studies in the pronunciation of English: A commemorative volume in honor of A.C. Gimson.* London: Routledge.

Bliatout, B.R., Downing, B.R., Lewis, J., & Yang, D. (1988). *Handbook for teaching Hmong-speaking students.* Folsom, CA: Folsom Cordova.

California State Department of Education. (1986). *A handbook for teaching Filipino-speaking students.* Sacramento, CA: California State Department of Education.

Chang, J-M, Lai, A.Y., & Shimizu, W. (1995). LEP parents as resources: Generating opportunity to learn beyond schools through parental involvement. In L.L. Cheng (Ed.), *Integrating language and learning for inclusion: An Asian-Pacific focus* (pp. 265–290). San Diego: Singular.

Cheng, L.L. (1989). Service delivery to Asian/Pacific LEP children: A cross-cultural framework. *Topics in Language Disorders, 9(3),* 1–14.

Cheng, L.L. (1990a). The identification of communicative disorders in Asian-Pacific students. *Journal of Child Communicative Disorders, 13,* 113–119.

Cheng, L.L. (1990b). Recognizing diversity: A need for a paradigm shift. *American Behavioral Scientist, 43,* 263–278.

Cheng, L.L. (1991). *Assessing Asian language performance: Guidelines for evaluating LEP students* (2nd ed.). Oceanside, CA: Academic Communication Associates.

Cheng, L.L. (1993). Deafness: An Asian/Pacific island perspective. In K.M. Christensen, & G.L. Delgado (Eds.), *Multicultural issues in deafness* (pp. 113–126). White Plains, NY: Longman.

Cheng, L.L. (1994). Difficult discourse: An untold Asian story. In D.N. Ripich, & N.A. Creaghead (Eds.), *School discourse problems (2nd ed.)* (pp. 155–170). San Diego: Singular.

Cheng, L.L. (1995a). *Integrating language and learning for inclusion: An Asian-Pacific focus.* San Diego: Singular.

Cheng, L.L. (1995b, July). *The Bilingual language-delayed child: Diagnosis and intervention with the older school-age bilingual child.* Paper presented at the Israeli Speech and Hearing Association International Symposium on Bilingualism, Haifa, Israel.

Cheng, L.L., & Ima, K. (1989). *Understanding the immigrant Pacific islander.* San Diego: Los Amigos Research Associates.

Chhim, S., Luangpraseut, K., & Te, H.D. (1987). *Introduction to Cambodian culture.* San Diego: San Diego State University Multifunctional Service Center.

Ching, T. (1990). Tones for profoundly deaf tone-language speakers. *Chinese University of Hong Kong Papers in Linguistics, 2,* 1–22.

Chinn, P. (1990, September). *Multiculturalism in California.* Paper presented at the Conference on Multicultural Deafness, San Diego, CA.

Chu, H. (1990, September). *The role of the Korean language on the bilingual programs in the United States.* Paper presented at the Asian Language Conference, Hacienda Heights, CA.

Chuong, C. (1990, September). *The speech island: A Vietnamese perspective.* Paper presented at the Asian Language Conference, Hacienda Heights, CA.

Damico, J.S. (1990). Descriptive assessment of communicative ability in limited English proficient students. In E.V. Hamayan, & J.S. Damico (Eds.), *Limiting bias in the assessment of bilingual students* (pp. 157–218). Boston: College Hill.

Diana v. California State Board of Education, No. C-70-37. (N. D. Ca. 1970).

Gardner, R.W., Robey, B., & Smith, P.C. (1985). Asian American: Growth, change, and diversity. *Population Bulletin, 40,* 1–44.

Gollnick, D.M., & Chinn, P.C. (1990). *Multicultural education in a pluralistic society.* New York: Merrill-Macmillan.

Goodman, K. (1986). *What's the whole in whole language?* Portsmouth, NH: Heinemann.

Heath, S.B. (1985, November). *Second language acquisition.* Paper presented at the American Speech-Language-Hearing Association Convention, San Francisco.

Ima, K., & Labovitz, E.M. (1990, March). *Changing ethnic/racial student composition and test performances: Taking account of increasing student diversity.* Paper presented at the annual meeting of the Pacific Sociological Association, Santa Ana, CA.

Ima, K., & Keogh, P-E. (1995). "The crying father" and "my father doesn't love me": Selected observations and reflections on Southeast Asians and special education. In L.L. Cheng (Ed.), *Integrating language and learning for inclusion: An Asian-Pacific focus* (pp. 149–177). San Diego: Singular.

Jha, M. (1995). *An introduction to Indian anthropology.* New Delhi, India: Vikas Publishing.

Jiobu, R.M. (1996). Recent Asian Pacific immigrants: The Asian Pacific background. In B.O. Hing, & R. Lee (Eds.), *The state of Asian Pacific America: Reframing the immigration debate* (pp. 59–126). Los Angeles: UCLA Asian American Studies Center.

Johnston, E.B., Weinrich, B.D., & Johnson, A.R. (1984). *A sourcebook of pragmatic activities.* Tucson, AZ: Communication Skill Builders.

Jordan, C., & Tharp, R.G. (1979). Culture and education. In A. Marsella, R.G. Tharp, & I. Cibrowski (*Eds.*), *Perspectives in crosscultural psychology.* New York: Academic Press.

Kanahele, G.H.S. (1986). *Ku Kanaka: stand tall: A search for Hawaiian values.* Honolulu: University of Hawaii Press.

Kim, B.L. (1981). *The future of Korean-American children and youth: Marginality, biculturality, and the role of the American public school.* Urbana-Champaign, IL: University of Illinois School of Social Work.

Kim, E.C. (1984, April). *Korean Americans in the United States: Problems and alternatives.* Paper presented at the Annual Conference of Ethnic and Minority Studies, St. Louis.

Kim, R.H. (1978). *Understanding Korean people, language, and culture.* Sacramento, CA: California State Department of Education, Bilingual Education Resource Series.

Knapp, L. (1972). *Nonverbal communication in human interaction.* New York: Holt, Rinehart, and Winston.

Langdon, H.W., & Saenz, T.I. (1996). *Language assessment and intervention with multicultural students: A guide for speech-language-hearing professionals.* Oceanside, CA: Academic Communication Associates.

Lewis, J., & Luangpraseut, K. (1989). *Handbook for teaching Lao-speaking students.* Folsom, CA: Folsom Cordova.

Lewis, J., Vang, L., & Cheng. L.L. (1989). Identifying the language-learning difficulties of Hmong students: Implications of context and culture. *Topics in Language Disorders, 9(3),* 21–27.

Ma, L.J. (1985). Cultural diversity. In A.K. Dutt (Ed.), *Southeast Asia: Realm of contrast.* Boulder, CO: Westview Press.

Melendy, H.B. (1977). *Asians in America: Filipinos, Koreans, and East Indians.* Boston: Twayne.

Meredith, W., & Cramer, S. (1982). Hmong refugees in Nebraska. In B. Downing, & D. Olney (Eds.), *The Hmong in the West: Observations and reports* (pp. 353–363). Minneapolis: Southeast Asian Refugee Studies Project, Center for Urban and Regional Affairs, University of Minnesota.

Meyerson, D.W. (1990). Cultural considerations in the treatment of Latinos with craniofacial malformations. *Cleft Palate Journal, 27,* 279–288.

Minami, M., & McCabe, A. (1991). Haiku as a discourse regulation device: A stanza analysis of Japanese children's personal narratives. *Language in Society, 20,* 577–599.

Minami, M., & McCabe, A. (1995). Rice balls and bear hunts: Japanese and North American family narrative patterns. *Journal of Child Language 1995, 22,* 423–445.

Mokuau, N., & Tauili'ili, P. (1993). Families with Hawaiian and Pacific islander roots. In E.W. Lynch, & M.J. Hanson (Eds.), *Developing cross cultural competence: A guide for working with children and their families* (pp. 301–318). Baltimore: Brookes.

Monzon, R.I. (1984). *The effects of the family environment on the academic performance of Filipino-American college students.* Thesis, San Diego State University.

Moraes, F., & Howe, E. (1991). *John Kenneth Galbraith Introduces India.* Calcutta, India: Rupa.

Norris, J.A., & Damico, J.S. (1990). Whole language in theory and practice: Implications for language intervention. *Language Speech and Hearing Services in Schools, 21(4),* 212–220.

Olsen, L. (1988). *Crossing the schoolhouse border: Immigrant students and the California public schools.* San Francisco: California Tomorrow.

Ortiz-Monasterio, F., & Serrano, R.A. (1971). Cultural aspects of cleft lip and palate treatment. In W.C. Grabb, S.W. Rosenstein, & K.R. Bzoch (Eds.), *Cleft lip and palate: Surgical, dental, and speech aspects* (pp. 130–141). Boston: Little, Brown.

Ouk, M., Huffman, F.E., & Lewis, J. (1988). *Handbook for teaching Khmer-speaking students.* Folsom, CA: Folsom Cordova Unified School District.

Rueda, R.S. (1993, July). *Meeting the needs of diverse students.* Paper presented at the Multicultural Education Summer Institute, San Diego State University, San Diego, CA.

Rumbaut, T., & Ima, K. (1987). *The adaptation of southeast Asian refugee youth: A comparative study.* San Diego: San Diego State University.

Shekar, C., & Hegde, M.N. (1995). India: Its people, culture, and languages. In L.L. Cheng (Ed.), *Integrating language and learning for inclusion* (pp. 125–148). San Diego: Singular.

Shekar, C., & Hegde, M.N. (1996). Cultural and linguistic diversity among Asian Indians: A case of Indian English. *Topics in Language Disorders, 16(4),* 54–64.

Strauss, R.P. (1985). Culture, rehabilitation and facial birth defects: International case studies. *Cleft Palate Journal, 22,* 56–62.

Takaki, R. (1989). Strangers from a different shore. Boston: Little, Brown.

Te, H.D. (1987). *Introduction to Vietnamese culture.* San Diego: Multifunctional Resource Center, San Diego State University.

Tolliver-Weddington, G. (1990). Cultural considerations in the treatment of craniofacial malformations in African-Americans. *Cleft Palate Journal, 27,* 289–293.

Trueba, H., Cheng, L.L, & Ima, K. (1992). *Myth or reality: Adaptive strategies of Asian newcomers in California.* London: Falmer Press.

University of California Linguistic Minority Research Institute (1996). LEP enrollments increase by almost 5% in 1996. *LMRI Newsletter, 6(1),* 1, Santa Barbara, CA: University of California.

U.S. Bureau of the Census. (1990). *Statistical abstract of the United States: 1990 (110th ed.).* Washington, DC: U.S. Bureau of the Census.

U.S. Bureau of the Census. (1995). *Statistical abstract of the United States: (115th ed).* Washington, DC: U.S. Bureau of the Census.

U.S. Department of Commerce. (1993a). *We, The American Asians.* Washington, DC: U.S. Department of Commerce.

U.S. Department of Commerce. (1993b). *We, The Asian and Pacific Islander Americans.* Washington, DC: U.S. Department of Commerce.

University of California Linguistic Minority Research Institute. (1996). *LEP Enrollments Increase Almost 5% in 1996.* Santa Barbara, CA: Author.

Wells, J.C. (1982). *Accents of English 3: Beyond the British Isles.* Cambridge, England: Cambridge University Press.

Additional Resources

The following publishers have developed resources focusing on APA populations:

Academic Communications Associates, Oceanside, CA
Communication Skill Builders, Tucson, AZ
Falmer Press, Philadelphia, PA
Longman Publishing, White Plains, NJ
Los Amigos Research Associates, San Diego, CA
Newbury House, Rowley, MA
Singular Publishing Group, San Diego, CA
Twayne Publishers, Boston, MA

4

□ □ □
□ □ □
□ □ □

American Indian Cultures: A Lesson in Diversity

Gail A. Harris

The fabric of culture is an intricate weave. Changing a basic fiber, such as a belief or a language, creates a change in the overall design. As interventionists, speech-language pathologists are agents of change. In the attempt to bring about change in an individual's communicative behavior, the speech-language pathologist may be unaware of the impact of intervention on the individual, the family, or the culture. Furthermore, when embarking on the treatment of individuals from a different culture, the speech-language pathologist may be unaware of how this experience may change his or her own beliefs and clinical practice.

This chapter discusses the current challenges in providing appropriate clinical and educational services to American Indian children. The information is offered to increase understanding of American Indian people, their cultural beliefs, language styles, and the general components of cultural diversity. Speech-language pathologists are encouraged to view assessment and treatment of communication disorders within a larger context and to expand their view of the client to include his or her background language, culture, and experiences. Without an understanding of cultural differences that contribute to perspectives toward health and disability, variations in child-rearing practices, and language-interaction patterns, clinical judgments and practices may lack precision and effectiveness within the multicultural context of American Indian communities.

The emphasis of this chapter on cultural differences as they affect language learning and use should in no way be interpreted to imply that genuine communicative disorders of various types and different levels of severity are absent from American Indian populations. The emphasis here is on assisting clinicians to more accurately identify and treat communication disorders within American Indian groups by increasing the clinicians' knowledge of culturally determined beliefs, child-rearing practices, and language-use patterns of American Indians.

Because of the diversity of languages and cultures of American Indian populations, characteristics of specific tribal groups are not addressed in depth. Rather, principles, beliefs, and practices that have some commonality among different tribes and that have a broader application are presented, and particular studies of specific tribal groups are discussed.

Diversity Among American Indians

Demographics

Referring to American Indians as a singular cultural group can lead to errors of generalization about language and culture and lead to misinterpretation of behavior within and among Indian tribes. Within and among Indian tribes, there are significant differences in adherence to traditional practices, acculturation within the dominant white culture, language structures, and language styles. In 1990, nearly 2 million individuals identified themselves as American Indians, and 50% of the American Indian population was younger than age 21 years (U.S. Bureau of the Census 1990). The U.S. Census Bureau reported American Indians among the populations of every state in the nation, with the largest concentrations in California, Oklahoma, Arizona, New Mexico, and North Carolina (U.S. Bureau of the Census 1990).

There are approximately 500 distinct and separate tribal entities, each with separate or collective governing bodies and distinct languages and cultures. Therefore, any general statement regarding these populations is nearly impossible and inappropriate. American Indian tribes have the status of sovereign nations. They have a unique government-to-government relationship with the federal government, which is experienced by no other minority group. With this unique governmental relationship comes a torrent of laws governing almost all aspects of American Indian life.

Reservation Status

There are 278 reservations and 209 Alaskan native villages in the United States. A large percentage of these are located in remote, rural areas isolated from population centers where comprehensive medical and rehabilitative services are routinely available. The vast size of some reservations and their great distance from metropolitan areas affect socialization, language patterns, and accessibility to health and rehabilitative services. For example, the Tohono O'odham reservation (formerly Papago), whose tribal headquarters is located approximately 80 miles south of Tucson, AZ, covers more than 2.5 million acres and is equivalent in size to the state of Connecticut. There are 12 separate districts or villages, with separate governance structures and dialectal variations of the O'odham language. The O'odham language is spoken by approximately 14,000 individuals (Mathiot 1973). This reservation is second only to the Navajo nation in size and number of native language speakers. The Navajo nation, equivalent to the size of the state of West Virginia, covers an area of 25,000 square miles and spans the boundaries of three states (Arizona, New Mexico, and Utah). The Navajo nation is reported to have approximately 160,000 members (Harris 1982).

The geographic isolation of many of the Indian reservations contributes to a number of difficulties in the delivery of special education and rehabilitation services. Indians who live on reservations often face limited access to services and difficulty recruiting and retaining special educational and related services personnel for their tribal programs. In addition, for both reservation and urban American Indians alike, ambiguities regarding agency responsibility for providing rehabilitation services often create duplications or lacunae in available services. The lack of adequately qualified, certified personnel; the historic lack of attention to special education and rehabilitative services by the Bureau of Indian Affairs and the Indian Health Service; and a number of environmental risk factors, including poverty, unemployment, and low levels of education attainment, contribute to the continued state of unmet prevention and intervention needs.

Urban Indians

More than half of the American Indian population resides in urban areas. Urban Indians are usually better educated, have lower unemployment rates, have higher family income levels, and have fewer dependent children than American Indians living on reservations (Miller 1975). Regardless of their location, many American Indians maintain traditional child-rearing practices and lifestyles (Miller 1975; Red Horse 1983). It is not unusual for parents to leave their jobs and for children to be taken from school to travel to the home reservation for important ceremonies at various times during the year. This reflects the continued involvement of American Indians in the traditional ways central to the American Indian family's existence, regardless of their apparent acculturation into mainstream society.

Cultural Variables of American Indians

American Indian inter- and intratribal cultural differences can be evaluated using the Brislin, Cushner, Cherrie, and Yong (1986) model of understanding culture and cultural differences. Among the cultural variables discussed in the model are work, values, rituals, superstitions, roles, space, time and language. The concepts included in the model provided by Brislin and associates (1986) are used as a framework for the discussion of American Indian cultures in the following sections.

World View

The background of the child is more complex than geographic location or language spoken. It includes values and world views that govern all aspects of life. Values refer to various end states that are considered desirable or important by many members of the culture. Values held by a culture shape the culture's political, economic, and aesthetic systems; underlie its religious beliefs; and influence its interpersonal relationships. Behaviors can be viewed as means to achieve the valued goals.

World view explains events, governs attitudes toward disabilities, guides child-rearing and caregiver-child interactions, dictates language behaviors, and determines the appropriateness of intervention techniques. There are great differences among tribes, and within tribes there is great variability in the level of traditional beliefs to which an individual or family adheres. One cannot judge the level of traditional beliefs of an individual or his or her family by age, reservation or urban status, or tribal affiliation. Adherence to traditional ways is a personal matter. Factors such as clan affiliation, society membership, formal education, intermarriage, urbanization, and technology have influenced the teaching and practice of traditional ways for some. For others, regardless of external indicators, traditional ways are at the core of existence.

Perhaps the most essential aspects of the American Indian world view are the appreciation of spirituality, the inter-relatedness of all life, and the concept of kinship.

Spirituality

There is a high degree of integration between the spiritual beliefs of American Indians and their beliefs regarding health and disabilities. Cultural orientation provides a classification scheme that separates health from pathology, normalcy from deviancy, and well-being from disease. For the American Indian, the triune nature of man—body, mind, and spirit—is central to the perceptions of wellness and disability.

In the traditional American Indian world view, there are no accidents. Nothing is impossible. Illness can be caused by lack of balance or harmony, mental or spiritual, manifested by the body. Harris and Bayles (1981) conducted a study of attitudes and perceptions of American Indian personnel in Head Start programs regarding communication disorders. Respondents indicated that certain communication disorders could be caused by witchcraft or violation of tribal taboos. Illness or disability may be related to an event or action involving the person affected or may be related to the actions of a family or clan member. These beliefs can affect the acceptance or rejection of a diagnosis, treatment regimen, or both. In addition, healing or treating one aspect of the individual without attending to other aspects of his or her well-being may be considered incomplete. Treatment from traditional Indian practitioners may be effectively coupled with medical treatment from physicians and therapists. Dukepoo (1980) reported that a lack of awareness, respect, and tolerance of culturally different beliefs and practices on the part of non-Indian practitioners not only precludes the delivery of quality care to American Indian patients but also serves as a primary deterrent to American Indians from seeking necessary health care services.

Acceptance of Differences

The terms *disability, impairment, handicap*, and *rehabilitation* are not easily translatable into American Indian conceptual or linguistic terms (Burgess, et al. 1979). Many Indian languages lack such words as *retarded* or *disabled*; instead American Indians use terms such as *incomplete* or *slow* (Locust 1986). A greater acceptance of differences has been reported among Indian tribes than in contemporary American society (Stewart 1975; Locust 1988). In some American Indian groups, for example, a child born with a disability is not evaluated negatively because it is assumed that the disability is by choice, because the child had the prenatal choice of how he or she wished to be born. Although there seems to be little question that a person with a severe disability is recognized as different in Indian communities, by and large, such differences are accepted within a wider range of tolerance.

Some American Indian families accept a child with disabilities as a gift from the Creator. For example, an Oneida father in an urban area of Wisconsin whose daughter had a neuromuscular disease explained that he viewed her slow development as a gift from the Creator. He related that he now had the opportunity to appreciate and be grateful for every small change in her growth and development. For rehabilitative personnel, this view can necessitate alterations in the manner, method, and sequence of rehabilitative procedures. Clinicians must have an appreciation of the family's perception of a child's disabling condition to appropriately interact with and serve families.

The Power of Words

According to the American Indian, the power of the spoken word is enigmatic. Because words are formed on a breath and breath comes from the location of the heart and is the Creator's breath, truth, honor, and the very power of life are intertwined in the spoken word. Words and thoughts have power—power to do harm and power to heal. Therefore, some American Indians maintain that mentioning or discussing disabling conditions can put the person or family at risk for greater difficulties (Locust 1988). The American Indian perspective highlights the necessity to be attentive to the words, tone, and manner in which family and case history interviews are conducted. Permission from the person or family should be granted before asking personal questions. A level of trust must be established between the clinician and the client and his or her family. Confidentiality must be assured and strictly maintained.

Religion

There is no equivalent word for *religion* in most American Indian languages (Locust 1986, 1988). Religion is not considered a separate activity that is somehow distant from day-to-day life. Spirituality—the relationship with the Supreme Creator and all creations—is pervasive in a traditional Indian world view.

Rituals and ceremonies are carried out to achieve the goal of establishing the relationship between man and nature (Brislin, et al. 1986). American Indian rituals can include simple daily practices or elaborate multiday ceremonial procedures. The importance of rituals in a culture is central to understanding and respecting that culture.

Diagnosis and treatment of disabilities in American Indian communities can involve rituals carried out by a medicine man or woman. In some American Indian communities, medicine people are afforded high levels of respect. They are not touched, a path clears where they are walking, and there is caution regarding chastising or defaming them. Their recommendations are important to the healing and rehabilitative process.

The Circle of Life

All life is considered sacred to American Indians, because all things and beings are created by the Supreme Creator. All life shares in the

Creator's essence and spiritual reality and is interconnected. Sacredness and ceremony mark critical periods of a child's life. Naming ceremonies for infants and puberty rights for adolescent girls are important aspects of traditional American Indian life.

The importance of the American Indian world view becomes most relevant to clinical practice when linear clinical medical beliefs collide with traditional circular beliefs of certain American Indian families. For example, families may choose to wait for treatment until culturally appropriate times. Due to the privacy and sacredness of certain practices, information may not be shared with the non-Indian service provider, and the family may be perceived as noncompliant.

On the other hand, families may assume that the speech-language pathologist or physical therapist is solely responsible for their child's rehabilitation. They may, therefore, expect a more holistic, personal relationship with clinicians in the treatment of their child than schedules and caseloads allow.

Kinship

Culture influences the behaviors associated with various roles one assumes within the family and the society. Understanding these role differences facilitates delivery of services to American Indian groups and ensures that the appropriate people are present for case history, diagnostic, and, in some instances, therapeutic procedures.

In an individualistic culture, such as mainstream Western culture, the individual is defined by his or her achievements or behaviors and is encouraged to set life goals. The individual speaks for himself or herself, and relationships with others are quick to form and can be short lived. In contrast, American Indian cultures place great value on the group (tribe) and the family. Within a collective culture, like those of American Indians, the individual is defined by his or her membership in the group (e.g., extended family or clan). Goals are set by the group for the individual, and the input and opinions of many are valued. In the collective culture, the group can speak for the individual. Relationships among people are slow to form but are lifelong. There is an emphasis on harmony and cooperation in the collective culture, for relationships within the group are paramount.

American Indian cultures are collective in nature. Many have a strong clan or kinship system. Decisions are made through a group process and can take longer to ensure adequate input. The involvement of the extended family in treatment of communication disorders may be required to ensure compliance.

The fundamental belief in the inter-relatedness of people and all living things is reflected in American Indian spiritual practices and familial relationships. These practices, which are not mythical so much as pragmatic, are based on group participation, observable inter-relationships, the cycles of things within nature, and the life experiences of the group members (Forbes 1979). The kinship or clan system is important for some American Indian tribes. It dictates appropriate marriage partners, ceremonial responsibilities, and child-rearing practices.

In a study of the families of Pueblo Indian children with developmental disabilities, Malach and her colleagues (1989) commented on the importance of the family's sense of supportive relationships with service providers. Their study indicated that the emotional support and respect of the service provider for the parents was considered the most important element in promoting the parent's empowerment and involvement in obtaining services for their disabled children. These personal relationships superseded the agency's or organization's status or the professional's title. Implications for training programs to include cultural differences and the importance of interacting with families as families first and clients second cannot be overstated.

Time and Space

Individualistic cultures (e.g., general U.S. population) are oriented to and often driven by "clock time," whereas collective cultures are often more attuned to "event time." When on clock time, a scheduled appointment time takes precedence over the current event, unless the current event is an emergency. Lateness is interpreted as a negative or disrespectful behavior. Approaching a day from the perspective of event time is quite different. One honors the time that it takes for a conversation or meeting to come to its full conclusion. "I'll see you in the morning," for example, is sometimes as committed to a time as a collectivist will be. The term *Indian time* emerged from within Indian country to refer to the lateness or uncertainty of when a meeting or event begins. It might help the non-Indian to view meetings and events as having an appropriate start time that has little to do with the clock. The meeting begins when the previous event is complete. The ceremonial begins when everyone is there. Working in Indian communities requires an understanding of and working within the community's concept of time.

A child who has been socialized in a world with the natural concept of time would not understand the need to complete assessments in a timely manner. His or her responses may be considered slow; therefore, he or she may be diagnosed as having a problem.

Space refers to how close people stand to one another. Generally, there is an unspoken distance of comfort operating within a culture. One knows when his or her space is invaded by either proximity or intensity. If a culture has rules that a person is not spoken to until he or she has entered a particular space, he or she may be perceived as quiet or unable to initiate communication. There is greater variability among Indian tribes regarding proximity and intensity. Careful observation of these factors can guide clinician behavior.

Family Structures and Relations

The family structure and relationships for some American Indian families differ greatly from familial characteristics of non-Indian cultures. The responsibility for raising and guiding American Indian children may be delegated to a number of different relatives or clan members, who serve important, specified functions. Depending on the tribal orientation, the paternal uncle or maternal aunt may have primary responsibility for supervising and instructing the child (Tafoya 1982). It is not unlikely for the child to live with these relatives while the child's biological parents are responsible for raising other children in the extended family.

These particular relationships are reflected in some Indian languages, in which cousins are referred to as "brothers and sisters" and uncles and aunts as "father" and "mother." Implications for speech-language pathologists lie in conducting family interviews and designing family-involvement practices. Decisions regarding care or early intervention for a child may be deferred to an individual other than the biological parent. In scheduling family conferences, parents should be encouraged to include all individuals who fill important roles in the child's life.

Disciplinary action may be the responsibility of another family member, the clan, or sacred societies. In the Hopi tribe, for example, an uncle may be the disciplinarian of a young child. In addition, the *kachinas* (men of the community who personify Hopi spirit helpers) instruct young children regarding proper behavior. Examples of proper behavior are attending to the needs of the community, obeying parents, and being respectful and obedient to elders. In some groups, discipline is often not individualized and is directed more toward the group. The misbehavior of one may therefore be used in a constructive manner to instruct all. The objective is to be a good Hopi and support one another to that end.

The practices of shared child rearing establish the basis of collective responsibility and form the foundation of tribal interconnectedness. Group orientation may conflict with individual performance expectations in the classroom or with clinical and decision-making demands placed on parents at parent conferences.

Child-Rearing Practices

Because most Indian groups are collective in nature, the child is viewed as a member of the extended group, not just the immediate family. Child-rearing practices socialize the child to function within the home culture and the larger community (Westby, in press). It is not unusual for an extended family member to play an active and significant role in a child's rearing, discipline, guidance, and decision making. In some communities, the aunt names the child, and the uncle is the chief disciplinarian. Culturally determined caregiver-child interactions and child-rearing practices provide the context for early language learning and later language behaviors. Differences in family structures and relationships, child characteristics, and adult-child interaction patterns affect the socialization process and subsequent clinical practice.

Characteristics of American Indian Children

Several studies of newborns have reported behavioral differences among minority groups. In studies comparing African American, white, Hopi, and Navajo infants, the Navajo infants were reported to have greater calmness, adaptability, consolability, and self-quieting behaviors than the other infant groups (Westby, in press; Brazelton, et al. 1976; Blout 1982). Other studies reported that Navajo infants were less irritable, demonstrated lower muscle tone, and began walking later than African American and white babies (Brazelton, et al. 1976; Blout 1982). These characteristics may establish behavioral norms and expectations that differ from non-Indian cultures.

In a review of the literature regarding cultural differences in caregiver-child interactions, Westby (in press) presented data indicating biologically based differences in motor development and temperament among infants from different ethnic and cultural groups. These differences may in part underlie different child-rearing practices and desirable child behaviors in a given cultural group. Desirable behaviors in one culture may not be considered optimal in another. Westby suggested asking caregivers if the child in question is "like your other children or is he [or she] different in some way?" to provide a more appropriate referent than formal standardized tools and scales (Westby, in press).

Adult-Child Interaction

In addition to child characteristics that contribute to variations in caregiver-child interactions, variations in the type, amount, and rhythm of maternal behaviors from different ethnic groups have been documented. In studies comparing Hopi, white, Navajo, and African American mothers, Navajo mothers demonstrated less attentiveness to infants, less reciprocal vocalization, fewer varieties of attention-getting behaviors, and fewer mutual gaze events than all other mother groups in the studies (Blout 1982; Callaghan 1981; Fajardo and Freedman 1981; Chisolm 1983).

Results of a study comparing the attitudes of Navajo and white mothers toward verbal and nonverbal behaviors of preschool children indicated differences between these two groups (Freedman 1974). Navajo mothers perceived extremely active verbal behavior as discourteous, restless, self-centered, and undisciplined. The same behaviors were judged by white mothers as exciting to observe, evidence of active learning, and advantageous for the child (Freedman 1974). One explanation for these differences may be the high-context nature of American Indian cultures. Within high-context cultures, much of the learning occurs through observations, compared with the emphasis on verbal transmission of low-context cultures. Since the emphasis is on learning through observations, attention to spoken words is reduced, and extremely verbal behavior in children may not be encouraged or reinforced (Westby, in press; Harris 1985a).

Early experiences and adult-child interactions can affect later speech-language performance, the appropriateness of normative observational and developmental scales, the parental perceptions of appropriate speech-language behaviors, and the appropriateness of intervention techniques with young, communicatively disabled children and their families.

Value of Work

In an individualistic society, there is emphasis on personal performance, and people are defined by their work. The individual's work provides status, and acceptance and rewards are determined by the amount of effort the individual expends. In a collective society, such as American Indian cultures, the rewards are divided equally among the members of the group. An individual's work is not central to his or her identity. A person's status is not determined by job title or role within the work place but is influenced by his or her standing within the community. In American Indian cultures, it is not unusual for highly honored and valued tribal members to have menial jobs within a school or medical system.

Languages

The language a group uses is central to its identity. This is particularly true in collective societies that emphasize relationships. Not only must one know the form of the language, but it is also important to know how a language is used in a culture (Brislin, et al. 1986).

The indigenous languages of the native peoples of North America are many and diverse. Although the precise number of American Indian languages is unknown, estimates are that approximately 200 distinct languages are still spoken in North America (Highwater 1975). The number of speakers of tribal languages varies greatly from language to language from many thousand to fewer than 50. American Indian languages can be divided into approximately 60 different language families. Highwater recognized no genetic relationships among them.

The classification of Native American languages into families is not without controversy. Highwater identified eight major linguistic families—Algonquian, Iroquoian, Caddoan, Muskogean, Siouan, Penutian, Athabascan, and Uto-Aztecan (Highwater 1975)—whereas Greenberg proposed that native languages of the Americas can be classified into just three families—Eskimo-Aleut, Na-Dine, and Amerindi (Greenberg 1987). Professionals are encouraged to become familiar with distinct linguistic features and cultural rules of use of the tribal languages of groups that are served. For the purposes of illustration and discussion, aspects of Navajo language are presented here.

Navajo Language Form

The Navajo language has intricate verb structures that focus more on aspect, motion, and state than on time. Witherspoon commented that Navajo seems to indicate a cosmos composed of processes and events as opposed to a cosmos of facts and things (Witherspoon 1977). Fletcher (1983) suggested that the lack of distinctive words to express color in Navajo may reflect a world view that seeks to create harmony and synthesis rather than separation and analysis.

Navajo Phonology

Phonologically, the Navajo language differs from English in vowels, consonants, and consonant combinations. Final consonants are uncommon in Navajo, and for this reason they are not easily heard or produced when the Navajo speak English (Cook and Sharp 1966). For example, there is no /ŋ/ sound in Navajo. It follows that the present progressive tense ending, expressed in English with -*ing*, may be difficult for these speakers.

Differences in the vowel systems of English and Navajo have been noted to create problems with minimally different pairs, such as *his* and *he's* in English. These phonologic differences, because of their morphologic importance, can create difficulties for native Navajo speakers in their use of English.

Navajo Morphology and Syntax

Navajo morphology and syntax present differences that can affect the Navajo's receptive and expressive language skills in English. Number is not expressed in noun forms but in verb forms in Navajo. The verb forms are for singular, dual, and plural (i.e., one, two, and more than two). Common errors include saying "three boy" and "we like all the ride." Gender or number distinctions in the third-person pronoun form do not exist in Navajo, which can result in confusion of pronouns *he* and *she* and possessives *his* and *her*.

The Navajo verb system is based on mode or aspect rather than tense. Navajo verbs deal more with states of completion, duration, or action than the time or tense of action. Tense is expressed by the use of adverbs of time. English tenses that can present difficulty for Navajo speakers are third-person singular present tense, the *-(e)s* ending, regular past and past participles, the *-(e)d* ending, and progressive verb forms *-ing* ending. A Navajo speaker's shift between the use of English present and past tense in describing past events may not indicate a lack of the concept of time but rather an interchanging of words with different forms that have the same meaning to the speaker (Fletcher 1983; Cook and Sharp 1966). A comparison of Navajo and English is presented in Table 4-1.

Navajo Language Use

Culture affects the dimensions of language use. Turn-taking behaviors, appropriate periods of pause and silence, and constraints on topic maintenance are influenced by culture. In addition, in some tribal communities who may be addressed by whom and what topics are appropriate to discuss at different seasons of the year are dictated by culture.

Silence is more than the absence of speech. It is a culturally governed practice that can indicate respect, thoughtful consideration of what has just been said, and evidence of culturally appropriate behaviors in situations that are unpredictable and ambiguous (Basso 1970). Although it is possible to convey all pragmatic functions through Navajo, the appropriateness of questioning, commenting, requesting, or commanding is culturally determined.

Indian English

As distinctive dialectical variations of English are spoken by other minority groups, different forms of English are spoken within American Indian communities that can be termed *Indian English*. The rules that govern these variations of English reflect the phonologic and syntactic influences of the tribal languages (Leap 1982a, b, in press; Fleisher 1982; Nelson-Barber 1982). The variations of Indian English among different

Table 4-1   Comparison of Navajo and English

Navajo	*English*
Phonologic (sound) system	
Vowel length distinguishes meaning.	Stress and intonation distinguish meaning.
Vowels occur in a nasal as well as an oral series, a feature that also distinguishes meaning. Inherent tone distinguishes meaning.	Sentence pitch distinguishes meaning.
Consonantal clusters have limited use, and none occur in the syllable final position.	A wide variety of consonantal clusters occurs in the syllable or word final position.
Only 11 simple consonants occur in syllable final position.	Almost all simple consonants can occur in the syllable or word final position.
Navajo has a simple vowel system.	English has a simple and a compound vowel system.
Navajo has 15 or more sounds that do not occur in English.	English uses six consonant sounds that do not occur in Navajo (v, f, dʒ, θ, r, ŋ) and have no close correspondent in Navajo.
Particles are used to express interrogation, surprise, incredulity, exasperation, and other emotional overtones.	Sentence pitch is used to express interrogation, surprise, incredulity, exasperation, and other emotional overtones.
Grammar and syntax	
Navajo is action oriented and has an intricate verb system. The environment acts on man.	English is object oriented and has many nouns. Man acts on things in the environment.
Navajo has a limited use of noun plurals to express number. Number is often implied by the verb form. Special verb stems are used.	Singular and plural numbers are usually expressed by the noun or pronoun subject.
Possession is expressed by personal pronouns prefixed to the noun or possessor noun added to the possessive prefix plus the possessed object (e.g., boy his-hat).	Possession is expressed by possessive pronouns (e.g., my book) or by suffixes (-'s and -s') added to the nouns.

Navajo	*English*
Postpositions follow the nouns or pronouns to which they relate (e.g., "rock on-it" meaning "on the rock"). Also, postpositions function as verbal prefixes (e.g., "something on-marking takes place" meaning "writing").	Prepositions precede the noun or pronoun to which they relate.
Certain suffixed elements are used to express relative definiteness. These suffixes are attached to the noun, a descriptor word, or the verb.	Articles (i.e., *the*, *a*, and *an*) are used to express relative definiteness.
Contrasting opposites are not used to the extent that they are used in English or in a manner corresponding to English (e.g., good: not good, agree: not agree, loved: not loved).	Contrasting opposites comprise a wide use of forms with opposite meanings (e.g., good: bad, agree: disagree, loved: unloved).
Modal prefixes and special forms of verb stems are the principal mechanisms used to mark mode and aspect (kind of action). These are more important than tense (time of action). Modes include the following: imperfective (action begun but not completed), perfective (action completed), progressive (action in process), usitative (action customarily performed), optative (action expressed as potential or desired). Aspects include the following: momentaneous, continuative, semelfactive (performed once), semeliterative (performed once again), durative (lasting or static), and repetitive (repeated action).	Verb tense (time of action) is most important. Aspect (kind of action) is also expressed by verb. Verb suffixes (-*ing*, -*ed*), auxiliary verbs (e.g., have, am), and modals (e.g., shall, will, did) are used. Tenses are past, present, and future. Aspects include completive (perfect), durative (imperfect), and repetitive.
Pronoun subject and pronoun object are expressed by prefixes to the verb. (Only the subjective and possessive person pronouns can occur alone.)	Pronoun subject, object, and possessor are expressed using words such as *I*, *he*, *him*, *us*, *its*, and *their*.

Table 4-1   *continued*

Navajo	English
There is no distinction of grammatical gender.	English distinguishes masculine, feminine, and neuter gender in third-person singular forms of the personal pronouns (e.g., *he, she, it, him, her, his, hers,* and *its*).
There is no adjective class per se. Neuter verbs perform a similar function (i.e., express a state, quality, or condition without direct reference to a preceding action).	An adjective class functions generally to qualify, describe, or limit the meaning of a noun. Adjectives can be made into nouns or adverbs by adding suffixes (e.g., warm, warmth, warmly).
Adverbial concepts are often expressed by prefixes incorporated within the verb. Navajo distinguishes between repetition (one more time) and reversion (return).	Adverbial concepts are expressed through words. The concepts again, another, some more are separate ideas. There is not always clear distinction between repetition and reversion (return).

Source: Adapted with permission from R.W. Young. (1967). *English as a second language for Navajos: An overview of certain cultural and linguistic factors* (pp. 146–154). Albuquerque, NM: Navajo Area Office, Division of Education, Bureau of Indian Affairs.

American Indian peoples are described by Penfield (1977) (Hopi, Mohave, Ute, and Navajo), Miller (1977) (Pima), Darnell (1979) (Cree), and Wolfram and colleagues (1979) (Laguna and San Juan Pueblos).

There are as many different forms of Indian English as there are different Indian languages and language traditions. Indian-English speakers acknowledge this fact frequently when they identify a person's tribal affiliation merely by calling attention to specific features in the person's spoken English (Leap 1982c, in press). The characteristics of Indian English can be summarized as follows: (1) Indian English retains the phonemic patterns and phonologic constraints characteristic of the community's tribal language, (2) Indian language syntactic rules may take priority over corresponding English syntax rules, (3) word formation and marking conventions in the Indian language may affect corresponding conventions in English, and (4) constructions found in other nonstandard variations of English are also found in Indian English (e.g., uninflected forms of *to be*) (Leap 1982c).

The syntactic characteristics of Indian English may be misinterpreted as a disordered production of the standard dialect. These differences, coupled with reported poor verbal performance of Indian children in the classroom, can, in part, explain the increased referrals and placement of American Indian children in special education and speech-language services.

The Native American Language Act: Public Law 101-477

In clinical exchanges with minority-language children, the techniques of acknowledging, expanding, and elaborating the child's utterance are vital elements of treatment. The implied respect and value of the language of the child is critical to his or her concept of self and to the therapeutic endeavor. The importance of respect for tribal languages was affirmed by Public Law 101-477, the Native American Language Act, which establishes as the policy of the United States the preservation, protection, and promotion of the rights of native Americans to use, practice, and develop Native American languages. The law acknowledges that the traditional languages of Native Americans are an integral part of their cultures and identities and that the continuation of their languages is vital to the preservation of our nation's indigenous cultures. Section 102(6) of the Act states that "there is convincing evidence that student achievement, community pride, and educational opportunity are clearly and directly tied to respect for and support of the first language of the child" (Indian Education Programs; Native American Languages Act 1990). For American Indian children, their first language may be the ancestral tribal language or the Indian-English dialect. Regardless, this first-language performance is the means of expressing their uniqueness and their solidarity with the group.

Implied in this conviction is the requirement that any changes that clinicians suggest and work toward in therapy must acknowledge the integrity of the first language system. The standard dialect of English should be presented in a manner that contrasts two systems, not devalues one for another.

Language Learning and Education

The Warm Springs Experience

Adult-child interaction in the development of language among American Indians was the focus of Susan Philips' longitudinal study of children from the Warm Springs Indian reservation in central Oregon (Philips 1983). The inquiry dealt with verbal and nonverbal interaction styles underpinning early language learning of Indian children and their later language behaviors in the classroom. Philips concluded that Warm Springs children are taught in their preschool years to communicate and attend to communicative acts in ways different from white middle-class children. Moreover, these differences made it difficult for Warm Springs children to comprehend verbal communication and interact appropriately in the classroom. Philips' subjects, like many American Indian children, tended to perform more poorly than their white counterparts on achievement tests, and their poorest performance area was language. Lombardi (1970), Kirk (1972), McShane (1980), and Mishra (1982) reported similar test bias—low performance on verbal IQ measures by children from other tribal groups.

Philips found that American Indian children on the Warm Springs reservation differed from non-Indian children in their use of the auditory and verbal channels of communication. She documented the differences between Indian children's classroom participant structures and those of white children. Differences were evident in turn-taking behaviors, topic maintenance and shift of topics, attention-getting behaviors, and behaviors that signal attention. Philips contended that these differences had their inception in the day-to-day interactions of the Warm Springs community.

The characteristics of Warm Springs that contributed to language differences are based on the reality of rural community life and tribal customs. These characteristics are similar to many reservation communities today. Warm Springs residents spend more time with others and less time alone. They have more face-to-face interactions. Few people live alone, and many daily activities, such as cashing a check and going to town, are done in pairs. Much of the activity of this reservation community is a collective effort. The residents work together in preparation for ceremonies and feasts, family events, and weddings. Talking is done in conjunction with physical tasks, such as cooking or crafts. Visiting is usually done in conjunction with work. Child care is shared among many adults and other children.

Warm Springs infants, like older children and adults, spent more time in the company of others. Even when a baby was asleep, he or she was rarely in a room alone cut off from auditory stimulation. For the Warm Springs infants, the use of cradleboards may have contributed to later behavioral differences.

A cradleboard is a wooden structure made for swaddling the infant. It is usually decorated across the top with a painted design or with turquoise. The infant is swaddled tightly in the cradleboard and spends wakeful and sleeping time there. The cradleboard is propped up so that the infant can see what is going on. At nap time, the child on the cradleboard is laid flat wherever he or she is, usually in close proximity to adults and in the midst of ongoing activities. In this manner, visual stimuli are cut off, while auditory stimuli are not.

This suggests that a visual orientation is considered more compelling for attention. In practice, the infant learns to filter out auditory stimuli.

These early childhood experiences may contribute to the reported elevated visual preference and skills of American Indian children (Philips 1983; Lombardi 1970; Kirk 1972; McShane 1980; Mishra 1982).

EARLY COMMUNICATIVE ACTS

Philips observed that although older members of the tribe talked to the infant, they rarely attempted to elicit sounds or words from babies and did not engage in reciprocal verbal exchanges with infants (Philips 1983). They appeared less likely to interpret the child's vocalizations as meaningful or to respond to them. This lack of perceived intention has been discussed as a factor influencing early language interaction patterns (Briggs 1984; Westby, in press).

Within the Warm Springs community, children have limited exposure to varied syntactic forms. Verbal interactions with young children were often in the form of commands (e.g., "Go get it"), and understanding was indicated through compliance. Adults played with infants, but with the desire to maintain calmness, not to excite, stimulate, or elicit laughter. Philips used these community characteristics to explain behaviors observed in classroom settings (Philips 1983).

CLASSROOM PARTICIPANT STRUCTURE

Participant structures include rule-governed speaking, listening, turn-taking behaviors, and performance in general. Philips' account of participant structures in the Warm Springs classrooms revealed four aspects of American Indian children's behaviors that could indicate their lack of comprehension of classroom discourse: (1) Indian children talked less than their white peers in official classroom interactions controlled by the teacher, (2) they exhibited a greater frequency of inappropriate responses, (3) they asked questions regarding teacher instructions more frequently, and (4) they asked peers to clarify what the teacher had said (Philips 1983).

In addition, Philips documented other culturally specific behaviors that could be misinterpreted as inattention and disengagement in communicative interactions. For example, the Warm Springs children exhibited less back channel work (i.e., affirmative head nodding, verbal interjections, and gazing into the face of the speaker) than white students to indicate attention and engagement in the communication process. In addition, Warm Springs students seemed to prefer group projects in which they had control of selecting themselves as speaker over both small and large group, teacher-directed instruction (Philips 1983).

Philips' comprehensive study of the effect of the child's home culture on classroom behavior gives a possible profile interpretation for elevated referral rates of American Indians for communication disorders.

Apparent lack of attention to the teacher, requests for repetition of directions and instructions, and a quiet nonverbal affect are common reasons for referral of American Indian children for speech-language services in schools. These behaviors could indicate a communicative disorder with auditory comprehension and verbal formulation components, or they could indicate different styles of interaction. It is important to determine if a mismatch of student behaviors and classroom procedures interferes with optimal interactions and learning or if a true disability exists.

Learning Styles and Communicative Competence

Data regarding American Indian children continually present a picture of children with normal or above-average intelligence who score well below their non-Indian peers on tests of auditory comprehension, auditory memory, and verbal communication skills while performing at much higher levels on visual motor, visual memory, and nonverbal performance IQ tasks (Philips 1983; Lombardi 1970; Kirk 1972; McShane 1980; Mishra 1982; Tomeoda, et al. 1984). Numerous reports in the literature indicate that Indian children are taught to watch and listen and to learn through observation. Within a high-context culture, children apparently are encouraged to demonstrate understanding through physical performance. These studies suggested the impact of cultural values and early socialization among American Indian children explains their observed learning and school performance (Philips 1983; Lombardi 1970; Kirk 1972; McShane 1980; Mishra 1982; Tomeoda, et al. 1984). There appears to be no empirical evidence to support the notion that American Indian children have basic cerebral differences that create distinctive learning patterns, although this position has been debated in the literature (Chrisjohn and Michaels 1989; Ross 1989; Rhodes 1990). More influential to the development of preferred learning style in American Indian children are characteristics of reservation lifestyles, language-use characteristics in the home, early child-caregiver interactions, and early learning experiences (John 1972; Brewer 1977; Cazden 1988; Appleton 1983; Tippeconnic 1989).

These characteristics, coupled with reported classroom discourse and test performance of American Indian children, suggest that American Indian children learn and demonstrate their learning in ways that differ from those expected in the mainstream American classrooms (Philips 1983; Tippeconnic 1989). Their approach appears more visual than auditory. They prefer group-interactive projects in which they control their verbal participation, over small- or whole-group, teacher-directed instruction (Blout 1982; Brewer

1977). Their learning process appears to be to learn through observation (i.e., watch, then do) in contrast with the trial-and-error learning of non-Indian children (Longstreet 1978).

A. Paul Ortega, lead medicine man for the Mescalero Apache tribe, commented on these differences from a cultural perspective, saying, "[t]he educational system tries to make them individuals instead of part of the whole" (AP Ortega, personal communication. June, 1987). The non-Indian focus on the individual and the fostering of competition and individual performance differ from the holistic approach to learning and the group association that are promoted by American Indian societies, creating a mismatch between preferred and expected behaviors in the classroom (Longstreet 1978; Erickson and Mohatt 1982; McCarty, et al. 1991; Au 1980; Wong-Fillmore, 1991; Gallimore 1985). This cultural mismatch appears to play a significant role in the underachievement of many minority students (Longstreet 1978; Erickson and Mohatt 1982; McCarty, et al. 1991; Au 1980; Wong-Fillmore, 1991; Gallimore 1985).

The cultural mismatch may be related to asynchronous interactions between teacher and child (Gallimore 1985). When expected behaviors differ from those exhibited, asynchronous interactions result. These asynchronous interactions can arise from various sources, including different participant structures and communication styles. Asynchronous teacher-pupil interactions are a primary cause of minority children's school problems.

Study of American Indian children's learning styles has led some to generalize that Indian children are nonverbal learners. Their learning styles have been characterized in the literature as "field dependent," "holistic," "nonanalytical," and "right-hemisphere dominant" (Chrisjohn and Michaels 1989; Ross 1989; Rhodes 1990).

In a study using an inquiry-based social studies curriculum in the northern Arizona Navajo community of Rough Rock, McCarty and her colleagues (1991) investigated the effects of alterations in the learning environment on language performance of Navajo students. They reported highly verbal behaviors among Navajo students in classroom discussions. These behaviors differed significantly from typical behaviors reported in the literature. McCarty and her colleagues concluded that the active student participation and verbalizations demonstrated in their study were a result of the degree to which the activity enabled the students to use what they knew to learn something new. They reported that the Navajo students responded positively to the inquiry curriculum because the material presented familiar scenes and cultural-linguistic content that tapped the students' backgrounds and experiences, thereby motivating them to express their ideas and to actively engage in the lessons.

Learning-style research among Indian students must be treated cautiously because it can lead to a stereotypic labeling of diverse groups into a collective whole. Attaching to a pan-Indian learning style such labels as *nonverbal, right-brained,* and *visual not auditory* can be precarious and discriminatory. One danger these generalities can create is the reduced performance expectations. Second, relying on explanatory models of culturally based learning- and interacting-style differences of children, which generally ignore the context of the interactions, focuses on the student with low performance and allows for a lack of scrutiny of the curricular or therapeutic environment in which these behaviors occur.

Health Status of American Indians

American Indian groups are ranked at the bottom of virtually every social status indicator with regard to health, income, and education (Toubbeh 1982). Twice as many Indian families live in poverty and are headed by women than in the general U.S. population (Toubbeh 1982). Only 8% of American Indians complete 4 or more years of college, compared with 16% of the general U.S. population (U.S. Bureau of the Census 1990). The interaction of social class, poverty, and yet unidentified factors affect the health status and access to health care of American Indians, especially those living in the remote and rural reservations.

American Indian Children with Disabilities

Rameriz and Johnson (1987) reported that between 1978 and 1986 the number of American Indian elementary- and secondary-school students enrolled in special education programs rose 41.8%. Of the approximately 37,000 American Indians receiving special education, almost 80% were identified as learning disabled or speech-language impaired. This reflected a 60% increase in those identified as learning-disabled, and a 50% increase in those identified as speech impaired during this 8-year period. These increases could be due to greater surveillance of disabilities, greater availability of services, and the effects of fetal alcohol syndrome (FAS) and otitis media (OM), or they could be artifacts of inappropriate diagnostic techniques and due to the lack of alternatives within the regular education system for students with learning and language problems.

Chinn and Hughes (1987) reported a consistently disproportionately high percentage of American Indian children in classes for the learning disabled, whereas their representation in classes for the gifted and talented was consistently low. Compared with non-Indian children, American Indian children were more often referred to special education for academic difficulties, for being quiet or a "loner," or for excessive absences. Non-Indian children were referred more often for physical or neurologic problems or nonconforming behaviors (McShane 1980).

Certain behaviors exhibited by American Indian children in educational settings appear to imply problems in communication and learning. These behaviors may indicate true learning or language disabilities or may be due to their bilingual background, standards of communication, and behavior fostered in the home, or the child's lack of awareness or lack of acculturation to the pragmatic expectations of mainstream American classrooms (e.g., maintaining eye contact, exhibiting questioning behavior, and large-group participation). Behaviors cannot be appropriately understood out of context because they are governed by cultural values and experiences. Two contexts should be considered: the cultural and linguistic background of the child and the cultural and linguistic context of the educational setting.

Otitis Media

Although improvement in the control of infectious diseases has been documented, OM continues to be one of the most prevalent health problems among American Indians. American Indians share with the people of the Pacific Basin the distinction of having the highest prevalence of otitis media in the world (Stewart 1986; Canterbury, et al. 1981). Toubbeh (1985) reported that the disease affects 15% of the American Indian reservation population at any point in time. The prevalence rate is 4–13 times higher than that of the general U.S. population. Canterbury and colleagues (1981) reported a higher incidence of all types of hearing impairments in Alaska native populations, stemming in part from an excessively high rate of OM. These findings are similar for American Indian populations outside Alaska as well (Stewart 1986).

Racial, anatomic, and familial variables have been studied with regard to the high rates of OM. Stewart (1986) concluded, from an extensive review of the literature, that anatomic and genetic variables associated with the common racial background of American Indians and Pacific islanders appear to influence the occurrence of OM and hearing loss in these populations. The significant variables cited by Stewart are the following: (1) Asiatic origin, (2) eustachian tube placement and insufficient middle ear aeration, (3) relative insufficiency of the immune system, and (4) age, with both extremes of the life span continuum disproportionately represented.

Fetal Alcohol Syndrome

FAS is a leading cause of birth defects and the third most common cause of mental retardation in the nation. FAS and fetal alcohol effect

(FAE) are major health problems threatening young American Indian children. FAS and FAE are sometimes referred to collectively as alcohol-related birth defects. FAS is a constellation of abnormalities related to teratogenic effects of maternal alcohol ingestion during pregnancy.

FAS was first discussed in the U.S. medical literature in 1973 (Jones and Smith 1973). Major characteristics of FAS include both prenatal and post-natal growth deficiency, central nervous system dysfunction (e.g., microcephaly, tremulousness), and craniofacial anomalies (e.g., cleft lip and palate, thin upper lip, short palpebral fissures, epicanthic folds) (Church and Gerkin 1988). Delays in gross and fine motor development; delays in language development; language disorders; hearing impairments; mental retardation; learning disabilities; and cognitive difficulties, behavior difficulties, or both are sequelae of FAS and FAE (Church and Gerkin 1988; Abel 1990; Flint 1983; Gerber 1990).

Diagnosis of FAS is a medical judgment best made by a dysmorphologist. Children with FAS display characteristics from the three main categories outlined previously, in addition to a history of prenatal alcohol exposure. For children who exhibit one or two, but not all, of the characteristics required for a diagnosis of FAS and whose mothers have a history of alcohol exposure during pregnancy, the term *FAE* is used. FAE should not be viewed as a less serious impairment. The mental retardation, delayed and disordered speech and language, hyperactivity, and learning problems associated with children with FAE present serious, lifelong challenges.

May and colleagues (1984) reported variable prevalence rates of FAS among Indian tribes, ranging from 1 in 97 to 1 in 749 live births on different reservations of the Southwest, compared with the national prevalence of 1 in 750.

The high prevalence of OM, FAS, and FAE among American Indian populations combined with environmental factors suggest an elevated risk for communication disorders among these populations. FAS and FAE are related to the occurrence of cleft palate, which is associated with deafness and hearing loss (Church and Gerkin 1988; Abel 1990; Flint 1983). The American Speech-Language-Hearing Association estimates that approximately 0.19 million American Indians have communication disorders (American Speech-Language-Hearing Association 1985).

Unique Challenges in Service Delivery to American Indian Populations

The complexity and challenges of providing appropriate assessment and intervention of communication disorders to American Indian children presents a pressing need for the application of new knowledge and innovative techniques. Response to the growing awareness of the inadequacies of traditional practices in assessing and providing services to American Indian and other minority-language children is long overdue. A holistic, nonreductionist approach to the assessment and treatment of communication disorders should attend to the dynamic interactions of acculturation, familial language use expectations, tribal cultural and linguistic characteristics, and the child's early development and educational experiences.

A basic dilemma exists with regard to providing speech-language services to American Indian populations. Often, American Indian parents are confused and concerned as to how best to prepare their children to succeed in the school system while maintaining cultural and linguistic integrity within the tribe and community. Speech-language pathologists have indicated a lack of confidence in their ability to serve minority populations (American Speech-Language-Hearing Association 1985). Appropriate instruments, materials specific to American Indian populations, and bilingual competence in the languages of American Indians are lacking. In addition, typical clinical approaches often do not include factors necessary to appropriately appraise dynamic language behaviors. Cultural differences may be identified as disorders. Assessment personnel may be unable to distinguish characteristics of normal language development of a bilingual child from language characteristics of children who require therapeutic intervention.

Assessment

Attention to cultural differences, the artificial use of language in testing situations, social aspects of testing, and limitations of assessment instruments and procedures can assist clinicians in addressing the many pitfalls in the assessment process.

The Artificial Use of Language

Many formal testing tools and procedures lack linguistic realism and create a situation that requires test behavior and artificial language use. The testing format and responses are inflexible and unlike real communication. This can be especially problematic in the assessment of American Indian children because of the differences in home and school learning and performance styles. American Indian children prefer to observe an activity repeatedly before attempting performance. When confronted with a formal testing situation in which minimal trials are permitted and instances of observing another perform the task are rare or nonexistent, the child may find himself or herself in a stressful situation. Dumont (1972), Philips (1983), and, more recently, McCarty and colleagues (1991) documented that for American Indian children, child-controlled engagement and freedom of interaction increased verbal participation. These researchers cautioned that American Indian children are less likely to display their performance skills on demand. Establishing rapport, including clear explanation of the testing procedure, may help with validity of testing.

Social Aspects of Testing

The social aspects of formal testing may be biased against American Indian children. The question-and-answer format of formal testing is often not characteristic of communication exchanges in American Indian homes. These children, therefore, may not know the "rules of the game" and, if they do, may choose not to play. The following anecdotal record of this author's first encounters with children from the Hopi reservation may illustrate the importance of this concept:

In 1973, I served as a consultant speech-language pathologist to the Hopi Indian Head Start program in their reservation high on the windswept mesas of northern Arizona. One of my first tasks as a new clinician was to administer articulation tests to Hopi Head Start children. I had spent a full day in the classroom and out on the playground with the children that I was going to test that day to "establish rapport" and also to observe their language and speech skills in multiple settings. Afterward, I took one of the boys into the classroom, sat on the floor with him, and began to administer an articulation test. He gave no response to the beautifully colored pictures of the standardized instrument. No matter how I modeled, cajoled, prompted: no response. Later that evening, I had dinner with a Hopi man who is an anthropologist and tribal judge. I related my experience to him. He smiled at me and said, "The boy knew it was a picture of a house, he knew you knew it was a picture of a house, and he was not about to tell you something that you already knew."

The language interactions in a formal testing situation lack authenticity. Clinicians ask questions to which they already know the answers. "Correct" responses are standard English in form and generally reflect the cultural perspective of life outside an American Indian community. The linguistic task characteristics of formal assessment, which include the methods of giving directions and the language structure of the test itself, may be biased against minority-language children. A typical response of a group of Southwest American Indian children when instructed to tell everything they can about an object is to label the object. When encouraged to elaborate, they generally repeat the label or say nothing at all. More expansive utterances are elicited from the children when they are involved in story-retelling tasks from pictorial representations or when they are allowed to describe or comment on their own ongoing activity or a recent event in the community (e.g., Hopi home dances or the Yaqui Easter Ceremonies). Wolfram (1983) explained that the more distant an individual's life experiences or everyday speaking style are from the content and style of the testing task, the greater the potential for task interference. The correct responses listed in test manuals reflect a cultural and linguistic orientation toward the dominant culture. An example of these biases was reported by Tomeoda and colleagues (1984) from a study of the performance of seventy-one 6-, 7-, and 8-year-old San Carlos Arizona Apache Indian children on the Test of Language Development (Newcomer and Hammill 1977). The Apache children did not perform significantly differently from the national sample on a nonverbal intelligence measure (i.e., the block design subtest of the Wechsler Intelligence Scale for Children–Revised), except the group of 8 year olds, which on average performed significantly better than the established norms. However, all of the Apache subjects performed significantly lower on all four language measures compared with the normative sample. Performance was best on the Grammatic Understanding subtest, whereas performance was poorest on the Grammatic Completion subtest, which required not only comprehension but also expression of English morphology and semantics. An error analysis revealed similar patterns, which appeared to be appropriate and acceptable given the subjects' experiential backgrounds but were considered error responses using standard scoring criteria. For example, in response to the task of defining a cow, Apache children typically responded "it bucks; you ride it," rather than the "correct" response of "it moos; it gives milk" (Tomeoda, et al. 1984).

Toronto and Merrill (1983) suggest that cultural and socioeconomic influences may determine test-taking behaviors and that values, motivation, and competitiveness differ among ethnic groups and socioeconomic classes. Differences among children's backgrounds, experiences, and interests and their willingness to be engaged in the assessment process warrant consideration when selecting, administering, and scoring assessment tools and when designing the entire assessment enterprise. For example, for some children there may be diminished pressure to please the examiner or to comply with the requests of the examiner (Witt, et al. 1988). Children may require more time to establish rapport with the examiner and more wait-time during the actual testing. What may be viewed as noncompliant behavior, inappropriate pause time, or a processing problem may in fact be a culturally appropriate behavior from the child's perspective. Traditionally, poor test performance has been assumed to reflect the child's lack of ability or knowledge. It may be that an interaction of the factors discussed affects test performance. Although the examiner may follow the standardized procedures and may be in total compliance with the dictates of formalized assessment, child factors, as well as task factors, may affect the child's performance.

Sensitivity to certain variables is required when assessing American Indian children. Clinicians should be aware that tribal social communication patterns may differ. For example, greetings are not always used when entering or leaving a room. In certain American Indian cultures, lack of a greeting is a sign of respect for the activities that are going on and a desire to not be obtrusive or interrupt. Although maintaining eye contact may indicate attending behavior and engagement in Western communication, for some American Indian groups, a child does not maintain eye contact out of respect for the communication partner.

The pragmatic rules of a community may require the contemplation of questions before responding. Latency of responses can be misinterpreted as a processing problem or an indication that the child does not know the answer, leading the examiner to proceed with another question without allowing adequate time for the child to respond (Philips 1983).

Assessment Tools and Practices

Speech-language pathologists continue to rely heavily on traditional assessment tools and practices to assess American Indian children. Other options are lacking, and the children have varied language skills in tribal languages. Many American Indian children are monolingual English speakers or are speakers of English and their tribal language. Due to the lack of bilingual speech-language pathologists fluent in tribal languages and a lack of bilingual assessment tools, generally English is assessed using the best tools available.

Harris (1985b) conducted a study of speech-language pathologists serving American Indian children in Arizona, Alaska, California, Michigan, New Jersey, New Mexico, New York, North Carolina, North Dakota, Oklahoma, Oregon, South Dakota, Texas, Utah, and Washington. Information regarding assessment tools and techniques was collected. Data indicated that standardized tests were used as part of the assessment battery by all 50 respondents. Most clinicians reported that they used standardized procedures in test administration and standardized norms for scoring and interpretation of results. More than one-third of the clinicians indicated that native language abilities were not assessed. Approximately one-third of the responding clinicians stated that they estimated local norms, whereas only 8% actually calculated them.

The efficacy of establishing local norms for standardized instruments has been controversial. Some believe this practice is prejudicial because it lowers performance expectations for groups of children. Others believe that appropriate diagnosis is achieved only when a child is compared with his or her community peer group. Evard and Sabers (1979) reviewed procedures for improving the validity of speech and language tests for use with ethnic or racial groups. These procedures included (1) developing a new test, (2) modifying existing test items or required responses on existing tests, and (3) developing new norms for existing tests. They determined that establishing local norms was the most efficient and effective method.

The development and application of local norms for existing tests for minority groups was implemented in a study by Evard and McGrady (1974). They found that with the use of local norms, the percentages of children from Tohono O'odham, Mexican-American, and African American families identified as speech-language impaired decreased. Bayles and Harris (1982) and Tomeoda and colleagues (1984) used a similar procedure in studies involving Tohono O'odham and San Carlos Apache Indian children in Arizona, respectively. The resulting local norms were found to be a useful standard in distinguishing a disorder from differences in language performance. To use a language test, clinicians can establish local norms by administering tests to at least 50 randomly selected children of the same age and calculating performance means and standard deviations. This facilitates comparisons of each child to his or her age mates and helps identify children with language problems. When a child scores below the mean of his or her age mates, further inquiry should be made about language competencies.

When standard English language tests are used, the clinician can analyze the most frequently missed test items to discover rules of standard English that are not used in the English dialect spoken by the tribe. For example, English personal pronouns express gender and case, two aspects that are absent in the Tohono O'odham language. This could explain the following sentences from the Bayles and Harris study (1982):

He shirt caught in his zipper.
He dropped his glasses and when him tried to zip his thing and it got stuck.
The boy's zipper got caught in her jacket.

Interpretation of Assessment Data
The variability within and among American Indian populations of language, levels of bilingualism, and characteristics of reservation communities prohibit the development of an American Indian test battery. However,

well-trained, skillful, sensitive clinicians can use the guidelines presented here and in other resources to provide more appropriate assessments. Computing and establishing local norms for a school or group may be perceived as too time consuming or costly. Use of established norms that compare an American Indian child's performance with a group to which he or she is dissimilar in experience or language background and using this comparison to determine the presence of a disorder, however, is an inappropriate and unsound practice.

The need continues for alternative methods in assessment of American Indian children and other minority-language children. These methods will vary for each language group because they must integrate what is known about characteristics of second language learners and characteristics of the child's home community.

Intervention

In introducing therapeutic goals to American Indian families, a clear link to the greater goal or purpose must be explained. In addition, as a collective society, relationships are slow to form and highly valued. The unfamiliar professional should establish rapport and build trust within the community as a preliminary step to any therapeutic interventions.

When compatibilities between school and home culture are increased, minority children's performances improve (McCarty, et al. 1991; Tharp 1989; Gallimore 1985). However, achieving this compatibility is no small undertaking. The Kamehameha Early Education Program (KEEP) has been a major source of theory, research, and demonstration of culturally compatible language arts programs for kindergarten through third-grade children in Hawaii and on the Navajo reservation (Tharp 1989; Gallimore 1985). Characteristics of the KEEP Hawaiian model required substantial alterations for effective implementation within the Navajo culture. These alterations were made in part to respond to four psychocultural variables that affect educational achievement—social organization, sociolinguistics, cognition, and motivation.

Social Organization

Typically, classrooms in North America are characterized by whole-group instruction provided by a teacher or leader. This system may be less effective for American Indian children than for children from the dominant culture. Implementation of the KEEP model within the Navajo classroom was more effective when small, sex-specific groups were formed. This organization reflects the cultural dictates of segregating boys and girls in play activities. Navajo teachers moved from student to student and engaged in individualized, quiet discussions (Tharp 1989). Inquiries about tribal mores regarding sex-specific groupings for activities can ensure speech-language therapy groups reflect appropriate social organization.

Sociolinguistics

Three components of sociolinguistics variables affect relationships, learning, and satisfaction in the classroom: (1) wait time, which is the amount of time given by teachers for student response, and wait time II, which is the amount of time following a student's response before the teacher again speaks; (2) rhythm, which is the tempo of material presentation, vocalizations, and vocal inflections of teachers and students; and (3) participation structures (Tharp 1989).

Wait Time

The different wait times of white and Navajo teachers with the same group of Navajo students indicate the significance of this sociolinguistic phenomenon. Navajo teachers allowed longer wait times than white teachers. What was perceived as a completed response by white teachers was often intended by the child as a pause that white teachers interrupted (Tharp 1989). The preference for prolonged wait time among Pueblo Indian children was also reported by Winterton (1976). Pueblo children participated twice as frequently in longer wait time classes than shorter wait time classes. Given the need to learn and practice language in an interactive context and the meaning attributed to silence in American Indian cultures, the significance of this finding is apparent.

Rhythm

The research on rhythm patterns used by American Indian children indicates that a slow, fluid tempo of material presentation resulted in more efficient and organized patterns of interactions and higher levels of rapport between teachers and students (John 1972; McCarty, et al. 1991; Gallimore 1985; Tharp 1989).

Participation Structure

Participation structures are discussed earlier in this chapter in the section "The Warm Springs Experience." The participation structures of Navajo and Hawaiian cultures differ greatly. In the KEEP study, Navajo children spoke for long periods in an individualized, discursive manner, circling around the central point. There was little interruption by fellow students (Tharp 1989). This is a typical pattern found among American Indian adults in business negotiations and spiritual teaching. When these participation structures are not honored, American Indian children may develop a pattern of short answers or silence.

Cognition

American Indian children appear to prefer a holistic pattern of learning stemming from early observation and learning experiences. KEEP researchers reported Navajo children's preference to listen to a story completely before asking questions or having a discussion. This preference can be maximized in therapy by presenting a complete context for learning-specific language forms (Tharp 1989).

Motivation

Motivation is critical to speech-language therapy outcomes. Important insights were revealed by the KEEP research findings. Navajo teachers maintained on-task behaviors by moving physically through the classroom, almost silently. The Navajo adults were more reserved in their affectionate displays but were highly respectful of children's individuality and sovereignty (Tharp 1989). Punishment, contingent rewards, or any openly manipulative behavior of others, including children, is a violation of cultural values (Bayles and Harris 1982). This perspective requires the clinician to be thoughtful in the selection of appropriate reinforcers and in behavior-management techniques in clinical settings.

Recommendations for Assessment and Intervention with American Indian Populations

Recommendations for the administration include the following:

1. The school administration, in conjunction with the tribe(s), should provide in-service training and cultural orientation to all new personnel. The in-service training should include a discussion of community characteristics, linguistic characteristics, and communication of community goals.
2. Administrators should accommodate the professional's need for classroom observations as part of orientation and ongoing assessment procedures. Time for these activities must be provided in personnel schedules.
3. If the language characteristics of the community warrant the use of interpreters, the school district or clinic should hire and provide training to an interpreter.

Recommendations for assessment include the following:

1. Classroom observations should be part of the assessment process.
2. Error analyses of responses to test items should be undertaken.
3. Calculation and use of local norms should be considered, if standardized assessment instruments are used.
4. For family conferences related to assessment, the clinician should (a) determine the need for an interpreter and discuss the interpreter of choice with the family and (b) indicate that the family may wish to invite other family members or a friend to the conference. These individuals may be able to provide information regarding the child and be supportive to the family.
5. The clinician should follow a collaborative model with classroom teachers. Teachers can assist in comparing a child referred for speech-language services to his or her cultural mates.
6. Speech-language pathologists can provide information regarding normal speech-language development in bilingual children, characteristics of the Indian dialect, and cultural considerations that can improve classroom language performance.
7. Assessment should be a multistage, multisituational process.

Recommendations for intervention include the following:

1. The clinician should seek out information regarding the linguistic characteristics (both on form and use) of the tribal language or dialect of English.
2. If part of intervention requires shaping a linguistic form that reflects the first language of the child, the clinician should approach this in a positive, contrastive manner by (a) selecting phonemes that are absent in the tribal language or dialect and that contrast with English and (b) linking the final consonants and consonant clusters with morphologic significance for instruction.
3. The clinician should stress functional, problem-solving language skills in therapy.
4. The clinician should involve tribal elders as cultural and linguistic informants and allies. He or she should invite them to share information and legends with the children. If tribal members judge that they are appropriate for the task, they will respond. If not, they will not.

Conclusion

If differences of world views, child-rearing practices, language acquisition and use, and the appropriateness of assessment and intervention strategies and the effects of these differences are ignored, errors in judgment can result. These errors have potential negative effects on a child's self-worth, emerging language, and creative communicative potential. Ignoring these differences can alienate the child from the educational or social system of schools because of the conscious or unconscious message relayed to the child regarding his or her home language, dialect, or culture.

Freire and Macedo (1987), education theorists, stressed the importance of legitimizing an individual's life experiences because these experiences are the foundation for all subsequent learning. They emphasized that the ability to name one's experiences or communicate through a distinctive voice is part of what is meant by "reading the world." Through the ability to read the world, the ability to read the word, or literacy, emerges.

One of the continuing challenges for American Indians is living in two worlds, the Indian world and the "white man's world." Chief Seattle stated that one cannot stay long with one's feet in two different canoes. Walking in two worlds is fraught with challenges and choices—choices of language, of values, and of behaviors. Because language is so strongly rooted within culture and tied to an individual's sense of self, change in this fundamental tool of communication affects both the individual and the larger culture.

In the Indian world, this understanding of self and the culture comes through language in the form of legends and through ceremonies. As specialists in communication, speech-language pathologists contribute to the individual's process of exploring the ideas expressed through language. When the work of a speech-language pathologist is understood in this context, the work will be respected by the members of the American-Indian culture as a vital learning process.

References

Abel, E.L. (1990). *Fetal alcohol syndrome*. Oradell, NL: Medical Economics.

American Speech-Language-Hearing Association. (1985). Clinical management of communicatively handicapped minority language populations. *ASHA, 27*, 29.

Appleton, N. (1983). *Cultural pluralism in education*. New York: Longman.

Au, K.H. (1980). Participant structures in a reading lesson with Hawaiian children: Analysis of a culturally appropriate instructional event. *Anthropology Education Quarterly, 11*, 91–115.

Basso, K. (1970). To give up on words...silence in Western Apache culture. *Southwest Journal of Anthropology, 26*, 213–230.

Bayles, K.A., & Harris, G.A. (1982). Evaluating speech-language skills in Papago Indian children. *Journal of American Indian Education, 1*, 11–20.

Blout, B.G. (1982). Culture and language of socialization: Parental speech. In D.A. Wagner, & H.W. Stevenson (Eds.), *Cultural perspectives on child development* (pp. 54). San Francisco: WH Freeman.

Brazelton, T.B., Koslowski, B., & Tronick E. (1976). Neonatal behavior among urban Zambians and Americans. *Journal of the American Academy of Child Psychology, 15*, 97–107.

Brewer, A. (1977). On Indian education. *Intergrateducation, 15*, 21–23.

Briggs, C.L. (1984). Learning how to ask: Native metacommunicative competence and the incompetence of field workers. *Language in Society, 13*, 1–28.

Brislin, R., Cushner, K., Cherrie, C., & Yong, M. (1986). *Intercultural interaction: A practical guide.* Beverly Hills, CA: Sage.

Burgess, B., & Adams, C.P. (1979). *Feasibility study report: Proposed research and training center for the habilitation/rehabilitation of Native Americans with neurosensory disabilities.* Lawrence, KS: Native American Research Associates.

Callaghan, J.W. (1981). A comparison of Anglo, Hopi, and Navajo mothers and infants. In T.M. Field, A.M. Sostek, P. Vietze, & P.H. Leiderman (Eds.), *Culture and early interactions* (pp. 115). Hillsdale, NJ: Erlbaum.

Canterbury, D.R., Dixon, C.L., & Gish, K.D. (1981) Hearing loss in Alaska. *Journal of the American Audiological Society, 17*, 18–24.

Cazden, C. (1988). *Classroom discourse: The language of teaching and learning.* Portsmouth, NH: Heinemann, 1988.

Chinn, P.C., & Hughes, S. (1987). Representation of minority students in special education classes. *Journal of Remediation and Special Education, 8*, 41.

Chisholm, J.S. (1983). *Navajo infancy: An ethnological study of child development.* New York: Aldine.

Chrisjohn, R.D., & Michaels, P. (1989). The right-brained Indian: Fact or fiction? *Journal of American Indian Education, Special issue, August,* 77–83.

Church, M.W, & Gerkin, K.P. (1988). Hearing disorders in children with fetal alcohol syndromes: Findings from case reports. *Pediatrics, 82*, 147–154.

Cook, M.J., & Sharp, M.A. (1966). Problems of Navajo speakers in learning English. *Language Learning, 16*, 21–29.

Darnell, P. (1979). *Reflections of Cree interactional etiquette: Educational implications.* Austin, TX: Southwest Educational Development Laboratory.

Dukepoo, F. (1980). *The elderly American Indian.* San Diego: San Diego State University Center on Aging.

Dumont, R. (1972). Learning English and how to be silent: Studies in Sioux and Cherokee classrooms. In C. Cazden, V. John, & D. Hymes (Eds.), *Functions of language in the classroom* (pp. 344–369). New York: Teachers College Press.

Erickson, F., & Mohatt, G. (1982). Cultural organization of participation structures in two classrooms of Indian students. In G. Spindler (Ed.), *Doing the ethnography of schooling* (pp. 94). New York: Holt, Rinehart, and Winston.

Evard, B.L., & McGrady, H.J. (1974, November). *Development of local language norms for Papago Indians, Mexican Americans, blacks, and Anglos.* Presented at the annual meeting of the American Speech-Language-Hearing Association, Las Vegas.

Evard, B.L., & Sabers, D.L. (1979). Speech and language testing with distinct ethnic groups: a survey of procedures for improving validity. *Journal of Speech and Hearing Disorders, 44,* 271–281.

Fajardo, B.F., & Freedman D.G. (1981). Maternal rhythmicity in three American cultures. In T.M. Field, A.M. Sostek, P. Vietze, & P.H. Leiderman (Eds.), *Culture and early interaction* (pp. 133). Hillsdale, NJ: Erlbaum.

Fleisher, M.S. (1982). The educational implications of American Indian English. In R. St. Clair, & W.L. Leap (Eds.), *Language renewal among American Indian tribes* (pp. 141–149). Roslyn, VA: National Clearinghouse for Bilingual Education.

Fletcher, J.D. (1983). What problems do American Indians have with English. *Journal of American Indian Education, 23,* 1–14.

Flint, E. (1983). Severe childhood deafness in Glasgow. *Journal of Laryngology and Otolaryngology, 97,* 421–425.

Forbes, J. (1979). Traditional Native American philosophy and multicultural education. In *Multicultural education and the American Indian.* Los Angeles: University of California Press.

Freedman, D.G. (1974). *Human infancy: An evolutionary perspective.* Hillsdale, NJ: Erlbaum.

Freire, P., & Macedo, D. (1987). *Literacy: Reading the word and the world.* South Hadley, MA: Bergin & Garvey.

Gallimore, R. (1985, June). *The accommodation of instruction to cultural differences.* Presented at the University of California Conference on the Educational Underachievement of Linguistic Minorities, Lake Tahoe.

Gerber, S.E. (1990). *Prevention: The etiology of communicative disorders in children.* Englewood Cliffs, NJ: Prentice-Hall.

Greenberg, J.H. (1987). *Language in the Americas.* Stanford, CA: Stanford University Press.

Harris, G.A. (1982). *Proposal to establish the Native American rehabilitation research and training center (NARTC).* Submitted to the National Institute of Handicapped Research. University of Arizona, Department of Family and Community Medicine, Tucson, AZ.

Harris, G.A. (1985a). Considerations in assessing English language performance of Native American children. *Topics in Language Disorders, 5,* 42–52.

Harris, G.A. (1985b). *Survey of speech language pathologists serving Native American populations.* Tucson, AZ: Native American Research and Training Center, University of Arizona.

Harris, G., & Bayles, K. (1981, November). *Speech-language pathology and audiology: Native American perspectives.* Presented at the annual meeting of the American Speech-Language-Hearing Association, Los Angeles.

Highwater, J. (1975). *Indian America.* New York: David McKay Company.

Indian Education Programs; Native American Languages Act. Public Law 101-477, 101st Congress, 2nd session, 30 October 1990.

John, V.P. (1972). Styles of learning—styles of teaching: Reflections on the education of Navajo children. In C.B. Cazden, V.P. John, & D. Hymes (Eds.), *Functions of language in the classroom* (pp. 331). New York: Teachers College Press.

Jones, K.L., & Smith, D.W. (1973). Recognition of fetal alcohol syndrome in early infancy. *Lancet, 2,* 999–1001.

Kirk, S.A. (1972). Ethnic differences in psycholinguistic abilities. *Exceptional Children, 36,* 112–118.

Leap, W.L. (1982a). Semilingualism as a form of linguistic proficiency. In R. St. Clair, & W.L. Leap (Eds.), *Language renewal among American Indian Tribes* (pp. 148–159). Roslyn, VA: National Clearinghouse for Bilingual Education.

Leap, W.L. (1982b). Role of the linguist in Indian bilingual education. In R. St. Clair, & W.L. Leap (Eds.), *Language renewal among American Indian Tribes* (pp. 19–30) Roslyn, VA: National Clearinghouse for Bilingual Education.

Leap, W.L. (1982c). The study of Indian English in the U.S. Southwest: Retrospective and prospect. In F. Barkin, & J. Ornstein-Galicia (Eds.), *Bilingualism and language contact: Spanish, English, and Native American languages* (p. 34). New York: Teachers College Press.

Leap, W.L. (in press). American Indian English. In L. Cole, & V. Deal (Eds.), *Disorders in multicultural populations*. Rockville, MD: American Speech-Language-Hearing Association.

Locust, C. (1986). *American Indian beliefs concerning health and wellness*. Tucson, AZ: Native American Research and Training Center, University of Arizona.

Locust, C. (1988). Wounding the spirit: discrimination and traditional American Indian belief systems. *Harvard Education Review, 58*, 315–330.

Lombardi, T.P. (1970). Psycholinguistic abilities of Papago Indian school children. *Exceptional Children, 36*, 485–493.

Longstreet, E. (1978). *Aspects of ethnicity*. New York: Teachers College Press.

Malach, R.S., Segel, N., & Thomas, T. (1989). *Overcoming obstacles and improving outcomes: Early intervention services for Indian Children with special needs*. Bernalillo, NM: Southwest Communication Resources.

Mathiot, M. (1973). English and Papago compared. In P.R. Turner (Ed.), *Bilingualism in the Southwest* (pp. 251). Tucson, AZ: University of Arizona Press.

May, P.A., Hymbaugh, K.J., Aase, J.M., & Samet, J.M. (1984). Epidemiology of fetal alcohol syndrome among American Indians of the southwest. *Social Biology Quarterly, 30*, 374–387.

McCarty, T.L., Wallace, S., Lynch, R.H., & Benally, A. (1991). A classroom inquiry and Navajo learning styles: A call for reassessment. *Anthropology Education Quarterly, 22*, 42.

McShane, D. (1980). A review of scores of American Indian children on the Wechsler intelligence scales. *White Cloud Journal, 1*, 3–10.

Miller, D. (1975). *Native American families in the city*. San Francisco: Institute for Scientific Analysis.

Miller, M.R. (1977). *Children of the Salt River: First and second language acquisition among Pima children*. Bloomington, IN: Indiana University Publications Language Science Monographs 16.

Mishra, S.P. (1982). The WISC-R and evidence of item bias for native American Navajos. *Psychology in the Schools, 19*, 458–464.

Nelson-Barber, S.S. (1982). Phonologic variations of Pima English. In R. St. Clair, & W.L. Leap (Eds.), *Language renewal among American Indian Tribes* (pp. 115–133). Roslyn, VA: National Clearinghouse for Bilingual Education.

Newcomer, P.L., & Hammill, D.D. (1977). *The test of language development*. Austin, TX: PRO-ED.

Penfield, S. (1977). *Some examples of Southwestern Indian English*. San Antonio, TX: Trinity University Press.

Philips, S.U. (1983). *The invisible culture: Communication in classroom and community on the Warm Springs Indian Reservation.* New York: Longman.

Rameriz, B.A., & Johnson, M.J. (1987). American Indian exceptional children: Improving practices and policy. In A.A. Ortiz, & B.A. Rameriz (Eds.), *Schools and the culturally diverse student: Promising practices and future direction* (pp. 128–140). Reston, VA: ERIC Clearinghouse, Council for Exceptional Children.

Red Horse, J. (1983). Indian family values and experiences. In G.J. Powell (Ed.), *Psychosocial development of minority group children* (pp. 258–274). New York: Brunner/Mazel.

Rhodes, R.W. (1990). Measurement of Navajo and Hopi brain dominance and learning styles. *Journal of American Indian Education, May,* 29–40.

Ross, A.C. (1989). Brain hemispheric functions and the Native American. *Journal of American Indian Education, Special Issue, August,* 72–76.

Stewart, J.L. (1975). *Unique problems of handicapped Native Americans.* Washington, DC: U.S. Government Printing Office.

Stewart, J.L. (1986). Hearing disorders among the indigenous peoples of North America and the Pacific Basin. In O.L. Taylor (Ed.), *Nature of communication disorders in culturally and clinically diverse populations* (pp. 237–276). San Diego: College Hill.

Tafoya, T. (1982). Coyote eyes: Native cognitive styles. *Journal of American Indian Education, 21,* 21–23.

Tharp, R.G. (1989). Psychocultural variables and constants: Effects on teaching and learning in schools. *Journal of the American Psychological Association, 44,* 1–11.

Tippeconnic, J.W. (1989). Preface. *Journal of American Indian Education, Special issue, August,* i.

Tomeoda, C.K., Lennertz, M.A., Fischler, R.S., & Feldman, C. (1984, November). *Performance of Apache children on the test of language development.* Presented at the annual meeting of the American Speech Language-Hearing Association, San Francisco.

Toronto, A.S., & Merrill, S.M. (1983). Developing local normed assessment instruments. In D.R. Omark, & J.G. Erickson (Eds.), *The bilingual exceptional child* (pp. 105–122). San Diego: College Hill.

Toubbeh, J. (1982). Native Americans: A multidimensional challenge. *ASHA, 24,* 395–397.

Toubbeh, J. (1985). Handicapping and disabling conditions in Native American populations. *American Rehabilitation, 11,* 3–9.

U.S. Bureau of Census. (1990). Populations and housing unit counts for identified American Indian areas and Alaska Native Villages. In *1990*

Census Population General Population Characteristics. Washington, DC: U.S. Bureau of the Census, Series PC 90-1B.

Westby, C. (in press). Cultural differences in caregiver-child interactions: Implications for assessment and intervention. In L. Cole, & V. Deal (Eds.), *Communication disorders in multicultural populations.* Rockville, MD: American Speech-Language-Hearing Association.

Winterton, W.A. (1976). *The effects of extending wait-time on selected verbal response characteristics of some Pueblo Indian children.* Ph.D. dissertation, University of New Mexico.

Witherspoon, G. (1977). *Language and art in the Navajo universe.* Ann Arbor, MI: University of Michigan Press.

Witt, J.C., Elliot, S.N., & Gresham, F. (1988). *Handbook of behavior therapy in education.* New York: Plenum.

Wolfram, W.A. (1983). Test interpretation and sociolinguistic differences. *Topics in Language Disorders, 3,* 21–35.

Wolfram, W., Christian, D., Leap, W.L., & Potter, L. (1979). *Variability in the English of two Indian communities and its effects on reading and writing.* Arlington, VA: Center for Applied Linguistics.

Wong-Fillmore, L. (1991). Second language learning in children: A model of language learning. In E. Bialystock (Ed.), *Language processing by bilingual children* (pp. 49). Cambridge, UK: Cambridge University Press.

5

Hispanic Cultures and Language

Hortencia Kayser

Hispanic is a term that has arisen in the literature in the past years and may still be misunderstood by the general population. A Hispanic, as defined by the U.S. Bureau of the Census (1996), is an individual of Spanish background. However, Hispanics can come from any race. Individuals who are Asian, white, or black can all be Hispanic if their language background is Spanish. For example, black and white people living in Puerto Rico are considered to be Hispanic. To say that Hispanics have one culture would be a simplification of that definition because Hispanics encompass a variety of cultures, just as they come from a variety of races. *Hispanic*, then, is a broad term used for convenience to identify individuals who come from a Spanish heritage and may or may not use Spanish as the language of the home.

It is important to note that not all Hispanics are recent immigrants. Some Mexican-American families trace their roots to the Spanish explorers or to the early settlements of the Southwest. Hispanic cultures and Spanish language in the Western hemisphere have been maintained for the past 500 years and continue to be a driving force in the United States.

The Hispanic population totaled more than 27 million in the United States in 1995. The Hispanic population grew by 28% between 1990 and 1994. In comparison, the total United States population grew only 6% during that same 4-year period. It is projected that the Hispanic population will number 31 million by the year 2000 and 63 million by the year 2030 (U.S. Bureau of the Census 1996).

In this chapter, the Hispanic cultures of those from Mexican, Puerto Rican, and Cuban descent are described, as these are the largest groups of Hispanics in the United States (U.S. Bureau of the Census 1996). This chapter reviews the literature as it relates to Hispanic culture and family roles and linguistic, assessment, and intervention considerations for Hispanic groups. Finally, a discussion of the perceptions of disabilities and diagnostic and intervention considerations are provided that take into account the cultures of these populations.

The Hispanic People

Hispanic individuals come from different cultural backgrounds, socioeconomic levels, and educational experiences. The Hispanic population in the United States has had a tremendous impact on the American culture, but Hispanics have yet to feel the impact of a truly equal society that allows them to benefit from its educational and economic riches. In general, Hispanics in the United States are likely to be less educated and to earn less annual income and are thus more likely to be below the poverty level than non-Hispanics. Fifty-three percent of Hispanics complete 4 or more years of high school, whereas the rate among non-Hispanics is 83%. Only 9.3% of Hispanics complete 4 or more years of college, whereas among non-Hispanics the rate is 23% (U.S. Bureau of the Census 1996). The 1995 median income of Hispanic families was $24,313; the median income was $41,864 for white, non-Hispanic families. These figures reflect a $4,000 increase for Hispanics and $10,000 increase for non-Hispanic white families in the time period between 1980 and 1995. Approximately 27% of Hispanic families were living below the poverty level in 1996, compared with 9.1% of white non-Hispanic families in 1995. Sixty-eight percent of Hispanic families were married couples, and 25% of Hispanic families were headed by single women (U.S. Bureau of the Census 1996). Language may be the barrier that has limited the Hispanic from the American dream.

The Family and Socialization Practices

Just as Hispanic cultures differ, so do the interactions of Hispanic families. Peñalosa (in press) and Erickson and Iglesias (1986) discussed the heterogeneity within Hispanic cultures that makes it impossible to easily characterize specific cultural interactions of Hispanic groups. Any scholar who attempts to assign characteristics to Hispanic families will soon meet an Hispanic family that does not fit the description.

What can be said is that the Hispanic family provides children with unique early experiences that influence their overall development. Hispanic children are exposed to environments that are characterized by unique cultural beliefs and care-giving practices that are different from those of mainstream English-speaking populations (Garcia Coll 1990). Children are socialized to meet competencies that adults believe they should have in their interactions with adults and other children. Hispanic adults try to teach their children cognitive, linguistic, motivational, and social abilities that are relevant to the Hispanic culture. Underlying these competencies is the Hispanic family's belief in the strength of the family.

Zayas and Palleja (1988) described this familialism in Puerto Rican homes. They suggested that the support for family integrity within Puerto Rican families gives shape and direction to the conduct of family members. Puerto Rican society emphasizes the importance of the nuclear and extended family and the cohesion among its members. According to Zayas and Palleja, the family governs the individual identities of its members and the collective identity of the family. The family influences the members' conduct not only within the family but also in public. Protecting other family members, advising them, and assuming responsibility for them are part of the rules of membership. Members learn to accept these responsibilities to preserve family integrity, tradition, and social and emotional equilibrium (Zayas and Pallaja 1988).

Two specific concepts that influence Hispanic relationships beyond the family include (1) the importance of individuals and their qualities as a person and (2) the importance of relationships (Kayser, in press). The specific qualities that Hispanics observe in their relationships include *respeto* (respect), *dignidad* (dignity), *personalismo* (character), *honor* (honor), and *confianza* (trust) (Harry 1992). These qualities transcend social class. A low-income person who has fulfilled obligations to family and community is respected. The mainstream belief that a professional should be respected because of skill rather than personal disposition is not always accepted by Hispanics. The person and his or her qualities cannot be separated.

Relationships are also important. Networking among community members and extended families makes up the community's system of trustworthy individuals. Hispanics trust people and rely on people. Thus, an Hispanic family may respect and trust the individual who also happens to be a professional but may not understand or trust the agency or organization.

Exposure to the American culture is an added dimension that complicates the description of an Hispanic family's interactional style and value system. An individual's culture changes as he or she is exposed to differing belief systems. The individual may drop beliefs of his or her family and take on those of the majority culture.

The family attitudes toward the mainstream culture may determine the acculturation of each individual. For example, Heath (1986) described Mexican-American families as either open or closed to the mainstream culture. If the family is closed, the children within the family are protected and, to some extent, isolated from the mainstream. The children do not have the opportunity to learn about mainstream values and communication functions. On the other hand, an open family allows its children to participate in the community through secondary institutions, such as the public library and the Boy Scouts. Interactions with the mainstream provide the children with experiences that eventually affect the family interactions and family expectations for the children.

Hispanics vary in the way individual families socialize and teach their children. These socialization practices bring the child into the community as a communicatively competent speaker. Specific studies have attempted to describe the socialization of children in Mexican families. Garcia Coll (1990) stated that mother-infant interactions among Mexican-American mothers are predominantly nonverbal. Field and Widnayer, as reported in Garcia Coll, reported that Cuban mothers talked more to their infants, had longer mean length utterances, and played more teaching games than Puerto Rican, South American, and African American mothers with their 3- to 4-month-old infants.

Steward and Steward, as reported in Garcia Coll (1990), studied the teaching interactions of Mexican mothers. They found that Mexican mothers presented little direct teaching, gave nonverbal instructions, used slow pacing and negative feedback, and used a high percentage of adult wording in their speech with infants. The Mexican mothers perceived themselves as mothers and not teachers. Laosa (1978) reported that the mother's level of formal education was a factor in the type of teaching strategies used with her children. The higher the mother's level of formal education, the more she used inquiry, praise, and teaching strategies. The lower the mother's level of formal education, the more she used modeling as a teaching strategy, and, for boys in particular, the more she appeared to physically punish and control. Ethnographic studies of first-generation Mexican families appear to confirm these reports. Valdes (1986) studied child socialization in Mexican families and found that parents emphasize observation and independence in learning. Children are encouraged to observe and participate in the performance of household tasks when the parent believes the children are ready to do so. It is assumed that children are able to judge when they are ready. It is also assumed that when children undertake a task, the performance is the best that they are able to manage at the time. Adults provide guidance if it is needed or requested, but the parent rarely offers much in the way of unsolicited verbal instructions.

Perceptions of Disabilities

Hispanics are a heterogeneous people. Those of Mexican descent have a mixture of European and Indian ideology and practices, whereas those from the Caribbean have a mixture of Native American, European, and African influences. The common basis for many Hispanics' belief system is Catholic ideology. Mexican Catholic ideology includes Indian practices, whereas Cuban and Puerto Rican Catholicism includes African religious beliefs (such as those of Yoruba), which are sometimes called *Santerismo* or *Espiritismo*. The greater the influence of African tradition the more the perspective reflects an animistic view (i.e., a belief that spiritual influences abound throughout the universe) (Harry 1992). These spirits can have a negative influence (e.g., illness), as well as a positive influence (e.g., wellness) on the individual.

Among Mexican Americans, there is a belief that an evil eye, or *mal ojo*, which is obtained by admiring an individual or envying the person, causes illness. *Curanderos*, or medicine women, are called to perform rituals and prayers and provide herbal medicinal teas to counteract the evil that affects the afflicted individual. There are beliefs that explain speech disorders, such as *susto*, a severe fright that can cause a child to stutter. If a pregnant woman views a full moon or an eclipse, the event is said to cause a cleft palate in the unborn child (Langdon 1992; Maestas and Erickson 1992). Table 5-1 summarizes Hispanic beliefs and perceptions about illness and its consequences.

The view of how a disability is obtained affects what is believed should be done to treat the disorder. Harry (1992) and Teller (1988) described Hispanics as having a fatalistic view of life. Reyes (1995) described this as an external locus of control—that is, an individual cannot and does not change what has happened to him or her.

Traditional folk medicine practices may be sought first, if the individual perceives that medical treatment is not effective. The use of folk medicine varies depending on the assimilation of the individual into mainstream views of disease and disability and the availability of the *curanderos.* Marin and colleagues (1983) reported that in East Los Angeles only a small percentage of respondents to their questionnaire on health services stated that they could find a *curandero* (7%), a *yerbero* (herbalist; 15%), or a *partera* (midwife; 2%). According to Teller (1988), folk medicine for diseases and disabilities is probably used in conjunction with, rather than instead of, Western medicine.

Bilingualism and Heterogeneity of Hispanics

Definition of Bilingualism

The term *bilingualism* has different meanings for different individuals. It has been defined with varying degrees of strictness regarding how proficient or competent a speaker must be to be considered bilingual.

Table 5-1   Hispanic Perceptions Concerning Disabilities

Families may believe in *curanderismo* (i.e., folk medicine using herbs, prayers, and rituals).

Families may resist institutionalization (i.e., individuals with disabilities may be cared for in the home).

A visible disability may be attributed to external causes (e.g., witchcraft or the moon).

Parents may believe that they are being punished for wrongdoing.

Families differ in their perceptions of disabilities.

Catholic parents may accept disabilities stoically because of a larger divine plan that is not comprehensible to humans.

Some families may hide a disabled child if the family takes pride in itself for health and vitality.

Children with disabilities may be indulged by family and friends.

Children with disabilities may not be expected to participate in treatment and their own care.

Families may not accept invisible disabling conditions (e.g., learning disabilities).

Families may use spiritualists to seek healing and dispel evil spirits.

Sources: A.G. Maestas, and J.G. Erickson. (1992). Mexican immigrant mothers' beliefs about disabilities. *American Journal of Speech-Language Pathology, 1(4),* 5–10; H.W. Langdon. (1992). *Hispanic children and adults with communication disorders: Assessment and intervention.* Gaithersburg, MD: Aspen; and C.A. Roseberry-McKibben. (1995). *Multicultural students with special language needs: Practical strategies for assessment and intervention.* Oceanside, CA: Academic Communication Associates.

Bloomfield (1935) defined a bilingual as an individual who has native-like control of two languages and exhibits no loss of the native language. At the other extreme, MacNamara's (1966) definition states that a bilingual individual possesses at least one of the language skills (i.e., listening, speaking, reading, or writing) in the two languages to a minimal degree. With this definition, the academic who acquires a reading ability in a second language is also considered a bilingual.

Baetens-Beardsmore (1986) distinguished between two types of bilinguals. He described the natural bilingual as one who, out of necessity and with no specific training, has learned two languages. Spanish-speaking children entering English-only educational programs are considered natural bilinguals if they have no formal instruction in English. In contrast, the academic bilingual is a person who chooses to take course work to learn a second language. These two types are distinguished only on the basis of how the second language is learned and do not address proficiency in the two languages.

A person who is beginning to learn and develop a sense for the second language is termed an *incipient bilingual.* This development of the language may be at the comprehension or expression levels. Baetens-Beardsmore (1986) stated that incipient bilingualism can lead to passive and active types of bilingualism. In passive bilingualism, there is comprehension and relatively little or no expression in the second language. Active bilinguals use two languages for communication with other bilingual or monolingual speakers of the respective languages.

Advanced bilingualism is described as *equilingual* and *ambilingual.* An ambilingual person is fluent in both languages in all domains of language and culture. Ambilinguals have no trace in their speech and language that indicates that they speak another language. The equilingual, or balanced bilingual, person has a mastery of two languages that compare with that of the monolingual speaker of each language but are not equal to the monoglot norm. That is, most listeners detect an influence from the other language when listening to an equilingual speaker. The equilingual is more common, whereas the ambilingual is rare.

Bilingualism is a relative concept, with no clear delineations and with many definitions. It can be defined strictly or minimally, depending upon the researchers' views. Descriptions of the bilingual's proficiency, rather than a bilingual categorization, assist the speech-language pathologist because there are two major influences on the bilingual's linguistic abilities—societal factors and individual factors.

Societal Factors Affecting Bilingualism

Bilingual communities can be described using several dimensions—historical, political, social, and psychological (Fishman 1966). One dimension may be strong in one community and not play an important role in the lives of bilingual people in a second community. An Hispanic community, such as San Antonio, TX, or Santa Fe, NM, may thrive on its historical contribution to the region. The political strength of the Hispanic community determines its economic and educational futures. If a community accepts both languages as equal and desirable socially, bilingualism flourishes. The psychological effects and attitudes from the majority culture have either a positive or negative effect on the use of the minority language in public.

The historical, political, social, and psychological dimensions do not operate independently; they interact in a complex manner to produce either a stable or transitional bilingual community. Stable Hispanic communities (e.g., San Antonio) continue to use both languages through many generations and continue to have new immigrants in the community that "feed" the minority language. A transitional bilingual community, on the other hand, is in transition toward English monolingualism. The transitional community consists of two generations of monolingual English speakers (e.g., parent and child). Many Hispanic communities in Northern California, Colorado, Arizona, New Mexico, and North Texas no longer use Spanish and speak only English.

The societal factors that help determine the type of bilingual community include whether the minority language population (1) is an immigrant or indigenous one, (2) is of recent origin or long standing, (3) is greater in number in relation to the majority language speakers, (4) is evenly distributed within the community, (5) is urban or rural, (6) is near or far from the country of the mother tongue, and (7) frequently visits the mother tongue country (Baetens-Beardsmore 1986; Miller 1984). The societal factors that operate in different communities help determine the opportunities that bilingual speakers have to hear, see, and use the minority and majority languages in public. These factors are different for each community, thereby producing unique circumstances for the development of bilingualism. Bilingual communities can be different from city to city and even within one city. The diversity of communities has an impact on whether the children learn the two languages simultaneously or consecutively or whether the presence of two languages is regarded as an advantage or a burden (Sanchez 1983).

Individual Factors Affecting Bilingualism

The bilingual speaker determines when to speak, what to speak about, and to whom to speak (Fishman 1965). Depending on the act of communication and the speakers involved in the event, place, or topic, the bilingual may choose one language over the other or use both (Fishman 1966). Speakers vary with regard to age, sex, ethnic group, class, rural or urban background, relative role status, in-group (e.g., friends) or out-group status, and, most important, the interlocutor's willingness to operate the linguistic conventions that would normally occur while these factors are present (Baetens-Beardsmore 1986; Miller 1984).

Bilingual speakers may be consciously or subconsciously influenced by the speaking situation in their choice of language. Hispanic youth recognize the status of teachers; therefore, they use one style of communication with students and change their language style, as well as the language, when addressing a respected teacher. These students also recognize that a different style of interaction should be used with one who is older; therefore, they may use Spanish exclusively with an older Hispanic adult. A frequent occurrence in young Mexican-American second-language learners is the unwillingness to speak their first language in school. Some of these children deny speaking Spanish and refuse to converse with another person unless it is in English. Another variable for language choice is the topic of conversation. Topics such as the home, religion, and relatives are preferably discussed in the home language. Topics for which the second language is preferred include work, education, and administrative affairs. Foreign students trained in American universities often use English easily to speak about their professional expertise but may not have the same ability in their first language. The reasons and purpose of the exchange also influence the choice of language. Place is another important variable. The bilingual child may use English only in the classroom but prefer his or her home language with friends on the playground.

The bilingual speaker is also faced with an internal battle concerning the development of a second language. Baetens-Beardsmore (1986) described this psychological state, or anomie, as a feeling of personal disorientation, anxiety, and social isolation. This phenomenon was first described by Child (1943), who observed symptoms of frustration in the children of Italian immigrants in New York. The children experienced conflicts of loyalties between the home language and the dominant culture. Child reported that, for these children, the conflict was resolved by withdrawing either from the outside culture or from the home language and culture. The latter brought about feelings of turmoil and severance from the family. Baetens-Beardsmore (1986) stated that this situation becomes more acute for the adolescent who is trying to develop a set of personality traits in two languages.

Anomie tends to occur in the bilingual individual who moves from one cultural group to another. McCloskey and Schaar (1965) suggested that anomie is highest among those of low education and low income and having low-prestige occupations. As the individual learns more about the second language, its cultural values, and norms, the standard expected from the second-language learner becomes higher. The individual is then faced with changing linguistic and cultural expectations from the second-language group, while the first-language community expects the person not to change and to react as though he or she has not assimilated. Both groups notice any failure to conform with either language and culture. These individuals eventually perceive themselves as different, and so may the two language communities.

Because of the societal and individual factors that determine the choice of one language over another, bilingualism is a multivariate phenomenon. The factors that influence the degree of bilingualism in an individual involve the community, the family, the child, and the outside influences of the majority language. The Hispanic population in the United States is a heterogeneous group because of the societal and individual factors that determine each individual's bilingualism.

Communicative Competency

Communicative competency for Spanish-speaking monolinguals and bilinguals is determined by the norms that are accepted by the community of speakers of the language(s). According to Kessler (1984), in becoming communicatively competent, bilingual children must learn the grammatical, sociolinguistic, discourse, and strategic competencies necessary to successfully communicate in their group. Grammatical, or linguistic, competence refers to the knowledge of the phonologic, syntactic, and lexical features of the language. Sociolinguistic competence refers to the knowledge of the cultural rules of language use and appropriateness for the context. Discourse competence is concerned with the skill to connect utterances to form conversations, narratives, and other speech events. Strategic competencies refer to the strategies used by the bilingual to compensate for breakdowns in communication that can result from imperfect knowledge of the rules or fatigue, memory lapses, distraction, and anxiety.

Communicative competence is the interaction of grammatical, sociolinguistic, discourse, and strategic competencies. For Hispanic bilingual individuals, the interaction of the two languages and exposure to the two cultures shape the bilingualism.

Linguistic Competency

Phonologic Development

Spanish and English appear to contain many of the same phonemes, but direct phonemic equivalents do not exist. English phonology is made up of 24 consonants and two semivowels, compared with 19 consonants and two semivowels in Spanish. Additionally, many of the Spanish consonants are unaspirated, which gives a perceptually different production of the consonants (e.g., *paper* versus *papel*). Stockwell and Bowen (1965) stated that English contains 17 syllabic nuclei (vowels), as compared with 10 frequently occurring nuclei in Spanish. There are also differences in the rules governing the combinations of sounds within each of the languages. Spanish clusters are fewer and less complex. Two sets of consonant clusters occur most frequently in both languages: consonant plus /l/ and consonant plus /r/. The /s/ clusters cannot appear in word or syllable initial position in Spanish but do appear in English (e.g., *school* versus *escuela*). Final consonant clusters rarely occur in Spanish but do occur in English. Medial consonant clusters occur in both languages (Stockwell and Bowen 1965). Since Spanish appears to have a simpler phonologic system than English, it stands to reason that Spanish-speaking children develop their sound system earlier than English-speaking children. The following paragraphs summarize the phonemic and phonologic development of Spanish-speaking children.

It appears that the majority of the Spanish phonemes are mastered by 4 years of age. Table 5-2 summarizes the phonetic development found in four studies. Acevedo (1989), Jimenez (1987), Linares (1981), and Terrero (1979) agree that /j/, /l/, /r/, /rr/, /s/, and /tʃ/ appear to be more difficult for these children to produce. Goldstein (1995) stated that by 3 years of age Spanish-speaking children use the dialect features of the community and have the vowel and the majority of the consonant systems in place.

The use of phonologic processes by Spanish-speaking children is a new area of research (see Goldstein 1995 for an extensive review of phonologic development in Spanish-speaking children). For Spanish-speaking children, it appears that developmental phonologic processes occur at or before 4 years of age. Becker (1982) reported consonant-cluster reductions, deaffrication, and nonphonemic substitutions, including tongue protrusions, occur before 4 years of age in monolingual 4 year olds. Diamond's (1983) 4-year-old bilingual subjects were highly intelligible but exhibited difficulty with liquids, clusters, and tongue protrusion. The only differences between Diamond's bilingual and Becker's monolingual subjects were the increased use of deaffrication by Spanish monolinguals and the increased usage of assimilation by the bilinguals. Goldstein (1995) summarized phonologic development by stating that Spanish-speaking children occasionally exhibit cluster reduction, unstressed syllable deletion, stridency deletion, and tap /r/ and trilled /rr/ deviations.

Morphosyntactic Development

It is difficult to study Spanish-language development in the United States because these children are exposed to English as well. The subjects may not be monolingual Spanish speakers, but may understand English and be incipient bilinguals. Children are exposed to their English-speaking age peers, an English-speaking community, and English-language programs on television. This English influence has a great impact on the development of Spanish in these children. To negate this English influence, researchers have collected data on children in Mexico or other Latin American countries. This has helped our understanding of the development of the Spanish language; however, using these data on Hispanic-American

Table 5-2   Spanish Phoneme Development as Reported by Four Researchers

	Age (years; months)[a]			
Phoneme	Acevedo (1989) (studied Mexican-Americans)	Jimenez (1987) (studied Mexican-Americans)	Linares (1981) (studied Mexicans)	Terrero (1979) (studied Venezuelans)
m	3; 6	3; 7	3; 0	3; 1
n	3; 6	3; 7	3; 0	4; 1
p	3; 6	3; 3	3; 0	3; 1
b	3; 6	3; 3	6; 0	3; 9
B	—	—	6; 0	—
k	3; 6	3; 7	3; 0	3; 1
g	3; 6	4; 7	3; 0	5; 5
t	4; 0	3; 3	3; 0	3; 1
d	4; 0	4; 7	4; 0	4; 9
d	>5; 6	—	4; 0	>5; 5
f	3; 6	4; 3	4; 0	4; 9
j	4; 6	3; 11	3; 0	5; 1
l	4; 6	3; 11	3; 0	4; 5 (M)[b] >5; 5 (F)[b]
x	5; 0	4; 7	3; 0	4; 1 (M)[b] >5; 5 (F)[b]
t	5; 0	4; 7	4; 0	5; 1
s	<5; 6	5; 7	6; 0	>5; 5
r	3; 6	4; 7	4; 0	>5; 1 (M)[b] 5; 5 (F)[b]
rr	>5; 6	>5; 7	6; 0	>5; 5
ñ	3; 6	4; 11	3; 0	4; 9
w	3; 6	3; 7	5; 0	—
ng	—	—	3; 0	—

[a]The ages indicate the point at which the subjects had mastered the respective phonemes, with mastery being at the 90% level.

[b]M and F refer to medial and final positions, respectively. These differences were reported if they spanned more than two age groups. Those ages not designated as corresponding to word position indicate the age at which the phonemes are mastered in all positions in which they occur.

Source: Data from D.M. Paulson. (1991). *Phonological systems of Spanish-speaking Texas preschoolers*. Thesis, Texas Christian University.

children is comparable to using English language standardized tests on bilingual children.

Table 5-3 gives an overview of Spanish language development by age, verb tense, and syntax, with examples for each area. This chart is not exhaustive of Gonzalez's (1983) work with Mexican-American children, but it is a summary of important milestones that clinicians can use in evaluating Spanish-speaking children.

Spanish-speaking children use single words before 2 years of age, two-word utterances by 2 years of age, and simple three-word constructions by 3 years of age. They are asking questions and using compound sentences with conjunctions by 4.5 years of age. According to Garcia, et al. (1984), by 4.5 years of age, the Spanish-speaking child should be using approximately 38 different syntactic structures. Normalcy among children varies greatly; therefore, the clinician should keep in mind the individual's style in language learning (Owens 1988).

The development of Spanish morphology is different from the development of English morphology. These differences appear in noun and article gender agreement, dialectal variations, and the linguistic complexity of the utterances. The use of the article in Spanish is different from English. The Spanish speaker must use the correct gender article for the noun that is to be expressed. If plurality is used, article, adjective, and noun must be marked. An example is the phrase *the red car*. In Spanish, the child must learn that *carro* (car) is a masculine word and must have a masculine article *(el carro rojo)*. If the phrase becomes plural (i.e., *the red cars*), the child must mark the article, noun, and adjective as plural: *los carros rojos.* Spanish-speaking children have difficulty with gender and number agreement as late as 6 years of age (Garcia, et al. 1984). The acquisition of article and gender agreement is affected by the complexity in use, the influence of English, and the possibility that some children are losing proficiency in Spanish. It is therefore unrealistic to insist that a child have article-noun agreement at a young age.

Complexity of language form is an area that is looked at in monolingual English-speaking children to determine if a language disorder exists. But with Spanish-speaking children who are exposed to English in uncertain amounts, complexity is not an indicator of a communication disorder. Leopold (1939) observed in his daughter Hildegarde an avoidance of difficult words and constructions in the weaker language. For Hildegarde, the weaker language shifted from German to English and back to German, depending on the child's dominant language environment (Leopold 1939). Avoidance of difficult words and constructions is a communicative strategy that bilingual children and adults use for efficiency and ongoing communication.

Table 5-3   Acquisition of Spanish Verb Tenses and Syntax

Age (years; months)	Verb Tenses	Syntax
2; 0	Present indicative (e.g., *son pollos* [they are chickens])	First sentences 2- to 3-word utterances
2; 6	Emergence of (1) preterit (e.g., *la agarra esta muchachita* [this little girl got it]) (2) present progressive (e.g., *me esta pintando los zapatos* [he's polishing my shoes]) (3) periphrastic (*ir a* + infinitive), past progressive, and imperfect (e.g., *van a tomar* [they're going to drink])	Indirect and direct object usage Transformations (i.e., yes-and-no and wh- questions and negation [no]) Advanced imperative forms (e.g., *dame el libro* [give me the book]) Conjunction *y* (and)
2; 9	—	Verb-subject-direct objective (e.g., *Comi yo blanquillos* [I ate eggs]) Verb-direct object-subject (e.g., *Perdio la llanta el bos* [the bus lost the tire]) Subject-verb-direct object (e.g., *Yo tengo zapatitos* [I have little shoes])
3; 0	Imperfect indicative (e.g., *caminaba asi* [walked like that]) Present subjunctive (e.g., *cuando acabemos* [when we finish])	Locate conditional clauses Comparisons (e.g., *alla* [over there], *Si* [if], and *mas* [more])
3; 3	—	Tag questions (e.g., ¿*verdad?* [right?]) Temporal adverbs (e.g., *cuando* [when])
4; 6	Functional use of present indicative, preterit, imperfect indicative, present progressive, present perfect indicative, present subjunctive, and past subjunctive (e.g., *Te dije que no lo hicieras asi* [I told you not to do it that way])	Conjunctives *pero* [but] and *y* [and] Comparison *como* [as]
5; 0	—	Relative clauses, noun clauses, temporal adverbial clauses (e.g., *antes que* [before], *hasta que* [until], *cuando* [when])

Source: Data from American Speech-Language-Hearing Association. (1983). *ASHA bilingual language learning system project.* Rockville, MD: American Speech-Language-Hearing Association.

Anderson (1995) reported that children may use the dialectal variation of the parent. That is, if the parent uses a nonstandard variety of Spanish (e.g., simpler or nonstandard grammar) that is acceptable for the community, the child may also use this dialect (see Anderson 1995 for an excellent and extensive review of Spanish morphosyntactic development in children).

Semantic Development

Development of an awareness of the meaning of words and the use of specific vocabulary is closely tied to the child's socialization within the family unit. Parents instruct their children on what they believe the child should know. Slobin (1983) described the social context of three Mexican-American families who used Spanish as the language of the home. He reported that the words learned were related to topics that adults believed the children should know. Slobin found four major topics: (1) labels for objects and names of individuals, (2) the identity of the donor of an object, (3) the location or activity of relatives, and (4) the birth of a new sibling. He stated that parents taught their children names of important family members and other individuals important to the family. This semantic knowledge was reinforced by the frequency with which this type of information was asked for outside the home by other people.

Quinn (1995) reported that 22-month-old Spanish-speaking infants responded differently than English-speaking children on the Sequenced Inventory of Communication Development (Hedrick, et al. 1990). The highest category of single words used by the children were in family members' names. This was followed by categories for animal names, household objects, verbs, foods, and social words. In a longitudinal study of the acquisition of language of a bilingual child, Fantini (1978) reported that his son Mario's first words were social words.

Specific information concerning concept development and vocabulary development in Spanish-speaking children is not fully known. It is known that Hispanics do not believe that knowledge of colors, numbers, and letters is important information for their children to know. Respect and politeness are emphasized, and with these ideals follow the socialization of rituals and specific formulas for social interaction. Specific vocabulary that is considered important by mainstream society may not be part of the Hispanic child's semantic knowledge.

Sociocultural Competency

Fantini (1978) provided an excellent description of the sociocultural rules that Hispanic children are often exposed to during early years.

These rules are not universal in all Hispanic homes, but some of the social norms that Fantini described are true for many Hispanics.

Fantini used observations and a diary to describe his son Mario's bilingual development. He described Mario's environment as permissive, with clear boundaries for behavior. Adults enjoyed and treated children as children, with no expectation of early independence. Mario was able to do things for himself, but it was not expected of him from the family. Mario's mother was accustomed to a certain degree of separation between adults and children. Mario was therefore taken to another room when visitors were present. Many Hispanic adults believe that children have time—usually a short period immediately after greetings—to speak in the presence of adults; consequently, children are not expected to participate in adult conversations.

Mario's early socialization to the appropriate adult-child routines began with the parents' phrase of *"di _____"* (*"say _____"*) such as *"di gracious," "di te quiero,"* or *"di hasta mañana."* The child was given the exact word or phrase to say, which depended on the circumstance. The child's early speech reflected these routines. His early words included *gracias* (thank you), *te quiero* (I love you), and *hasta mañana* (see you tomorrow). As he grew older, increased stress was placed on proper verbal interaction—that is, when and when not to talk to whom. The instruction was described as direct correction of improper etiquette. For example, he was reprimanded when he interrupted adult conversations, and he had to wait until the end of lengthy discussions to gain his turn (Fantini 1978).

Fantini (1978) described four styles of speech that Mario used with adults, siblings, and peers: intimate, peer talk, "baby talk," and adult-style speech. Mario used the intimate style in interactions with the family. In this style, diminutives (e.g., *perrito* for *perro* [dog]) and terms of endearment were common. This style was used to show affection and appeared to be limited to Spanish only. When Mario attempted to show affection to an English-speaking teacher, he switched to Spanish to express his feelings. Mario's peer talk used more direct commands, many expressive interjections, imitated utterances, songs, and recitations. Courtesy terms and diminutives were absent. This style was in direct contrast to the adult style, which included courtesy and etiquette terms and frequently used titles of respect. When talking to younger children, Mario used baby talk, with extreme variations in intonation, a high-pitched voice, and frequent diminutives.

Fantini (1978) provided a wealth of descriptions of the sociocultural interactions of Mario with other speakers. What is made clear from the study are the differences in expectations for the Hispanic child.

Discourse Competency

Conversation

Heath (1986) stated that there are two universals concerning discourse. First, not all adults believe that children should be included in conversational talk. Adults are likely to speak directly to children to teach them to talk. Second, instruction and running narratives do not occur routinely in many cultures. The idea or belief that language is the future goal is a Western school idea. Conversational norms vary from culture to culture. Among Mexican families, children show their respect for adults by not considering themselves equal to the adult during adult-child interactions. Peers are considered to be equal conversational partners. This rule appears to be maintained even into adulthood. Children do not interrupt the adult conversations and are allowed to participate in these adult interactions only when the family views the growing young adult as a full adult. The age of admittance into important family decision making and adult conversations varies with each family.

Narratives

Heath (1986) stated that every society allows its young to hear and produce at least four basic narrative genres: recast, event cast, accounts, and stories. The distribution and frequency of these narratives vary greatly, as does the degree of elaboration. Each society determines how much children participate in learning these genres.

The recast is a narrative that brings to present attention experiences of the past. The child retells an event. This report has consecutive chronology and a consistent point of view. There is a high value on verbal imitations of events. This type of narrative is seen in the classroom when the teacher asks for summaries. Heath (1986) found that Hispanic children use this type of narrative with peers to retell an event with specific purposes in mind. The child may role play and retell an event in the present tense.

Event cast is a verbal reply or explanation of activity scenes that are either in the current attention of the listener, are being planned, or will take place in the future. In mainstream culture, a mother may narrate an event before it takes place or while it takes place, or the clinician may outline what is going to happen. Event casts are susceptible to metalinguistic or metacognitive commentaries. The adult may stop talking and talk briefly about language or think of what is said. Language is segmented. Schools encourage this type of narrative. Heath (1986) found that the event cast rarely occurs in Hispanic families.

Accounts are early narrative forms whereby children spontaneously share what they have experienced. Children must learn on their own that each account must carry within it a predictable progression that allows the listener to anticipate what is coming. This type of narrative is judged by its truth value and organization. In school, show-and-tell is an example of an account. Among Hispanics, Heath (1986) found that accounts were used when children talk of their experiences to a visiting family member.

Stories have a focus and a definite structure. Mainstream listeners expect stories to contain some fictionalized segments and reshaping of language (e.g., the use of *Once upon a time...*). Mainstream society uses books to generate stories. For Hispanics, stories are often oral, with a moral emphasis or emphasis on socially acceptable behavior. These stories may be fictional, but often the content surrounds details of family members.

Gutierrez-Clellen (1995) stated that many of the problematic narratives of Spanish-speaking children may be related to differences in contextual or background knowledge rather than ability. Clinicians and teachers should not assume that children have a knowledge of school narratives and treat deviations from the norm as disorders.

Code Switching

Code switching is the alternating use of two languages at the word, phrase, and sentence level with a complete break between languages in phonology. This phenomenon is developed and encouraged in children who live in bilingual communities. Child code switching begins early in children and is different from adult code switching. McClure (1981) noted that Mexican children produce different kinds of code switching depending on age. Young children tend to mix codes by inserting single items from one language into the other. Usually English nouns, followed by adjectives, have the highest frequency of mixing into Spanish utterances. For example, a child might say, *"Quiero comer un hot dog"* ("I want to eat a hot dog") or *"Me gusta la red pelota"* ("I like the red ball"). At 3 years of age, code switching is used to resolve ambiguities, clarify statements, and attract attention (e.g., *"Mira aqui, look here"*). At 6 years of age, mode shifting, such as moving from narration to commentary, is seen through code switching. At 8 years of age, code switching is used for emphasis, commands, and elaboration. For example, during an English dialogue a child may emphasize a negation, saying, *"Te dije que no"* ("I told you no"). By the time bilingual children are 9 years of age, code switching may occur at the phrase and sentence levels (McClure 1981). For example, a child may say, "Give me the pencil *que tiene un arco*" ("that has a rainbow").

Genishi (1976) found that children generally chose the language that the interlocutor spoke better. If the addressee was English dominant or monolingual, the children used English only. On the other hand, if the addressee was Spanish dominant or monolingual, the children used Spanish only.

Hudelson (1983) described the functions of code switching in an 8-year-old boy named Beto during an art activity in his bilingual classroom. Beto used both languages for questioning, informing, persuading, controlling, playing with language, initiating and maintaining social interaction, and personal self-expression.

Zentella (1983) studied bilingual Puerto Rican children in two New York bilingual classrooms (third grade, ages 7–10; sixth grade, ages 11–13). Zentella stated that these children knew the rule "follow the leader," which is expected of capable bilinguals beyond the age of 5 years—for example speak English when the adult speaks English. These children could accurately determine the language preference of peers and would use English, Spanish, or both. Zentella stated the children used more intrasentential (within sentence) code switching during the interviews with the researcher and more extrasentential (between sentences) code switching among themselves. She found that these children were skilled by the age of 8 years at code switching if the addressee switched codes, using their abilities in two languages for communication. She also noted that the children readily interacted in Spanish with Hispanic staff members and English with non-Hispanic bilingual teachers. The children identified all non-Hispanics as English speakers. Zentella stated that it was considered abnormal to speak Spanish to a non-Hispanic. She also noted that switching to mark ethnicity and group membership appeared later.

School-age bilingual children who learn the second language when they enter school learn that there are social rules concerning code switching depending on who the listener is, the listener's bilingual language abilities, and the function of the communication event. Some children of school age learn English because of both necessity and their situation and therefore switch codes. Valdes-Fallis (1978) suggested that monolingual Spanish-speaking children who are in a monolingual English classroom normally remain silent in the classroom unless forced to speak. The child may begin to speak in English but switch languages as an emergency attempt to continue communication. English is understood to be the norm for the classroom; therefore, code switching may not be heard by the monolingual teacher. Bilingual children do not alternate between two languages with those who speak only one of the languages. It is reasonable to assume that children who begin to switch codes follow the adult rules for when it is appropriate to switch codes.

Code switching among children is an area of research that has not yet provided a complete picture of how children learn to alternate between two languages. The occurrence of code switching among children with language impairments has also not been studied.

Strategic Competency

Children are known to have a variety of strategies to help them learn a language. Peters (1977) discussed the analytic versus gestalt strategies of the young language learner; Nelson (1973) referred to the referential versus the expressive strategies used by children; and Snyder-McLean and McLean (1978) discussed the metalinguistic strategies of children for language learning. Imitation has been used as a strategy in the acquisition of words, morphology, and syntactic-semantic structures (Bloom, et al. 1974). These same strategies appear in children who are learning two languages. Corder (1967) suggested that bilingual children have two strategies: learning strategies and communicative strategies. Communicative strategies are used to communicate effectively, whereas learning strategies are mental processes to help construct the rules of the language. Similar to Corder's communicative and learning strategies are Wong-Fillmore's (1979) social and cognitive strategies. Social strategies include joining groups and acting as if one understands, using choice words to give the impression of expressive abilities in the language, and counting on friends for help when a topic is not understood. Cognitive strategies include the assumption that speech is related to the context, guessing, analysis of repeated phrases, and focusing on the big picture rather than the finer parts of the language. Older children use a number of other strategies, such as imitation, deferred practice, asking informants, reading, observation, using a dictionary, silent practice, asking for repetition, and many others. All are strategies, whether social, learning, or cognitive, that the second language learner uses to become communicatively competent.

Assessment

A communication disorder in an Hispanic individual who actively uses two languages is not difficult to determine when the disorder is severe and the client has identified himself or herself as communicatively impaired. Frequently, the diagnosis is made by the family, the community, or peers. The Hispanic client may stutter, complain of hoarseness, be difficult to understand, or not speak at all. It is important to distinguish a language difference from a language disorder. When a school-age child is not performing at the English monolingual level of academic performance, there is concern that the student may have a language-learning disability. The student may appear disordered when attempting to speak English. Nonfluencies or morphosyntactic, semantic, and pragmatic errors can be perceived as stuttering or a language impairment. A native language assessment is necessary because communicative disability affects both languages and can therefore be detected.

The diagnostic assessment of individuals who are bilingual in Spanish and English has been discussed by Ambert and Dew (1982), Gavillan-Torres (1984), Ortiz and colleagues (1986), Dew (1987), and Kayser (1989). All have proposed that the assessment of bilingual individuals include (1) a determination of the language status of the speaker, (2) an assessment battery of tests, and (3) documentation of linguistic and cultural differences and of the socioeconomic status of the client. These researchers recommended that tests be used; however, they also recommend nonstandard procedures in using these test instruments. This section briefly outlines this assessment process involved in acquiring knowledge of the client's background and acculturation into mainstream culture.

Language Status

Language status relates to the client's proficiency in using each language by domain. The language status of the client may be assessed through the use of language samples in both languages, observations, and questionnaires. Observations of the client's language proficiency can be made through the use of observational techniques as described by Omark (1981): the focal child, scan sampling, and matrix completion techniques. These procedures can be used to quantify language behaviors, such as the frequency of the use of each language for different contexts. The specific language behaviors that are of interest to the speech-language pathologist can be noted and observed over time and compared to those of age and language history peers. Questionnaires can be completed by a parent or other caregiver in addition to a second informant (e.g., teacher). The observations and questionnaires from the two informants should provide a language-status profile of the client. Language behaviors can then be identified, observed, and confirmed through observational techniques.

Assessment Battery

The purpose of the diagnostic assessment is to determine whether a communication disorder exists. For the bilingual Hispanic, this purpose is broadened to include the determination of whether the communication difficulty is a result of a language difference or a language disorder. Three alternatives for improving language assessment have been recommended by researchers in minority language assessment (Erickson and Iglesias 1986; Kayser 1989, 1995; Mattes and Omark 1984; Taylor 1986; Vaughn-Cook 1983; GT Weddington, unpublished data, 1987). These include (1) modifying the testing procedures, (2) adapting or revising existing tests, and (3) using a language sample.

Using a standardized procedure on a test with an Hispanic client provides the minimal rather than the maximum ability of that individual. Taylor (1986, 1992) stated that the testing situation is a social event that may not be familiar to the minority client. The procedures normally used in a test situation may be foreign and not part of the experiences of the client. With this situation, the standardized procedure does not provide the maximum linguistic ability of the client. Modifications in the testing procedures provide the individual with a variety of response modes, thereby providing the speech-language pathologist with information that is far above the minimal knowledge of the client. Table 5-4 lists those procedures that have been recommended by Erickson and Iglesias (1986) and Weddington (unpublished data, 1987). Erickson and Iglesias suggested that it should be the clinician's goal to obtain a dynamic assessment of the individual's ability to modify his or her behavior or ability to learn during the testing process rather than to obtain a static measure from a standardized test.

Adaptation of existing tests developed for English-only speakers should be done with caution, if at all. Adapting a test requires changing the tasks and content of the original test instrument to adapt to the cultural and linguistic differences between the two languages. This changes the validity and reliability of the original instrument. Because the test is normed on a different population and a different language, the norms from the existing test cannot be used. Adapting a test requires the efforts of a team of professionals who know the population and the Spanish language. Adapting a test takes time, but the efforts in evaluating the content and tasks may be well rewarded (Kayser 1989).

The language sample should provide examples of language content, form, and use by the client in natural contexts. Kayser (1989) suggested three contexts (home, school, and clinic) with three different interlocutors (siblings, peers, and clinician). Language samples that provide a variety of participants (i.e., known and unknown and intimate and nonintimate), settings (e.g., home and school), functions (i.e., informal and formal), forms (e.g., play, storytelling, and jokes), and topics (e.g., experiences and academic achievements) enable the clinician to differentiate between the language used by a nonimpaired bilingual and that used by a language-disordered bilingual client (Fantini 1978). The language samples should be reviewed to determine whether the errors in phonology, syntax, semantics, and pragmatics could be a result of the influence of the first language. Experienced clinicians recognize features that are common Spanish influences in the use of English by bilinguals. Limited variations in form and content and restricted use of English and Spanish in all

Table 5-4   Modification of Testing Procedures

1. Reword instructions.
2. Provide additional time for the child to respond.
3. Continue testing beyond the ceiling.
4. Record all responses, particularly when the child changes an answer, explains, comments, or demonstrates.
5. Compare the child's answers to dialect or to first-language or second-language learning features. Rescore articulation and expressive language samples, giving credit for variation or differences.
6. Develop several more practice items so that the process of taking the test is established.
7. On picture vocabulary recognition tests, have the child name the picture in addition to pointing to the stimulus item to ascertain the appropriateness of the label for the pictorial representation.
8. Have the child explain why the "incorrect" answer was selected.
9. Have the child identify the actual object, body part, action, photograph, and so forth, particularly if he or she has had limited experience with books, line drawings, or the testing process.
10. Complete the testing in several sessions.
11. Omit items that the child may miss because of age, language, or culture.
12. Change the pronunciation of vocabulary.
13. Use different pictures.
14. Accept culturally appropriate responses as correct.
15. Have parents or another trusted adult administer the test items.

Sources: Data from G.T. Weddington, unpublished data, 1987; and J.G. Erickson, and A. Iglesias. (1986). Assessment of communication disorders in non-English proficient children. In O. Taylor (Ed.), *Nature of communication disorders in culturally and linguistically diverse populations* (pp. 181–218). San Diego: College Hill.

contexts with different listeners are characteristic of bilingual individuals with language impairments. Normal bilingual individuals display variety in form, content, and use of language in their normal communication within the community (Kayser 1989) (see Kayser 1989 and Kayser and Restrepo 1995 for further discussions of the analysis of language samples).

Documentation of Linguistic and Cultural Differences and Socioeconomic Status

The Individual's with Disabilities Education Act of 1997 requires that sociocultural and socioeconomic status not be the reason for the identification of the need for special education. Differences in background and experiences with the mainstream culture do not constitute a disability. Documentation of the child's background and experiences is made through observations, questionnaires, and interviews with the family (Ambert and Dew 1982). The types of questions for interviews with the family that could be asked have been suggested by Mattes and Omark (1984) and Saville-Troike (1978). Information concerning the family's language use, length of stay in this country, frequency of visits to the mother-tongue country, educational level, literacy, and community and work experiences provide a profile of cultural and environmental influences on language learning.

An assessment of the communicative abilities of the bilingual Hispanic should include the determination of language status for both languages, an alternative and dynamic assessment battery, and the examination of variables that document linguistic and cultural differences and the socioeconomic status of the client.

Assessment Practices and Suggestions

Speech-language pathologists are trained to provide diagnostic evaluations for communication disorders using quantitative and qualitative procedures. Speech-language pathologists who regularly assess Hispanic clients have identified common practices that should be part of a nonbiased assessment of this population. This section discusses procedures for testing clients and reporting assessment data.

Testing Procedures

The speech-language pathologist uses standardized procedures for administering tests, which are described in the test manual. When testing a Spanish monolingual or bilingual client, a number of procedures may be necessary that are not discussed in these test manuals. The following are practices to avoid when testing a Spanish-speaking monolingual or bilingual client:

1. Do not use only standard American English–normed reference instruments with the Hispanic client. The majority of normed referenced instruments are developed for English-speaking people from mainstream America. The norms are not valid for non–English-speaking clients (Kayser 1989, 1995).
2. Do not use only formal standardized tests to determine whether the client has a communication disorder. A language sample provides a better description of the communication abilities of the client than tests (Kayser 1985).

3. Do not give multiple measures to obtain low scores to qualify a student for services. Identification of a communication disorder on the basis of a test that the clinician believes confirms the assumption of a disorder is unethical (Kayser 1985; Meitus and Weinberg 1983).

4. Do not use on-the-spot translations of instruments. Translation into another language requires skill and training (Kayser 1989, 1995; Langdon 1988). Any testing done in the minority language should be done with an instrument that has been adapted with the consensus of a team of professionals (Kayser 1989, 1995). The report should clearly state that the test was adapted and explain the nature of the adaptation.

5. Do not use two languages simultaneously in the assessment. The purpose of the assessment is to determine the client's ability in one language. When both languages are used simultaneously, the clinician is unable to determine the extent of the client's communication abilities in each language separately.

6. Do not use only one elicitation technique for the language sample (e.g., narratives). A variety of language elicitation techniques should be used with a minority language client (Cornejo, et al. 1983). The exclusive use of only one procedure, such as conversation or narrative, is biased in nature.

Reporting Procedures

The procedures used are rarely reported in the speech and language evaluation report (Ortiz, et al. 1986). This information is important for the documentation of the testing context. The following reporting procedures are recommended:

1. Report any test adaptations. Any changes should be documented so that repeated administration of the test instrument can provide information concerning the client's performance. The clinician should not report the published norms.

2. Report the nature of the evaluation. The report should state whether an interpreter was used for the testing and whether the interpreter was trained to administer the test. The language of testing should also be reported, as well as the language order (e.g., English first, Spanish second).

3. Report norms when appropriate. A test can be administered in the standardized procedure, but the norms may be inappropriate for the client being tested. This should be reported. Norms that have been developed outside the United States are inappropriate for U.S.

Hispanics. A test that is translated into Spanish is not the original test; therefore, the norms should not be reported for translated instruments.

Additional Suggestions

The suggested procedures for the evaluation of an Hispanic client can produce a formidable collection of data to review to determine whether a communication disorder exists. The clinician should review the following suggestions while examining test data:

1. Identify parent or client concerns (hearing, oral, or peripheral). The clinician can be relatively sure that a communication disorder exists if the parents refer a child for assessment.
2. Obtain a complete language history of the client's experience with both languages.
3. Identify possible neurogenic etiology. The characteristics of acquired aphasia, dysarthria, apraxia, and traumatic brain injury should be considered. Do not assume that all observed language and speech differences are the result of second language influence or are characteristic of the language.
4. Collect all relevant information. Information collected from questionnaires and interviews, as well as personal observations of the child's interaction in a variety of contexts, assist in the identification of a communication impairment.
5. Observe sequencing, memory, and attention span. Clients with language impairments have difficulty in these areas in both languages. Also, the clinician should consider the familiarity of the test items to the client. If a Spanish-speaking child does not know numbers, the clinician should not use digits to test these abilities. The clinician should compare the client's performance with that of age and language-history peers.
6. Consider the possibility of language loss. Children can lose their ability to speak the first language as they are exposed to English. If school language dominance records document this phenomenon, the child's communicative abilities in both languages may appear impaired or depressed. This does not mean the child is language impaired.
7. Observe the variety of forms, use, and content in different contexts. Hispanic children with language impairments have restricted abilities in both languages, regardless of the context (Kayser 1989, 1990, 1995).
8. Observe code switching and language mixing as the client talks with other bilingual speakers. A bilingual child does not switch codes or

mix languages with a monolingual speaker of either language.

9. Observe whether the disorder exists in both languages. The communication disorder exists in both languages whether it is articulation, fluency, voice, or language. The features of the disorder differ depending on the influence of the language being tested.

10. Observe possible cultural differences that affect testing. The clinician must become culturally sensitive to the norms and behaviors of the Hispanic population served. This sensitivity comes through reading about the people and their culture and participating in the important life events of the community.

These suggestions are provided to assist clinicians in their evaluations of Hispanic clients and to increase accountability in the assessment process. The valid and appropriate evaluation of Hispanic clients involves more than the translation of tests. Clinicians who integrate these considerations into their assessment processes know that they have done their best to serve the Hispanic population.

Intervention

Miller (1984) stated that no one person can tackle the language problems that the Hispanic client may have in the first and second languages. A group of professionals working with an Hispanic client may have different and specific goals in the overall development of the client. Coordinating these services should be the role of the speech-language pathologist. The clinician should monitor the student's overall progress in both languages. Data from the contributing professionals (e.g., specialists in English as a second language, reading, bilingual education, or language arts) can be compiled by the speech-language pathologist so that all staff involved can recognize the contributions of other staff members and support the goals of others in their own interactions with the student.

Speech-language pathologists should be familiar with bilingual education, the use of native language instruction and intervention, and counseling. These three factors greatly improve treatment efficacy for children from Spanish-speaking backgrounds.

Bilingual Education and the Language of Instruction

There has been considerable debate concerning the language of instruction for minority-language children in the United States. The issues that surround the language of instruction and bilingual education have been discussed in terms of legal, political, social, economic, and cultural ramifications for three decades. The debate is focusing now on those children with language impairments who come from a non-English–speaking background. This debate has caused some confusion in the general public about the relative effectiveness of English-only instruction versus native-language instruction. This confusion may have its source in the two different bilingual education systems that are found in the United States and Canada. A description of these two systems is therefore warranted.

Many Canadian programs are additive-immersion bilingual education programs. Children who speak the majority-language (English) enter kindergarten classrooms that are taught in French, the minority language. As the children progress through the grade levels, they are increasingly exposed to English, the home language, until they are receiving half of their education in English and half in French. The goal of these programs is to maintain the home language while helping children to acquire a valued second language. There are four important sociocultural features to such additive-immersion programs: (1) They are intended for children from the majority-group language (i.e., English), (2) teachers and administrators value and support the children's home language and culture, (3) the child and parents value their home language and culture, and (4) acquisition of the second language by the participants and parents is regarded as a positive skill (McLaughlin 1985). The success of additive-immersion bilingual education programs is believed to be due in large part to these features. Programs that share such features are found in target schools in major cities in the United States and throughout Canada and are considered to be enrichment programs for majority-language children (Hakuta 1986).

In contrast, the United States has several predominant curriculum designs for bilingual education for non–English-speaking children. These include (1) the maintenance model, which is designed to develop bilingualism and biliteracy, (2) the transitional model, which is designed to use the non-English language to facilitate learning of English through curriculum content, (3) the English as a second language model, which is usually a component of the first two models, and (4) the high-intensity model, which is found in middle and high schools where students are expected to learn English rapidly (Fradd 1987). Transitional bilingual education is the model mandated by the Bilingual Education Act of 1968 and the *Lau vs. Nichols* decision (Lau v. Nichols 1974). Minority-language students are to be instructed in their home language until they are able to receive exclusive instruction in English (Hakuta 1986). These children receive instruction beginning in kindergarten in the home language. As they progress through the grades, they are increasingly exposed to the majority language (English). After these children are determined to have adequate proficiency in English, they are transferred to English-only instruction.

The Canadian programs have received positive evaluations through research that supports the effectiveness of additive immersion (Lambert and Tucker 1972; Swain and Barik 1978). In contrast, the effectiveness of transitional bilingual education in the United States has not been documented adequately (Hakuta 1986; McLaughlin 1985). Thus, there is the opinion that immersion should be used with minority language children, at least partially, because it has been documented to be effective in Canada. However, Hakuta (1986) stated that neither transitional bilingual education nor immersion would be effective with minority-language children in the United States. As long as education is a subtractive rather than an additive experience (i.e., one of assimilation at all cost and without respect for the child's home language and culture), minority language children will not succeed in either of these models. This seems especially true for children who are having difficulty acquiring their first language.

Unlike the student population in the French-immersion programs, the minority-language student in the United States typically does not have the same sociocultural, economic, political, or language status as the English-speaking student when entering bilingual education or English-only classrooms. Native-language instruction, therefore, has been the focus for minority-language students in the United States. The stated purpose of native-language instruction has been to provide comprehensible input so that the child understands the nature and demands of the learning task (Krashen 1981). If the child is instructed in the unfamiliar language, the child's level of learning of the curriculum is expected to be compromised by the child's lack of comprehension of the second language.

Language of Intervention

Despite such legal mandates as the Individual's with Disabilities Education Act, myths remain about the ability of children with language impairments to learn more than one language and about the use of the first language in helping minority-language children acquire English as a second language. The historical argument has been that the children need to learn English to be able to communicate in the language used predominantly in the school and society (Barclay 1983; Juarez 1983). Ortiz (1984) added that among education and special education personnel, there is a belief that children become confused when both English and the home language are used for instruction. There is the assumption that bilingualism is difficult and not accessible for the individual with a language and learning impairment. It is believed, therefore, that these children are better served by English-only education and language intervention.

Recent research in speech-language pathology in the United States supports the hypothesis that the development of the native language is instrumental in helping minority-language children with language impairments to develop skills in both the native and the majority language (Kiernan and Swisher 1990; Perozzi 1985; Perozzi and Chavez-Sanchez 1992). Experimental single-subject designs by Perozzi (1985) and Kiernan and Swisher (1990) support the use of the first language before instructing in the second language and suggest that a bilingual curriculum is better than teaching only in English.

Despite such research and legal mandates, the use of the native language with children from language minorities is still not practiced widely in speech-language pathology or in classrooms. The paucity of knowledgeable professionals and legislation that encourages English-only classrooms for students may be primary factors in not promoting parent programs to develop the home language of the child. Parents are important in the child's social-behavioral and language development. Parents are also very important for children who have language impairments.

Miller (1984) suggested that there is no set rule for determining which language should be used for intervention and that each client should be seen as an individual. It seems reasonable that if the client prefers the home language, treatment should be in the home language.

After children and adults become active users of two languages, the choice of a language for treatment depends on several factors. Ortiz (1984) stated that possibly 12 factors determine the choice of language for instruction. These factors include the preference of the parent and client, the age of the student, the type and severity of the communication problem, and the availability of bilingual personnel. Other factors that should be taken into consideration are length of residency in the United States, motivation for learning the new language, attitude toward mainstream English speakers, and instruction in English. Innate abilities, such as language aptitude and general intellectual abilities, should also be considered. Factors that determine the continuance of therapy include the time allocated for treatment and progress in therapy in the chosen language. After the language of intervention has been determined and implemented, the next decision to be made is the content for intervention.

Miller (1984) suggested that the core content of remediation for bilinguals does not need to differ from that used with the monolingual child. The goal is communicative competence and independence. The differences between the monolingual and bilingual should be considered in planning and executing intervention. Miller further recommended that the clinician treat only those aspects of other-language influence that impair intelligibility and not treat locally current norms or features related to the dialect or influence of the first language on English. The speech-language pathologist needs to know the community to be able to identify these community norms. Miller also suggested that language therapy in English begin with those features of the language that the child already commands and that are structurally identical or near identical in both the child's first language and English. These features include syntax, morphology, and vocabulary. Examples include family kinship terms, verbs, common nouns, and adjectives.

Counseling the Family

Speech-language pathologists must learn to accept cultural differences and recognize that the Hispanic families they work with have their own values, sets of beliefs, and concerns for the future (Heath 1986). Each family is a unique unit. Counseling begins, therefore, by obtaining information about the family history or background. This includes the educational level of the parents, acculturation or assimilation of the family, the existence of an extended family within the area, and roles and expectations for each family member. The family background information helps in understanding the world experience of the family and child, as well as equips the clinician with knowledge on how to focus counseling with the family.

Counseling should address three areas: the rights of the client, future bilingualism, and the family's contribution to facilitating communicative competency in the client. The family may not be aware that individuals with disabilities have rights, potential, and skills that can be developed (Miller 1984). The family should be informed that the client has a right to nonbiased assessment, family involvement in the process of assessment and treatment, and appropriate treatment (Ambert and Dew 1982). The family and the client must recognize that their contribution in the treatment of the communication impairment is necessary and desired by the clinician. The family's input is important so that treatment goals and objectives are appropriate and feasible in the home environment.

Counseling parents in the area of bilingualism may be difficult for many clinicians who are not familiar with the literature concerning child bilingualism. Frequently, clinicians suggest that parents talk more and only in English. These suggestions are inappropriate recommendations to Spanish-speaking families. Three concepts are important to explain to the family concerning their child's success in achieving bilingualism and success in the academic arena: the threshold and interdependence hypotheses in language development, language use within Hispanic versus mainstream homes, and open-versus-closed family interactions with the mainstream society.

Cummins (1989) proposed the threshold level and the developmental interdependence hypotheses. In the threshold level hypothesis, Cummins suggested that a minimal level of language proficiency must be reached to avoid cognitive deficits. If a child has low linguistic skills in the first language, a similarly low level of language ability will be present in the second language. Parents, therefore, should provide sufficient maintenance and support of the home language to obtain a similar level of competency in the second language. The developmental interdependence hypothesis proposes that if the outside environment provides stimulus for maintenance of the first language, intensive exposure to a second language in the school leads to rapid bilingual development with no detrimental effects on the first language. Both concepts should be explained to the parents. Parents must support the language development of their children through continued maintenance and use of the home language.

Language use within the Hispanic family environment is different from that in mainstream families. The importance of conversational and narrative skills within the family cannot be emphasized enough. These discourse genres exist within the Hispanic home, but the rules for their use are different. Discussion of these home rules with the parents and the clinician's explanations of what is expected from children in mainstream society help the parents understand that there is more to language than talking to their child. Rules on how greetings are accomplished, who can start a conversation, what topics can be discussed, what is tolerated in taboo words during conversation, and what is appropriate for differing age groups are all important areas of discussion with the family. These discussions assist the clinician in planning treatment programs that consider the differences in the sociocultural roles and rules of who can speak to whom, when, and where.

The third area of counseling that should be addressed with the parent is the notion of open-versus-closed family interactions with the mainstream society. Parents should be made aware that the child's exposure to different language usages comes from interactions with people from outside the family and the immediate community. The mainstream ways of requesting, asking questions, using politeness formulas, and asking for clarifications are all possible language usages that the Hispanic child can learn when allowed to interact with the English-speaking community. The parent must be counseled to understand that withholding this interaction produces a lack of opportunity in English-language learning for the child. Parents may listen to these suggestions from the clinician, but the true acceptance of these recommendations will be evident in the child's participation in secondary institutions and in interactions with the community.

Conclusion

There is much to learn about the Hispanic populations in the United States. They are a heterogeneous population that is changing constantly with contact with mainstream American society. The complexity of bilingualism and biculturalism makes the task of assessment and treatment of the Hispanic client difficult and challenging.

References

Acevedo, M. (1989, November). *Typical Spanish misarticulations of Mexican-American Preschoolers.* Presented at the annual meeting of the American Speech-Language-Hearing Association, St. Louis.

Ambert, A., & Dew, N. (1982). *Special education for exceptional bilingual students: A handbook for educators.* Milwaukee, WI: University of Wisconsin, Midwest National Origin Desegregation Assistance Center.

Anderson, R.T. (1995). Spanish morphological and syntactic development. In H. Kayser (Ed.), *Bilingual speech-language pathology: An Hispanic focus* (pp. 41–74). San Diego: Singular.

Baetens-Beardsmore, H. (1986). *Bilingualism: Basic principles* (2nd ed.). San Diego: College Hill.

Barclay, L.K. (1983). Using Spanish as the language of instruction with Mexican-American Head Start Children: A re-evaluation using meta-analysis. *Perceptual and Motor Skills, 56,* 359–366.

Becker, M.C. (1982). *Phonological analysis of speech samples of monolingual Mexican four-year-olds.* Thesis, San Diego State University.

Bloom, L., Hood, L., & Lightbown, P. (1974). Imitation in language development: If, when and why. *Cognitive Psychology, 6,* 380–420.

Bloomfield, L. (1935). *Language.* London: Allen & Urwin, 1935.

Child, I.L. (1943). *Italian or American? The second generation in conflict.* New Haven, CT: Yale University Press.

Corder, S.P. (1967). The significance of learner's errors. *IRAL, 5,* 161–170.

Cornejo, R.J., Weinsten, A.C., & Najar, C. (1983). *Eliciting spontaneous speech in bilingual students: Methods and techniques.* Las Cruces, NM: Educational Resources Information Center.

Cummins, J. (1989). A theoretical framework for bilingual special education. *Exceptional Children, 56,* 111–119.

Dew, N. (1987). *From assessment to instruction: What do we do with the data?* Presented at Educating Exceptional Language Minority Students, Bilingual Special Education, Austin, TX.

Diamond, F.L. (1983). *Phonological analysis of Spanish utterances of normally developing bilingual Mexican-American Children.* Thesis, San Diego State University.

Erickson, J.G., & Iglesias, A. (1986). Assessment of communication disorders in non-English proficient children. In O. Taylor (Ed.), *Nature of communication disorders in culturally and linguistically diverse populations* (p. 181). San Diego: College Hill.

Fantini, A.E. (1978). *Language acquisition of a bilingual child: A sociolinguistic perspective.* Putney, VT: Experiment Press.

Fishman, J.A. (1965). Who speaks what language to whom and when? The analysis of multilingual settings. *La Linguistique, 3,* 67–88.

Fishman, J.A. (1966). *Language loyalty in the United States.* The Hague: Mouton.

Fradd, S.H. (1987). The changing focus of bilingual education. In S.H. Fradd, & W.J. Tikunoff (Eds.), *Bilingual education and bilingual special education: A guide for administrators* (pp. 1–44). Boston: College Hill.

Garcia Coll, C.T. (1990). Developmental outcome of minority infants: A process-oriented look into our beginnings. *Child Development, 61,* 270–289.

Garcia, E.E., Maez, L.F., & Gonzalez G. (1984). *A national study of Spanish/English bilingualism in young Hispanic children of the United States.* Los Angeles: California State University, National Dissemination and Assessment Center.

Gavillan-Torres, E. (1984). Issues of assessment of limited–English-proficient students and of truly disabled in the United States. In N. Miller (Ed.), *Bilingualism and language disability* (pp. 131–153). San Diego: College Hill.

Genishi, C. (1976). *Rules for code-switching in young Spanish-English speakers: An exploratory study of language socialization.* Thesis, University of California at Berkeley.

Goldstein, B.A. (1995). Spanish phonological development. In H. Kayser (Ed.), *Bilingual speech-language pathology: An Hispanic focus* (pp. 17–40). San Diego: Singular.

Gonzalez, G. (1983). Morphology and syntax. In J. Gillette, & N.P. Anderson (Eds.), *Bilingual language learning system.* Rockville, MD: American Speech-Language-Hearing Association.

Gutierrez-Clellen, V.F. (1995). Narrative development and disorders in Spanish-speaking children: Implications for the bilingual interventionist. In H. Kayser (Ed.), *Bilingual speech-language pathology: An Hispanic focus* (pp. 97–128). San Diego: Singular.

Hakuta, K. (1986). *Mirror of language: The debate on bilingualism.* New York: Basic Books.

Harry, B. (1992). *Cultural diversity, families, and the special education system: Communication and empowerment.* New York: Teachers College Press.

Heath, S.B. (1986). Social cultural contexts of language development. In Leyba, C.F. (Ed.), *Beyond language: Social and cultural factors in schooling language minority students* (pp. 143–186). Los Angeles: Evaluation Dissemination and Assessment Center, California State University, California State Department of Education, Bilingual Education Office.

Hedrick, D., Prather, E., & Tobin, A. (1990). *Sequenced inventory of communication development.* Los Angeles: Western Psychological Services.

Hudelson, S. (1983). Beto at the sugar table: Code switching in a bilingual classroom. In T.H. Escobedo (Ed.), *Early childhood bilingual education* (pp. 64–76). New York: Teachers College Press.

Jimenez, B.C. (1987). Acquisition of Spanish consonants in children. *Language, Speech, and Hearing Service in the Schools, 18,* 357–363.

Juarez, M. (1983). Assessment and treatment of minority–language-handicapped children: The role of the monolingual speech-language pathologist. *Topics in Language Disorders, 3,* 57–65.

Kayser, H.G. (1985). *A study of speech-language pathologists and their Mexican-American language-disordered caseloads.* Ph.D. dissertation, New Mexico State University.

Kayser, H.G. (1989). Speech and language assessment of Spanish-English speaking children. *Language, Speech, and Hearing Services in the Schools, 20,* 226–244.

Kayser, H.G. (1990). Social communicative behaviors of language-disordered Mexican-American students. *Child Language Teaching Therapy, 6(3),* 255–269.

Kayser, H.G. (1995). *Bilingual speech-language pathology: An Hispanic focus.* San Diego: Singular.

Kayser, H. (in press). Outcomes measurement of culturally and linguistically diverse populations. In C. Fratalli (Ed.), *Measuring outcomes in speech-language pathology.* New York: Thieme Medical Publishers.

Kayser, H., & Restrepo, M.A. (1995). Language samples: Elicitation and analysis. In H. Kayser (Ed.), *Bilingual speech-language pathology: An Hispanic focus* (pp. 268–288). San Diego: Singular.

Kessler, C. (1984). Language acquisition in bilingual children. In N. Miller (Ed.), *Bilingualism and language disability: Assessment and remediation* (pp. 26–54). San Diego: College Hill.

Kiernan, B., & Swisher, L. (1990). The initial learning of novel English words: Two single-subject experiments with minority-language children. *Journal of Speech and Hearing Research, 33,* 707–716.

Krashen, S. (1981). *Second language acquisition and second language learning*. New York: Pergamon Press.

Lambert, W.E., & Tucker, G.R. (1972). *Bilingual education of children: The St. Lambert Experiment*. Rowley, MA: Newbury House.

Langdon, H.W. (1988, June). *Working with an interpreter/translator in the school setting. Dimensions of appropriate assessment for minority handicapped students: Recommended practices*. Presented at the State Conference for School Superintendents, Tucson, AZ.

Langdon, H.W. (1992). *Hispanic children and adults with communication disorders: Assessment and intervention*. Gaithersburg, MD: Aspen.

Laosa, L.M. (1978). Maternal teaching strategies in Chicano families of varied educational and socioeconomic levels. *Child Development, 49*, 1129–1135.

Lau vs. Nichols, 414 U.S. 563, 39 L Ed 2d 1, 94 Sup. Ct. 786. (1974).

Leopold, W.F. (1939). *Speech development of a bilingual child: A linguist's record* (4 Vols.). Evanston, IL: Northwestern University Press.

Linares, T.A. (1981). Articulation skills in Spanish-speaking children. In R.V. Padilla (Ed.), *Ethnoperspectives in bilingual education series. Vol. III. Ethnoperspectives in bilingual education research: Bilingual education technology* (pp. 363–367). Ypsilanti, MI: Michigan State University.

MacNamara, J.T. (1966). *Bilingualism and primary education: A study of Irish experience*. Edinburgh: Edinburgh University Press.

Maestas, A.G., & Erickson, J.G. (1992). Mexican immigrant mothers' beliefs about disabilities. *American Journal of Speech-Language Pathology, 1(4)*, 5–10.

Marin, B.V., Marin, G., Padilla, A.M., & de la Rocha, C. (1983). Utilization of traditional and non-traditional sources of health care among Hispanics. *Hispanic Journal of Behavioral Sciences, 5(1)*, 65–80.

Mattes, L.J., & Omark, D.R. (1984). *Speech and language assessment for the bilingual handicapped*. San Diego: College Hill.

McCloskey, N., & Schaar, J.H. (1965). Psychological dimensions of anomy. *Sociology Review, 30*, 14–40.

McClure, E. (1981). Formal and functional aspects of the code-switched discourse of bilingual children. In R. Duran (Ed.), *Latino language and communicative behavior* (pp. 69–95). Norwood, NJ: Ablex.

McLaughlin, B. (1985). *Second-language acquisition in childhood: School-age children (Vol. 2)*. Hillsdale, NJ: Erlbaum.

Meitus, I.J., & Weinberg, B. (1983). *Diagnosis in speech-language pathology*. Baltimore: University Park Press.

Miller, N. (1984). *Bilingualism and language disability: Assessment and remediation*. San Diego: College Hill.

Nelson, K. (1973). *Structure and strategy in learning to talk.* Monographs of the society for research in child development 38(1–2). Chicago: University of Chicago Press.

Omark, D.R. (1981). Pragmatics and ethnological techniques for the observational assessment of children's communicative abilities. In J.G. Erickson, & D.R. Omark (Eds.), *Communication assessing bilingual exceptional children: In-service manual.* San Diego: Los Amigos Research Associates.

Ortiz, A.A. (1984). Choosing the language of instruction for exceptional bilingual children. *Teaching Exceptional Children, Spring,* 208–212.

Ortiz, A.A., Garcia, S.B., Wheeler, D.S., & Maldonado-Colon, E. (1986). *Characteristics of limited English proficient Hispanic students served in programs for the speech and language handicapped: Implications for policy, practice, and research.* Austin, TX: The University of Texas, The Handicapped Minority Research Institute on Language Proficiency.

Owens, R. (1988). *Language development: An introduction (2nd ed.).* Columbus, OH: Merrill.

Peñalosa, F. (in press). Chicano English. In L. Cole, & V. Deal (Eds.), *Communication disorders in multicultural populations.* Rockville, MD: American Speech-Language-Hearing Association.

Perozzi, J.A., & Chavez-Sanchez, M.L. (1992). The effect of instruction in L1 on receptive acquisition of L2 for bilingual children with language delay. *Language, Speech, and Hearing Services in Schools, 23,* 348–352.

Perozzi, J.A. (1985). A pilot study of language facilitation for bilingual, language handicapped children: Theoretical and intervention implications. *Journal of Speech and Hearing Disorders, 50,* 403–406.

Peters, A. (1977). Language-learning strategies: Does the whole equal the sum of the parts? *Language, 53,* 560–573.

Quinn, R. (1995). "Early intervention? ¿Qué quiere decir éso?/"...What does that mean? In H. Kayser (Ed.), *Bilingual speech language pathology: An Hispanic focus* (pp. 75–96). San Diego: Singular.

Reyes, B. (1995). Considerations in the assessment and treatment of neurogenic communication disorders in bilingual adults. In H. Kayser (Ed.), *Bilingual speech-language pathology: An Hispanic focus* (pp. 153–182). San Diego: Singular.

Sanchez, R. (1983). *Chicano discourse.* Rowley, MA: Newbury.

Saville-Troike, M. (1978). *Guide to culture in the classroom.* Roslyn, VA: National Clearinghouse for Bilingual Education.

Slobin, D. (1983). *The acculturation and development of language in Mexican-American children [final grant report NIE-G-81-0103].* Washington, DC: National Institute of Education.

Snyder-McLean, L., & McLean, J. (1978). Verbal information-gathering strategies: The child's use of language to acquire language. *Journal of Speech and Hearing Disorders, 43,* 306–325.

Stockwell, R.P., & Bowen, J.D. (1965). *The sounds of English and Spanish.* Chicago: The University of Chicago Press.

Swain, M., & Barik, H. (1978). Bilingual education in Canada: French and English. In B. Spolsky, & R.L. Cooper (Eds.), *Case studies in bilingual education* (pp. 22–71). Rowley, MA: Newbury.

Taylor, O.L. (1986). *Nature of communication disorders in culturally and linguistically diverse populations.* San Diego: College Hill.

Taylor, O.L. (1992, April). *Research designs and methodologies that NIDCD should encourage and support for intramural and extramural research on people of Color.* Paper presented at the Working Group: Research and Research Training Needs of Minority Persons and Minority Health Issues, National Institute on Deafness and Other Communication Disorders, National Institutes of Health, Bethesda, MD.

Teller, C.A. (1988). Physical health status and health care utilization in the Texas Borderlands. In S.R. Ross (Ed.), *Views across the border* (pp. 147). Albuquerque, NM: University of New Mexico Press.

Terrero, I. (1979, November). *Spanish phonological acquisition.* Paper presented at the annual meeting of the American Speech-Language and Hearing Association, Atlanta.

U.S. Bureau of the Census. (1996). *Statistical abstract of the United States: 1996 (116th ed.).* Washington, DC: U.S. Bureau of the Census.

Valdes, G. (1986, April). *Brothers and sisters: A closer look at the development of "cooperative" social orientation in Mexican-American children.* Presented at the 37th Annual Convention of the California Association of School Psychologists, Oakland, CA.

Valdes-Fallis, G. (1978). *Code switching and the classroom teacher. Language in education: Theory and practice (Vol. 4).* Arlington, VA: Center for Applied Linguistics.

Vaughn-Cook, F.B. (1983). Improving language assessment in minority children. *ASHA, 25,* 29–34.

Wong-Fillmore, L. (1979). Individual differences in second language acquisition. In C. Fillmore, D. Kempler, & W. Wang (Eds.), *Individual differences in language ability and language behavior* (pp. 202–228). New York: Academic Press.

Zayas, L.H., & Palleja J. (1988). Puerto Rican families: Consideration for family therapy. *Family Relations, 37,* 260–264.

Zentella, A.C. (1983). Ta bien, you could answer me en cualquier idioma: Puerto Rican code-switching in bilingual classrooms. In T.H. Escobedo

(Ed.), *Early childhood bilingual education: An Hispanic perspective* (pp. 36–62). New York: Teachers College Press.

Additional Resources

American Speech-Language-Hearing Association (1985). Clinical management of communicatively handicapped minority language populations. *ASHA, 27,* 29.

Cole, L., & Snope, T. (1981). Resource guide to multicultural tests and materials. *ASHA, 23,* 639.

Deal, V.R., & Yan, M.A. (1985). Resource guide to multicultural tests and materials. *ASHA, 27,* 43.

Hamayan, E.V., & Damico, J. (1991). Limiting bias in the assessment of bilingual students. Austin, TX: PRO-ED.

Kayser, H. (1995). *Bilingual speech-language pathology: An Hispanic focus.* San Diego: Singular, 1995.

Langdon, H.W., & Cheng, L.L. (1992). *Hispanic children and adults with communication disorders: Assessment and intervention.* Gaithersburg, MD: Aspen.

Mattes, L.J., & Omark, D.R. (1991). *Speech and language assessment for the bilingual handicapped (3rd ed.).* Oceanside, CA: Academic Communication Associates.

Mattes, L.J., & Omark, D.R. (1991). *Assessment of the bilingual bicultural child.* Baltimore: University Park Press.

McLaughlin, B. (1984). Early bilingualism: Methodological and theoretical Issues. In M. Paradis (Ed.), *Early bilingualism and child development.* Amsterdam: Swets and Zeitlinger.

Roseberry-McKibbin, C.A. (1995). *Multicultural students with special language needs: Practical strategies for assessment and intervention.* Oceanside, CA: Academic Communication Associates.

Wilber, C.J., & Lister, S. *Medical Spanish: The instant survival guide (3rd ed.).* Boston: Butterworth–Heinemann.

6

Delivering Speech-Language and Hearing Services in the Arab World: Some Cultural Considerations

W. Freda Wilson

Arab people throughout the world are proud of their long and prodigious history. Over the centuries they created great empires, established powerful centers of civilization, and made tremendous contributions to the arts and sciences. Moreover, the Middle East, the cradle of Arab civilization, has become one of the world's major melting pots of humanity. At the heart of the Arab world, and at the forefront of its accomplishments, is the Arabic language. With the emergence and development of Islam, the fastest growing religion in the world, the Arabic language has increased in importance and significance. In recent times, Arabic language continues to maintain its noble status; however, complex social and cultural issues in the present-day Arab world directly impinge on the language and its users.

Today's Arab world includes such diverse countries as Egypt, Jordan, Syria, Lebanon, Iraq, Saudi Arabia, Sudan, Algeria, Morocco, and Tunisia, as well as a number of smaller Arab nations (Hsourani 1991). Within this vast land are cosmopolitan cities such as Cairo in Egypt, Jeddah in Saudi Arabia, and Beirut in Lebanon, but much of the area in the Arab world is desert, and a majority of Arabs still live in rural areas (Shipler 1987).

The Middle East is a predominately Arabic-speaking region that is populated primarily by Arabs. This notion requires clarification, however, because the term *Arab* itself is not strictly definable. In a purely semantic sense, no people can be classified as Arab because the word connotes a mixed population with widely varying ethnologic and racial origins. Some people of Negro, Berber, and Semitic origins identify themselves as Arab (Wilson 1996). Hence, *Arab* is best used within a cultural context (Lamb 1987). Arab countries are those 18 countries in which the primary language is Arabic and the primary religion is Islam. Consequently, the Middle East makes up the greatest portion of the Arab world, a world that reflects one of the most amazing achievements in history: the development and growth of Islam from an embryonic phenomenon into a vast sphere of influence and civilization.

According to Lamb (1987) and Mansfield (1992), approximately 200 million Arabs occupy the Arab world. Roughly 2 million Arabs live in the United States, and more than 5 million Arabs live in Europe and other countries in the Arab Diaspora. Since the mid-1960s, the number of Arabs living outside of the Arab world has increased significantly. The United States, Germany, Brazil, Israel, England, France, Canada, and Sweden have among the largest populations of Arabs living outside of the Arab world.

During this period, the paradox of parallel modernization and political turmoil has influenced language, learning, and speech-language and hearing services in the Middle East. The hugely increased revenue flowing into the oil-producing Arab countries has facilitated the early phases of the development of speech-language and hearing services, while the turmoil of civil and regional wars has created populations of patients of all ages who desperately need communication disorders management. Additionally, age-old traditions of consanguinity contribute to a variety of communication problems among Arab speakers.

Arab World and Arabic Speakers

Arabs and Arab Lifestyles

People who practice Arab culture, who speak Arabic natively, or who have a solid kinship to the Arabic language and Islam can be defined as Arabs. Although *Arab* originally referred to the nomadic tribes of the Arabian Peninsula in southwestern Asia, the nomadic nature of Arab people has resulted in considerable ethnic diversity. Hence, the label "Arab" does not denote a single race of people.

Most Arab households are large, because several generations live together as an extended family, with the oldest male as the head of each family. Many Arabs continue to follow traditional ways, although modernization is rapidly changing their lifestyles. Historically, Arab cities, villages, and nomadic groups have remained interdependent. People in cities produce finished goods, villagers provide agricultural produce, and nomads supply animals that transport these products among the three kinds of communities.

Due to the uniformity of these lifestyles, Arabs are especially unique in their ability to maintain their cultural identity wherever they are located.

Geographic Diversity

The land of the Arab world lies in northern Africa and southwestern Asia. It ranges from Mauritania in the west to Oman in the east. The Arab countries from Egypt and Sudan eastward comprise the region of the world known as the Middle East. The Arab world throughout the ages has been an international crossroads. As a result, it has often come under foreign rule and influence. Vast deserts and mountainous terrain cover more than half of the Arab world, resulting in most Arabs living in selected areas. Due to the shortage of water in the Arab world, most Arabs live in the Fertile Crescent valley of the Nile, Euphrates, and Tigris rivers or along the Mediterranean Sea.

The Middle East contains four main geographic regions that cut across national and political divisions. These are the northern tier, the Fertile Crescent, the largely desert south, and the western area. The northern tier, which encompasses Turkey, northern Iraq, and both the northern and western sectors of Iran, consists mainly of mountains and semiarid plateaus. Much of the northern tier depends on both irrigation and light rainfall to support agriculture. The major language groups in the northern tier include Arabic, Kurdish, Turkish, and Farsi (Isenberg 1976). The primarily desert southern lands include the United Arab Emirates, Oman, and the two Yemeni Republics (North and South). The Fertile Crescent consists of the Gulf States of Qatar, Saudi Arabia, and Jordan. The Fertile Crescent forms the southern border of the northern tier. It stretches northward through Israel and Lebanon, then arches across northern Syria to the valleys of the Euphrates and Tigris rivers in Iraq. The primary languages spoken in the Fertile Crescent and the southern sectors of the Middle East are Arabic, Hebrew, and dialects of Aramic, Berber, and Nubian origin (Isenberg 1976). Djibouti, Ethiopia, Sudan, and Egypt capsule the western areas of the Middle East. The languages of this vast area include French, Arabic, and Aramaic.

Limited Natural Resources

The total of Middle Eastern natural resources are limited. The majority of Middle Easterners are farmers or laborers, although a great deal of the land space in the Middle East is unfit for agricultural use (Hitti 1985). Because the oil wealth of the Middle East has benefited only a fraction of the Arab population, many inhabitants of the Arab world have speech, language, and hearing problems due to lack of medical, educational, and human resource services. These inhabitants are often born into communities that do not systematically provide these services. According to Isenberg (1976), the reality of limited natural resources in the vast majority of the Middle East explains why the Arab world must be considered among the underdeveloped sectors of the world. Limited resources, too few trained professionals, and lack of access negatively influence speech, language, and hearing integrity among large populations of Arab speakers.

Ethnic Diversity Among Arab Speakers

The Arab world, due to its ancient and current history, remains a diverse melting pot of humanity, largely due to Islamic pilgrimages. Because national languages and speech-language and hearing dynamics are influenced by past histories of invasions, conquests, slavery, and, most important, the onset of Islam, the inhabitants of the Arab world are characterized by a multiplicity of racial groups, all struggling to coexist in a collision of cultures. The most useful method for classifying Middle Easterners is according to the language they speak, the religions they embrace, and the traditions they honor (Mansfield 1992). This categorization allows for four major national groups: the Turks, the Iranians, the Israelis, and the Arabs. The extremely close relationships and overlapping of linguistic, cultural, racial, and sociologic factors of all these groups foster many of the chronic problems of Middle Eastern society.

Arab Speakers and Religion

Arabic or dialects of Arabic are spoken by 160 million people. The dialects are grouped into five geographic categories: (1) North African (Moroccan, Algerian, Tunisian, Libyan, and Mauritanian), (2) Egyptian/Sudanese, (3) Syrian/Levantine (Lebanese, Syrian, Jordanian, and Palestinian), (4) Arabian Peninsular (Saudi, Yemeni, Adendi, Kuwaiti, Gulf, and Omani), and (5) Iraqi. North African dialects were influenced by the Berbers and the language of the colonists from other North African countries. The Egyptian/Sudanese dialect is understood by most Arabs because it is the dialect used in Egyptian movies, television, and radio, which are seen and heard throughout the Arab world. Arabian Peninsular dialects spoken in Saudi Arabia, Yemen, Aden, Kuwait, Gulf, and Oman are considered the closes to Classical Arabic. They are the dialects closest to the language of the Koran and are considered by Arabs to be the most prestigious of the dialects. Egyptian, Syrian/Levantine, and Arabian Peninsular dialects are mutually comprehensible. North African, Iraqi, and Gulf dialects are difficult for others to understand (Wilson 1996; Almaney and Alwan 1982).

Written Arabic is different from spoken Arabic. Written Arabic, or Classical Arabic, is the language of the Koran. It is more complex, is grammatically more difficult, and has a considerably larger vocabulary than spoken Arabic (Wilson 1996). To be truly literate in Classical Arabic requires many years of study. Even after 5 or 6 years of study, the average Arab may be functionally illiterate in Classical Arabic (Wilson 1996). Because of its difficulty, good command of Classical Arabic is admired in the Arab culture. Because the dialects have no prestige, a person who does not know Classical Arabic may be thought not to know Arabic, even if he or she is able to speak the local dialect well (Ferguson 1971).

In many ways, the Arab world is a religious empire. Except for a small, aged generation of Jews and a small handful of Christians, religious minorities do not exist. Between 90% and 94% of the people are Muslims, and most speak or read Arabic, or both. However, Arabs from Pakistan, India, and Iran speak Urdu, Hindi, and Farsi, respectively.

Throughout the history of the Middle East, religion has probably been both the most important bond and source of conflict dividing the inhabitants (Davidson 1991; Hitti 1985). The majority religion of the Middle East is Islam; the largest minority religion is Christianity. Both religions have played an important role in shaping the Middle East. The Arabic language has had a tremendous influence on the shaping and development of the modern Middle East. This is largely due to the fact that the language of the Holy Koran is Arabic. Many links exist between Islam and Arabic. Arabic is the only official vessel for the transmission of Islam. Therefore, the purity and sanctity of Islam as a religion is strongly correlated with maintaining purity of linguistic integrity within the Arabic language. It is significant that Arabic is the medium of familial, societal, and national communication.

More than 95% of Arabic speakers in the Middle East are Muslim, and their standards for spoken and written Arabic are extremely high. Some are strict orthodox Muslims (Hitti 1985), whereas others are more liberal. All regard their religion in a way that is difficult for the Western mind to grasp. The Arabic language is revered by Arabs as divine, or holy, because the Prophet Mohammed revealed the Word of God in the Holy Koran in Arabic. (Clinical implications are presented in Chapter 14.)

Arabic Speakers and Culture

Arabic speakers typically use "national" versions of contemporary modern Arabic (CMA) in their everyday communication. Most Arabic speakers have both formal and informal vernaculars that reflect social class, ethnographic background, and nationality. Typically, dialectal variations among native Arabic speakers reflect socioeconomic status, educational level, and nationality. French, English, and Turkish, as well as Spanish to a lesser extent, are language groups that have infiltrated CMA.

Socially, Arabic speakers use formal versions of CMA in business, academic, and religious settings. Typically, informal or colloquial Arabic is only used in informal communicative events that occur within family communication events. Since traditional Arab culture restricts interactions between nonrelated males and females, the use of informal Arabic is generally limited to family settings or intimate communication. Traditional Arab culture requires that "good" communicators use standard contemporary modern Arabic (SCMA) (Lamb 1987). SCMA refers to the hypothetical reference point for natural primary level (spoken) and standard secondary level (written) Arabic used by literate Arabic speakers. SCMA is derived from the Arabic of the Holy Koran and is spoken by the educated elite. In addition, native Arabic speakers are required to use formal or standard Arabic with their elders, authority figures, and religious leaders.

According to cultural mores, native Arabic speakers engage in lively interactive episodes of verbal communication that strongly adhere to highly stylized linguistic forms and rituals. Arab speakers, across and within various national and language groups, integrate Islamic and Arabic influences in all aspects of their communication. Younger communicators are expected to defer to their elders but are never excluded from participating in communication events. Typically, Arabic speakers engage in intense, interactive communicative dialogues that allow several speakers to talk at one time.

Arab speakers strive to speak eloquently and to use their language creatively. A communication disorder may be perceived as having a greater social penalty for Arab speakers than it does for English speakers (Wilson 1996).

Linguistic and Cultural Issues of Arab Speakers in the Diaspora (United States, Canada, Europe, Sweden, and Other Countries)

Since the Arab world consists of a number of diverse countries, immigrants and political refugees that form the Arabic-speaking Diaspora represent a myriad of dialectal and cultural variations. Several countries in sub-Saharan Africa with large Muslim populations (e.g., Somalia, Djibouti, Mauritania) and 18 Arabic-speaking countries (i.e., Algeria, Bahrain, Egypt, Iraq, Jordan, Kuwait, Lebanon, Libya, Morocco, Oman, Qatar, Saudi Arabia, Sudan, Syria, Tunisia, United Arab Emirates, North Yemen, and South Yemen) are among the countries represented (Lamb 1987). Thus, the Arab speakers that speech-language pathologists, audiologists, and educators may encounter in schools, hospitals, and other settings are likely to be diverse in both linguistic and cultural backgrounds. Moreover, Arab speakers of Egyptian, Syrian, Palestinian,

Lebanese, and Iraqi descent are likely to have higher levels of literacy in their native national language (i.e., Arabic or Farsi), as well as more English proficiency than other Arab speakers (Lamb 1987). On the other hand, both North and South Yemen, Sudan, Saudi Arabia, Kuwait, Bahrain, and Morocco have inhabitants with lower levels of literacy in Arabic and other languages (Lamb 1987).

Wherever Arab speakers are found in the Arab Diaspora, the Arabic language is more than a medium of communication; it is an object of worship—an almost metaphysical phenomenon that bonds men and women to their God. Arabs, however, also view the mastery of other languages, such as English and French, to be important to economic prosperity. Therefore, Arabs in the Diaspora usually demand that their children be bilingual and that Arabic or their national language be the dominant language, regardless of where they live. Naturally, this position poses problems for some children who may have psycholinguistic deficits or differences that can negatively influence bilingualism. Therefore, careful, culturally and linguistically fair assessment and treatment services must be rendered based on comprehensive probes into the cultural and linguistic backgrounds of the clients. The family or appropriately informed family representatives must team with the speech-language pathologist, audiologist, or educator and work with an Arab speaker to facilitate maximum and appropriate cultural input.

Educational and Clinical Implications

Because there are only approximately 100 Arab speech-language and hearing professionals worldwide (Wilson 1993), those with communication disorders in the Arab world (i.e., the Middle East and other locations where significant numbers of Arabs live such as Europe, Canada, and the United States) face a dearth of services. Collectively, these professionals include native Arabic, Hindi, Urdu, Farsi, and French speakers. Approximately 66% of Arab speech-language pathologists and audiologists (SLP/As) reside in the Middle East, whereas the other 33% live in the Arab Diaspora (Wilson 1993). Consequently, only these 100 Arab SLP/As and other non-Arab speech-language pathologists, audiologists, and educators must work with Arab speakers who have communication and educational problems. This professional pool must meet the formidable challenge of not only providing the services but also of generating culturally and linguistically appropriate clinical and educational materials for a large number of Arab speakers who have communication disorders.

Linguistic, social, cultural, national, gender, and educational issues contribute to the constellation of variables that influence the management of the communication of native Arab speakers. These variables must be dealt with in a timely fashion to facilitate better speech-language, hearing, and educational services for Arab speakers. Therefore, considerable research, materials development, and SLP/A personnel training are needed to improve the availability and quality of speech-language and hearing services to Arabs.

Demographics and Their Implications in Speech-Language Pathologist and Audiologist Service Delivery

A significant percentage of speech-language– and hearing-impaired individuals of Arab descent live in metropolitan areas worldwide. In the United States and the Arab Diaspora, families continue to engage in connubial practices based on strict tribal or family lineage. Consequently, it is thought that intermarriage is linked to a large number of the communication disorders found in Arab communities. Economic disparity, limited access to services, lack of trained native Arab SLP/As, and limited educational support systems result in large numbers of underserved, communicatively impaired individuals in the Arab world. To increase the variety and range of SLP/A services to those in the Arab world and the Arab Diaspora, the needs of the communicatively impaired must be examined from a worldwide perspective.

Different World Views and Belief Systems Among Arab Communicators

Arabs' limited knowledge about speech, language, and hearing often interferes with effective SLP/A service delivery in the Arab world and Arab Diaspora. *World view* refers to a set of belief systems and principles by which individuals understand and make sense of the world and their place in it. If SLP/As are to effectively serve communicatively impaired Arabs, fundamental differences between the belief systems of those of Arab descent and those of non-Arab culture must be acknowledged.

Mansfield (1992) observed that the Western world is characterized by reductionism and enriched by the expansiveness of modern technology. Conversely, Arab world view focuses on knowledge of the world and application of a lifestyle that is undergirded by the doctrines and influences of Islam. That is, Arab world sensibilities are driven by Islam, the Arabic language, family lineage, and a collective family-based culture. Another salient difference in world view is reflected in Arab versus non-Arab values. For instance, those of Arab descent typically value extended family, groupism, present time, holistic thinking, and religious roots (frequently Islamic-based doctrines). Each of these values must be viewed as a part of the Arab mosaic that has meaning only as a sum total. At the core of the Arab's world view is the belief that all aspects of life are integrated or related to spirituality, even the secular aspects of everyday-life activities.

Since belief systems extend beyond systems of thinking to integrate traditional knowledge, SLP/A professionals who engage in service delivery to Arabs must incorporate culturally appropriate tribal and traditional mores into the constructs of their treatment models. For example, traditional Arab stories, proverbs, songs, and literature should be incorporated into treatment materials regardless of the language of treatment. Useful and common sources of Arab literature known to most Arabs, Muslims, or non-Muslims are stories or conversations that report the actions or sayings of the Prophet Mohammed.

The Acculturation Paradox in the Management of Arab Speakers

Historically, Arabs in the Middle East and the Arab Diaspora have been expected to maintain their Arab culture both inside and outside of the Arab Diaspora. When those of Arab descent leave their cultural conclaves, they face particularly difficult cultural conflicts. In addition, when levels of acculturation vary significantly among parents, children, communities, and SLP/A service providers, stress develops. The end product is multicultural discord and identity diffusion (Alireza 1991). The communicatively impaired patient of Arab descent without culturally appropriate services may experience coercive assimilation (Alireza 1991) or, more simply, cultural collisions. Coercive assimilation, unmanaged, leads to issues of alienation and cultural identity confusion. Naturally, cultural alienation in the SLP/A treatment process makes successful communicative management difficult. Acculturation stress and its subsequent alienation disturb cultural exchanges and the mediation of information exchange essential to good SLP/A management. *When acculturation stress issues exist in the SLP/A process, a body of information is at risk.* Acculturation-related stressors may be significant factors that interfere with successful management of the communicatively impaired Arab population.

The range of levels of cultural maintenance is extremely wide among communicatively impaired Arabs. The speech-language pathologist or audiologist who treats the communicatively impaired Arab must recognize that some choice exists in current levels of acculturation for any Arab person or family. Variation in acculturation among those of Arab descent is typically influenced by lifestyle choices; geography; marriage patterns; and native-language retention, loss, or bilingualism. Cole (1989) reported acculturation variability as a spectrum of family systems, including the traditional, neotraditional, bicultural, and acculturated. Specifically, this variability is grounded in changes in modality behaviors, which include language, tribal lineage, folk practices, and religious-based mores.

The Role of Parents in the Speech-Language Pathologist/Audiologist Management of Arab Speakers

The extended family is very important in the Arab world; often, three generations live together in one household (Sharifzadeh 1992). Because of the emphasis placed on strong Arab families in the Middle East and the Arab Diaspora, parent involvement in the SLP/A treatment process is critical. The relationships, role, and scope of Arab parents in the SLP/A treatment process must be clearly defined and continuous. Arab children are greatly cherished, and their education, growth, and personal development are of great importance to all segments of their nuclear and extended families. Typically, the parents and family members of communicatively impaired Arab patients go to great lengths to provide their family members with any necessary medical, educational, and rehabilitative services needed. Arab families may be uncomfortable using SLP/A services provided by non-Arabs, however. They may perceive social organizations as attempts to replace the traditional functions of the extended family (Wilson 1996). They may be unwilling to talk about a disorder or disability, resulting in difficulty in obtaining an accurate or complete case history (Wilson 1996; Sharifzadeh 1992). If an Arab family member has a communication disorder, the family would likely seek help; however, because the family perceives its role as that of caring for the disabled family members, it would not accept a long-term intervention program (Wilson 1996).

SLP/A management schemes that involve clients or families of Arab descent must be sensitive to gender issues of a cultural nature. Depending on fundamentalist religious influences, certain roles in the management of patients may only be assigned to men or women. The more traditional family structure is patriarchal, with the male expecting to control all interactions between family and the clinician. The father or male may make decisions regarding treatment, but the mother may be responsible for the child's development and for carrying out treatment suggestions (Wilson 1996). Although Arab families expect their children to succeed in school, boys are expected to excel, whereas girls are expected to get a modest education (Wilson 1996). Critical gender preferences must always be determined at the onset of the treatment process. Careful consideration of Arab cultural factors enhances the opportunities for successful cross-cultural communication management.

The Role of Cultural Variables in Assessment and Evaluation

Because of the complexity and range of cultural differences among Arabs, SLP/A diagnostic processes must assume that assessment of

Arabs from the Middle East and the Arab Diaspora must place culture at the forefront of evaluation. The speech-language and hearing assessment of Arab speakers requires alternative, culturally relevant models that acknowledge the differences in narrative socialization and consider cultural factors that are fundamental to Arab culture (Guittierrez-Clellen and Quinn 1993) For example, among Arab families, attachment and parent-child bonding are important. The families encourage interdependence among children and family members so that the mutual bonding necessary for adult life can occur. This may be in conflict with the goal of independence in the intervention program (Wilson 1996). Less physical contact between mother and child, later development of self-help skills, and later bedtimes to allow time to be with parents are typically in contrast with what is expected of American children (Wilson 1996). In addition, language socialization practices may differ between American and Arab children. Arab children are discouraged from talking loudly and from talking during eating (Wilson 1996). Globally, the assessment of the speech, language, and hearing of Arab speakers must acknowledge all aspects of the speakers' language or languages within naturalistic environments (Damico 1993).

Since SLP/As have pursued information and cross-cultural research, systemic concerns must be addressed in language assessment and intervention. For instance, according to Wilson (1975), Butler (1989), and Damico (1991, 1993), the speech-language pathologist who assesses the communication of the Arab speaker must address critical factors, such as normal second-language acquisition, dialectical influence, and cross-cultural interference. Thus, the successful assessment of the communication of Arab speakers poses some rather interesting challenges. The core validity of virtually all existing tools and instruments is yet to be standardized for Arab speakers. Limited contemporary Arabic, Urdu, and other language tools and instruments exist. Of the instruments in existence, however, only a few have been standardized (Crago 1990; Butler 1989). Consequently, the most useful techniques and tools available for the communicative assessment of Arab speakers are naturalistic descriptive instruments (i.e., language sampling, narrative probes, and behavioral assessments).

Culturally Appropriate Service Delivery for Individuals of Arab Descent

Any SLP/A model of service delivery for Arab speakers must integrate Arab culture as a central component of the management process. The assessment and intervention process must validate Arab culture, individual human potential, and the linguistic reference of the Arab speaker's national community or country (e.g., Arabic, Urdu, English). This SLP/A service-delivery model must be comprehensive and address the ecologies of home, school, community, and any other cultural factors that might be relevant to the patient. For example, Arabs place a greater emphasis on memorization in education than Americans. Arab children may sing songs or recite poetry or nursery rhymes in a language they do not speak or understand. Because many Arabs are accustomed to rote learning and drill, they may not be responsive to indirect or facilitated language intervention in a naturalistic environment (Wilson 1996). *The culturally appropriate service-delivery model for SLP/A management of Arab speakers must clearly validate Arab culture as a central component of the service delivery process.* Wilson (1996) and Nydell (1997) have suggested several nonverbal and verbal cultural variables that should be observed and practiced when providing clinical services to those of Arab cultures:

1. Sit with good posture to show respect. Do not lean against the wall or put your hands in your pockets. Do not show the soles of your shoes when sitting with legs crossed.
2. Arab men shake hands when greeting or parting. The handshake may appear to be prolonged according to Western practices. Some Arab men will not shake hands with a female.
3. Greetings are long and formalized, with ritualized, predetermined expressions, and have a required response. Some formalized exchanges can last 5 or 10 minutes.
4. Formal dress is expected as an indication of professional respect.
5. Use of the left hand is considered rude. When handling objects, they should be placed in the right hand, and not on a table or counter.
6. Arabs are frequently late for appointments or do not keep the appointment at all.
7. Arabs usually maintain a conversation distance of 2 feet, in contrast to the usual American distance of 5 feet. Males frequently touch each other and use many gestures during conversation. Males do not usually touch females during conversation, especially one that is not a close friend or family member.
8. During conversations, Arabs maintain steady eye contact with the listener.
9. A positive response (a "yes") to a request may be an expression of good will, not an indication that the request will be carried out. Noncommittal answers usually mean "no."
10. The Arabic language is rich with forms of assertion; exaggeration; and rhetorical devices such as metaphors, similes, and proverbs. Repeated words and overassertion are used in most routine exchanges for emphasis and to convince the listener that what is being said is actually meant. Emphasis and repetition should be used in counseling to stress meaning.

The ecosystem approach, advocated by several researchers (Wilson 1975, 1990; Damico 1993; Robinson and Cook 1990), emphasizes the importance of pushing culture to the frontline in the delivery of services to Arab speakers. An ecologic assessment system takes into account patient culture, ethnicity, socioeconomic status, attitudes, self-concept, and learning style. This is critical to SLP/A service delivery and management of Arab speakers. SLP/As who serve speakers of Arab descent must develop new skills, including the following:

1. Use of descriptive situational assessment and intervention techniques within the context of interactions between the Arab speaker's culture and the culture of the speech-language pathologist or audiologist
2. Incorporation of literature and research data characteristic of the Arab speaker's background
3. Proactive application of the Arab speaker's culture to the diagnostic and treatment process

Finally, the ecosystemic and dynamic assessment methodologies propagated by several researchers (Wilson 1975; Taylor and Payne 1983; Crago 1990; Butler 1989) offer valuable mediums in the culturally fair assessment and treatment of Arab speakers. For a variety of reasons, detailed infusion of appropriate cultural factors into the SLP/A management process is vital to the treatment of Arab speakers in both the Middle East and the Arab Diaspora.

References

Alireza, M. (1991). *At the drop of a veil*. Boston: Houghton Mifflin.

Almaney, A.J., & Alwan, A.J. (1982). *Communicating with Arabs*. Prospect Heights, IL: Waveland Press.

Butler, K.G. (1989). From the editor, language assessment and intervention with LEP children: Implications from an Asian/Pacific perspective. *Topics in Language Disorders, 9(3)*, iv–v.

Cole, L. (1989). E pluribus pluribus: Multicultural imperatives for the 1990s and beyond. *ASHA, 31(8)*, 65–70.

Crago, M.B. (1990). The development of communicative competence in Inuit children of Northern Quebec: Implications for speech-language pathology. *Journal of Childhood Communication Disorders, 13(1)*, 54–71.

Damico, J.S. (1991). Descriptive assessment of communication ability in LEP students. In E.V. Hamayan, & J.S. Damico (Eds.), *Limiting bias in the assessment of bilingual students* (pp. 157–218). Austin, TX: PRO-ED.

Damico, J.S. (1993). Clinical forum: Adolescent language. Language assessment in adolescents: Addressing critical issues. *Language, Speech and Hearing Services in Schools, 24*, 29–35.

Davidson, E. (1991). *Islam, Israel and the last days*. Eugene, OR: Harvest House.

Ferguson, C.A. (1971). *Language structure and language use.* Standford, CA: Stanford University Press.

Guittierrez-Clellen, V.F., & Quinn, R. (1993). Assessing narratives of children from diverse cultural/linguistic groups. *Language, Speech and Hearing Services in Schools, 24,* 2–9.

Hitti, P. (1985). *The Arabs: A short history.* Chicago: The Gateway Edition: Regency Gateway.

Hsourani, A. (1991). *A history of Arab peoples.* Cambridge, MA: Belkcap Press of Harvard University Press.

Isenberg, I. (1976). *The Arab world.* New York: Wilson.

Lamb, D. (1987). *The Arabs: Journeys beyond the mirage.* New York: Random.

Mansfield, P. (1992). *The Arabs.* New York: Penguin.

Nydell, M.K. (1997). *Understanding Arabs: A guide for westerners.* Yarmouth, ME: Intercultural Press.

Robinson, C.A., & Cook, V.J. (1990). Alternative assessment: Ecological and dynamic. *NASP Communique, 18(5),* 28–29.

Scharifzadeh, V. (1992). Families with Middle Eastern roots. In E.W. Lynch, & M.J. Hansen (Eds.), *Developing cross-cultural competence: A guide for working with young children and their families.* Baltimore: Brookes.

Shipler, D.K. (1987). *Arab and Jew: Wounded spirits in a promised land.* New York: Penguin.

Taylor, O.L., & Payne, K. (1983). Culturally valid testing: A proactive approach. *Topics in Language Disorders, 3(3),* 8–20.

Wilson, M.E. (1996). Arabic speakers: Language and culture, here and abroad. *Topics in Language Disorders, 16(4),* 65–80.

Wilson, W.F. (1975). *Dialect-fair evaluation of the syntax of kindergarten children.* Ph.D. thesis, University of Illinois at Urbana-Champaign.

Wilson, W.F. (1990). *Prevalence of communication disorders: A comparative survey.* Paper presented at RCLMSS Seminar. Riyadh, Saudi Arabia: King Saud University Press.

Wilson, W.F. (1993, November). *The role of speech-language pathology and audiology in the management of handicapped children in Saudi Arabia.* Presented at the First International Conference of the Saudi Benevolent Association for Handicapped Children. Saudi Annals of Medicine. Riyadh, Saudi Arabia.

Additional Resources

Nydell, M.K. (1997). *Understanding Arabs: A guide for westerners.* Yarmouth, ME: Intercultural Press.

Scharifzadeh, V. (1992). Families with Middle Eastern roots. In E.W. Lynch, & M.J. Hansen (Eds.), *Developing cross-cultural competence: A guide for working with young children and their families.* Baltimore: Brookes.

Wilson, M.E. (1996). Arabic speakers: Language and culture, here and abroad. *Topics in Language Disorders, 16(4),* 65–80.

II

Communication Disorders and Development in Multicultural Populations

7

□ □ □
□ □ □
□ □ □

Culturally Diverse Families and the Development of Language

Dolores E. Battle and Noma Anderson

The acquisition of language is a dynamic and complex cultural act. Children acquire language within the context of the family. There is a dynamic interaction among cultural beliefs; family values, expectations, and experiences; and child-rearing, which influences the language development of young children. There are, of course, biological, physical, intellectual, and socioemotional underpinnings to language acquisition. These structural and constitutional requirements for the development of interpersonal and intrapersonal communication provide the mechanisms for speech and language. The child's linguistic and cognitive development are greatly influenced by cultural forces.

The basic unit of American culture is the family. Children acquire language within the context of the family. The language systems acquired by children reflect the family's language behavior, norms, and expectations. This is true for families from all areas of the globe, all socioeconomic classes, and all cultural groups.

A family consists of dynamic relationships and intrafamily interactions, as well as dynamic relationships and interactions between the family and the family's social support network of friends, religious organizations, and those in the community. Cultural variables within and between families are the keys to understanding family relationships. Cultural variables important to understanding families involve the culture's understanding of the structure of families, the culture's view of the importance of individuals and groups in society, and the roles of those within families. It is also important to consider the family's relationship to others in the community.

The belief in the importance of the family in the development of the young child is a tenet for best practice in speech-language pathology. The Individuals with Disabilities Education Act of 1997 (IDEA) requires that speech-language pathologists serve communicatively handicapped and at-risk children in a culturally sensitive manner. It also requires that service providers move from involving parents in child-centered service to a focus on family-centered service (Crais 1991). Early intervention programs for children with special needs must be family centered and provided by culturally competent service providers.

IDEA requires that speech-language pathologists function within the philosophical framework of family-centered care. Family-centered care is a philosophy and approach to health care and early intervention that requires intervention within the context of the lifestyle and values of the family (Shelton, et al. 1989). Speech-language pathologists must work within the context of the family's values and priorities. The family facilitates language development in infants, toddlers, and preschool children. Families, rather than professionals, are the decision makers regarding the child. Part C of IDEA reinforces the importance of intervention within the context of the family by requiring that families and professionals develop an Individualized Family Service Plan (IFSP) that addresses the needs of the family in the development of the child.

The term *cultural competence* (Roberts 1990) refers to the need for professionals to honor the cultural diversity of families in the provision of services. It is the ability to honor and respect the beliefs, interpersonal styles, attitudes, and behaviors of the families receiving service. For speech-language pathologists to achieve cultural competence, they must understand the culture, values and beliefs, child-rearing practices, parent-child interactions, and communication behaviors of the families they serve. It is extremely important that speech-language pathologists recognize and appreciate the tremendous cultural and linguistic diversity among families.

Culture influences world view, development, and behavior. Although many aspects of culture are explicitly transmitted within the family and community from one generation to another, much of one's cultural view is implicit. It is also critical for the clinician to keep in mind that there is a tremendous diversity between and within cultural groups. Family units must be regarded as individual units within a cultural group, in the same way that each person in a family must be regarded as an individual. Each family must be regarded as a cultural unit with its own values, beliefs, and practices, which may be shared with the larger cultural group or may be unique to that family. The extent to which a family can be characterized by the values and practices of a culture varies with each family.

It is important for the speech-language pathologist to be knowledgeable of the influence sociocultural factors can have on the language-acquisition process. The need to have an understanding of the influence of sociocultural factors poses a tremendous challenge to the discipline of speech-language pathology because of the lack of specific information about cultural diversity in families related to language development. It is critical for speech-language pathologists to work effectively with linguistically different families and to do so with respect for and an appreciation of each family's uniqueness. For this to occur, the sociocultural variables within the family that affect the development of language must be understood.

To properly aid a family in the development of language in young children requires an understanding of the development of language and also of the role that the family plays in the development of language. While writing this chapter, it became evident that few developmental studies have been conducted that research language acquisition by infants and toddlers from linguistically diverse families, with the exception of the studies in the development of language in African American children. In a recent study, Robert, et al. (1997) used the Communication and Symbolic Behavior Scales (CSBS) to profile the communication and social and symbolic activity of African American 1 year olds. Although sex differences occurred, the results indicated that this sample's CSBS scores were similar to those in the standardization sample. Unlike many other studies involving culturally and linguistically diverse children, this study controlled for socioeconomic variables known to affect language development (e.g., family's income level, age of mother at the birth of the child, and whether the child was in a single- or two-parent family). There is a dearth of well-controlled research involving Asian and Asian-Pacific, Hispanic, and Native American families and their role in child-language development. This is surprising given the increasing number of linguistically diverse children identified as disabled or at risk and the tremendous activity in language acquisition research for white middle-class children.

Culturally Diverse Families

The Changing Face of Families

Many changes in American society have affected the traditional family. According to data from the Children's Defense Fund (Hanson, et al. 1990), although the overall percentage of children in the United States is decreasing, the proportion of children from culturally and linguistically diverse families is increasing. From 1970 to 1994, the number of white families increased by 10%. During the same period, the number of African American families increased by more than 50%. From 1980 to 1990, the number of Hispanic families increased by more than 100% (U.S. Bureau of the Census 1995). During the 1980s, immigration to the United States of families from Asia, the Pacific Rim countries, the Caribbean, and Central and South America has increased tremendously. In addition, the number of families immigrating from Eastern Europe and the African nations is anticipated to increase at least until 2010. According to the Children's Defense Fund (Hanson, et al. 1990), there will be 25% more children from diverse cultural, linguistic, and ethnic groups in the United States by the year 2000 than there were in 1985. The percentage of nonwhite children will increase from 28% in 1985 to 33% in 2000. By 2030, there will be 53% more children from diverse cultural, linguistic, and ethnic groups than there were in 1985, and the percentage of nonwhite children will increase from 28% to 41%. Conservatively, 3% of these children will be communicatively disabled, and a much larger proportion will be at risk for disabilities.

The impact of changes in the American family on the development of language has not been studied widely. Little literature is available on the language development of children in families headed by male or female single parents. Studies of parent-child interaction in relation to language development have focused primarily on the middle-class mother in white two-parent families.

Language is a reflection of culture. The formulation of indigenous cultural behavior is thought to be through interaction within the family. To understand the development of language, it is necessary, therefore, to understand the function of the family interaction. Speech-language pathologists must become sensitive to the changing nature of families in this country and the impact these changes have on the understanding of language development. The speech and language development of culturally and linguistically diverse children, including the more than 1 million foreign-born children living in the United States, cannot be understood apart from an understanding of family systems and structures, the importance of individuals and groups in families, the roles within the family structure, and the dynamics within families.

Families as Systems

A family is a dynamic system consisting of many parts intricately bound together with a common purpose, usually the care and development of young children (Donahue-Kilburg 1992). Each family functions as a system consisting of several components that are essential and related to one another (Satir 1972). There is a constant action, reaction, and interaction between the parts of the system. When any one part is changed or altered, the system reacts and is forever changed. According to Satir (1972), the family system has the purpose of protecting and socializing its members through its cultural rules and child-rearing practices. It has its way of dealing with and adjusting to changes that affect the system.

Each family unit, or system, consists of several subsystems of people who interact with one another. Such systems include the adult partners, whether married or unmarried; the parent and child; the siblings, or child and child; and the extrafamily subsystems of family and nonfamily members (Turnbull and Turnbull 1986). Other subsystems can develop, depending often on the circumstances, such as mother-child with disability and father-children without disabilities.

Although all families have common characteristics, they also have differences. The boundaries of the system may be different across cultures. They may be rigid, based on power and well-defined rules and roles within the system. On the other hand, the boundaries may be more flexible, with self-worth of the individual being more important than the rules and roles.

Each family system operates according to rules that help maintain its stability and identity. The family system is defined by the degree of cohesiveness, adaptability, and the independence of its members (Turnbull and Turnbull 1986). As described by Lund (1986), these rules define who can participate in an activity, whom the members of the family can relate to, and what functions family members share with others not in the family. In families with rigid boundaries, power, role definition, and expectations for care are defined within the family. Revealing family matters to those not in the family, as in obtaining a case history or letting nonfamily members participate in child care, is problematic for families with rigid boundaries. Clients may not respond to questions or suggestions that are seen as overstepping the boundaries established for the family.

Families with more diffuse boundaries are likely to seek assistance beyond the immediate family. These families may have no difficulty turning all responsibility for the care and development of the child or client over to a nonfamily member. They may not be willing to assume a shared responsibility for the client care.

Structure of Families

Census data show that the structure of the traditional American family has changed from 1980 to 1995. There are many childless and single-parent families. Between 1980 and 1990, the percentage of married-couple families declined from 60.2% to 55.1%. Nine out of ten single-parent families are headed by women, except in Alaska, where nearly one in three single-parent families is headed by a male (U.S. Bureau of the Census 1996).

Galvin and Brommel (1982) define the family as a network of people who live together over a long period of time bound by ties of marriage, blood, or commitment, legal or otherwise. The definition encompasses numerous configurations and interaction patterns. The U.S. Bureau of the Census (1995) defines the *family* as "a group of two or more persons related by birth, marriage, or adoption and residing in the same household." It further defines a *subfamily* as a married couple and their children, if any, or one parent with one or more never-married children younger than age 18 years. Subfamilies are further divided into related and unrelated groups. Related subfamilies are related to, but do not include, the householder. Unrelated subfamilies include those such as guests, lodgers, or resident employees and their spouses and children, none of whom is related to the householder. In 1994, there were 37 million legal family groups of all races and ethnicities living in the United States (U.S. Bureau of the Census 1995).

The concept of family in the 1990s is different from that of earlier decades and different from what is included in the legal definition. Family units can be headed by one parent or two. The single parent can be a man or a woman. The parents can be of the same or opposite sex. The family can consist of socially bonded groups of married or unmarried adults brought together for some common purpose, such as a foster care unit or a group-home living unit. A family can have biological children, step children, adopted children, or any combination of the three. It can have no children. Children can belong to one family unit or two, as is the case when the parents marry other partners and the child spends time with each of the newly formed families.

Duvall (1985) described eight stages of family structure that depend on the interaction of the presence or absence of children; the age of the oldest child; the grade of the oldest child in school; and a combination of age, occupation, and status factors of the adults. Duvall's earliest stages, involving families with either no children or families with infants, toddlers, school-age children, and youths, have been most widely studied. Most studies of family structure have focused on the family's role in child development and socialization, including the development of language. Duvall's middle stages refer to families in which the children are reaching young adulthood and leaving home to begin their own families. He does not include in his structure families with adult children living at home or returning to the family home. The former group can include children with disabilities who do not live in group homes or institutions. The latter group can include those returning home because of the stresses resulting from the birth of a child with disabilities. Duvall's latter groups involve families that have been reduced to one by the death of the spouse. He does not refer to families that include an elderly parent in the home of their adult children whose own children have left the home. The impact these alterations in the traditional structure of the family has on the development of language has not been well studied.

Each family unit and culture defines the structure of the family differently. The operational definition of what constitutes a family is different for families from different cultures.

Nuclear Family

Nuclear families, the prototypical family in Western cultures, usually include children and their parents. In the traditional nuclear white middle-class family, the mother is the primary child-care agent. She is considered the prime communicant with the child and is thus the prime agent for transmitting cultural norms and linguistic behaviors to the child. If the child has a disability, it is usually the mother who has primary responsibility for obtaining services for the child.

Extended Family

In some cultures, *family* means the extended family, which is a group of relatives living in a nearby area who have considerable contact with the nuclear family. It includes all of the person's relatives, such as grandparents, cousins, aunts, and uncles. The extended family can also be used to designate a community of children and adults living together informally or in a more organized fashion, such as in a kibbutz or religious unit. Subgroups can be formed from any group of family members, such as parents, siblings, or grandparents. Child-care functions can be shared by members of the extended family or any subgroup, such as between co-wives, older siblings, or first- or second-generation grandparents. In an extended family, the people who share the child-care functions become the prime communicants with the child. Cultural values and linguistic behaviors are thus transmitted by several people, not necessarily the mother.

The African proverb, "it takes a whole village to raise a child" is reflected in African American and American Indian family structures. African American families are most often extended families characterized by strong kinship bonds and are most often headed by a woman. African American families often extend the concept of family to include selected close friends of the family. These members of the selected family are frequently called *cousin*, *aunt*, or *uncle*, although there is no true familial relationship. The entire community may be included in the concept of family, as evidenced by the use of the terms *brother* and *sister*, *soul sister*, and *brothers and sisters in Christ*.

Most white middle-class families are nuclear families. A child is born to the nuclear family. In African American families, on the other hand, a child is born to the extended family. Older siblings, aunts, grandparents, or selected family members (usually an older female) assume care of the child and give advice to the young mother regarding child-rearing practices and how to develop language in the young child (Westby, in press). It is not uncommon for the parents or the grandparents of young African American mothers to accompany them to receive clinical services or to participate in decisions regarding the welfare of the child, especially when the child has disabilities.

African American families, as well as other extended families, consider it the family's responsibility to care for both children and the elderly with disabilities. It is not uncommon for disabled adults and the elderly to be cared for at home, rather than be placed in group-living conditions or other types of institutional care. This includes the elderly who acquire disabilities due to stroke or other diseases. The elderly are usually cared for at home, rather than being sent to day-treatment facilities, senior centers, or other centers of care for older adults (Taylor 1985).

Among American Indian and Alaskan natives, the extended family is an important component of tribal life. The concept of family is defined broadly to include extended family as well as the immediate family (Joe and Malach 1983). Other members of the family's tribe may be included as well. In many cases, extended family members, including grandparents, may hold primary responsibility for the care of young children (Joe and Malach 1983). The American Indian family structure is open and assumes village-like characteristic (Red Horse 1983). Children are reared by tribal relatives who may live in separate households. The children may move between family homes with frequency, depending on who is best equipped to rear the child at the time.

In the American Indian extended family, all family members, including the Indian child, are considered equals. There is a horizontal class of relationships. For example, within the Chippewa tribe, the children of one brother may be considered the children of another brother. Responsibility for the transmission of cultural values within the extended family varies with cultures. The Chippewa "father" is responsible for teaching the child skills to earn a living, whereas the grandfather is responsible for transmitting philosophy, religion, knowledge of how to live a good life, and the meaning of things in the way of the world. If either parent believes that some form of punishment is warranted, an uncle is often given the responsibility of carrying out the task (Basso 1972).

The extended family is also an important concept in Asian cultures, especially among the Chinese (Cheng 1991). Asian-American families extend over one to three generations closely allied. Connections are maintained between families that have immigrated to the United States and those who have remained in the home country. Families sacrifice to make frequent trips to the homeland to establish and maintain the bond between the generations. Although many Asian-American family members live in a single household, the father is the autocratic head of the family and is responsible for the management of domestic affairs within the family and the behavior of the family members. In Chinese-American families, the nuclear family frequently resides separately from but close to relatives, while maintaining a close relationship between the husband and wife and grandparents (Char 1981). Newly arrived immigrants reside with or close by family members, relying on the family to aid in assimilation and acculturation.

In Hispanic cultures, the extended family is highly valued. The family is responsible for the care of young, elderly, and disabled family members. They are not likely to seek assistance from those outside the family without the approval and consent of the family. It is common for members of the family to accompany those seeking assistance from individuals outside the family and to participate in decision making involving the welfare of the child or the disabled or elderly person. Mexican-American families are dedicated to the nuclear, as well as the extended, family (Ehling 1981). Cousins frequently relate to one another as sisters and brothers. Words used to define first cousin in Spanish are *primo hermano* (literally translated "cousin brother"). The traditional Puerto Rican family also includes the nuclear and the extended family. In the nuclear family, the father is the sole family provider and decision maker. Both the father and the maternal grandmother assist the mother in household duties, whereas the maternal grandmother continues to support her daughter throughout the daughter's child-bearing years (Lacay 1981). New immigrants make frequent trips to Puerto Rico to maintain the connection with the family. Members of the family brought to the United States live with cousins or aunts. The children are enrolled in school, and the adults seek better opportunities for work. The frequent travel to Puerto Rico often affects the development of English in young children because they change frequently from an English-speaking to a Spanish-speaking society.

The fundamental unit in native Hawaiian culture is the *ohana* (family), or relatives by blood, marriage, and adoption (Handy and Pukui 1977). Emphasis is placed on the needs of the family unit rather than on the needs of any individual family member (Mokuau and Tauili'illi 1992). Native Hawaiian families are strongly interdependent extended families, in which many individuals within the family system share child-care responsibilities. Although the parents have the primary care, other members of the family, including the grandparents and other elder members of the family, provide child care. Until recently, the first-born (*hiapo*) child of the family was "given" to the grandparents and other infants were "given" to other relatives who asked for them (Pukui, et al. 1972). The child then was reared in a home where he or she could depend on the support not only of parents but also of the grandparents and elders. Although the practice does not continue today, Hawaiian children retain a strong bond with their grandparents.

The strong kinship bond is also present in the extended family of Filipino families. The boundaries of the family are extended to include god-parents, or *compadres*. A *compadre* can be a close friend or relative of the family who assumes a parental relationship with the child. The godparent sponsors the child in religious ceremonies; shares responsibility for the child's religious training, education, and financial needs; and contributes to the education of the child. They become incorporated into the extended family system and participate in decisions and concerns related to clinical services provided to the child. It is not uncommon for a Filipino family to extend to 100 or more individuals or "relatives" (Chan 1992).

Multigenerational Families

Multigenerational families, similar to extended families, include children, parents, grandparents, and often great-grandparents. In the Middle East, extended multigenerational families are important, and it is common for as many as three generations to live in the same household (Sharifzadeh 1992). In many African American families, elderly parents, their children, and their children's families live together and share in the roles defined for the traditional family (Hofferth 1984; Taylor 1985; Mutran 1985; Johnson and Barer 1990). Mutran (1985) reported the results from a national sample that indicated that African American families are more involved in exchanges across generations than white families. Johnson and Barer (1990) reported that elderly African Americans are more active with family and friends and are more likely to receive support from relatives.

Multigenerational families are becoming more common among U.S. families; however, the arrangements are often temporary. Adult children may return home with their own children due to divorce and separation. Elderly parents or grandparents may be taken into the family home after the death of a spouse or to care for young children while the parent or parents work. The stresses of multigenerational families in a society that is accustomed to the nuclear family have not been studied for their impact on child language development.

Importance of Individuals in Family Groups

Families are dynamic systems of individuals living in groups. In most Western cultures, the individual is more important than the group. Individual achievement is praised, and individuals are considered to be responsible for their lives. The goal of the family is to socialize the child toward independence at the earliest age possible, so that the child can establish his or her identity and family in adulthood.

Almost all non-Western cultures, including Asian and Pacific islanders, Hispanics, and Native Americans, place greater value on the group than on the individual. Among these groups, historical lineages, ancestors, interdependence among family members, and the submergence of self for the good of the family are highly valued (Kim 1985). When the family views the group as more important than the individuals within the group, decisions are made according to how they will affect the group. Individuals consider their behavior, whether good or bad, as a reflection of the group. No member of the group is expected to take glory. Inappropriate behavior brings shame or discredit to the family. The family is consulted in all matters of importance, before decisions are made. In Native-American tribal families, individuals are seen as extensions of the tribe. All children belong to the tribal family and cannot be reared or adopted by nontribal members without the permission of the tribal leaders. Families travel great distances to be present at important family events and ceremonies. The need to be present for the family supersedes all other obligations.

Roles Within Families

Although the legal definition of a family is important for the purpose of the Census count, because the family is a social unit, it is more advantageous to define the family by the social interactions and relationships within the unit. The roles of members within families vary across cultures. Different roles and expectations within families can have a significant impact on the delivery of speech and language services.

In the Hispanic family, roles are defined by gender. Young men or boys are socialized to be independent at earlier ages than young girls and to bond with male subgroups within the extended family. When a Hispanic male is disabled or becomes disabled later in life, the role expectation within the family system is altered. Blame may be placed on his mother for bringing the problem to the family. The family may deny the problem. The family may choose not to seek services rather than reveal to nonfamily members that there is a problem with a male member of the family.

Machoism exists in Mexican and Puerto Rican families, with the oldest man being the head of the household. Men are expected to be dominant and to have greater authority than women. In Asian families, there is a strict adherence to role status with unquestionable obedience to the authority of the elders and men. In African American and Filipino families, the roles of men and women are more egalitarian.

The customary roles within the family are defined by those in the family unit and may be altered when the traditional father or mother is absent. Sometimes, in cases of role reversal, the father serves the functions traditionally reserved for the mother or vice versa. Roles can be shared among members of a family when traditional role functions are shared. Although some families appear to be dysfunctional when compared with a traditional family, they may function in ways that work well for that particular family unit.

Cross-Cultural Child-Rearing Practices

Not only does the concept of the family differ from culture to culture, but also cultures have child-rearing practices that differ from those of middle-class America.

Sleeping Patterns

Cross-cultural differences exist in sleeping patterns and feeding patterns. In Chinese families, for example, it is not unusual for infants to sleep in the parents' bed or in the same room as the parents. Whiting and colleagues (Whiting, et al. 1958) reported that only five of their sample of 56 world societies have sleeping arrangements similar to that of mainstream America, in which the mother and father share the same bed and the baby sleeps alone. The practice of having the infant sleep alone in a crib or cradle was found in less than 10% of the world societies (Whiting, et al. 1958). Even when the infants had cradles of their own, the cradles were generally placed near the mother's bed within easy reach. Only in Western societies, most notably in middle-class American families, did infants have bedrooms of their own. Western sleeping patterns may be a reflection of the culture's view toward the need for the child to develop independence at the earliest age. Sleeping through the night in one's own room is a way of being socialized toward independence. On the other hand, cultures in which children and adults share the family bed or the family bedroom may be a reflection of the view that the family or group is more important than the individual.

Feeding Patterns

Feeding practices also vary with cultures and may also reflect the culture's view toward independence. In many societies, the infant's most intense relationship is with the person who nurses him or her. In industrialized Western societies, scheduled interval bottle feeding is typical. Bottle feeding separates the child from the mother and is a small step toward independence. In non-Westernized and nonindustrialized countries, continuous breast-feeding on demand is the traditional pattern. Feeding may occur as many as 30–40 times a day, as a means of soothing or comforting the distressed child. The mother, in many of these cultures, does not talk to or play with the child while feeding. She may continue to talk with others who are present in the area. Rather than engage in face-to-face interaction with the child, the mother may hold the child so that he or she faces outward between feedings (Whiting and Whiting 1960).

In North America, weaning from the breast or bottle generally occurs between 6 and 15 months of age, as the child progresses toward independence and walking. Weaning in some cultures, especially in the Third World, does not occur until the child is 3–4 years old or when the next child is born. Puerto Rican children, for example, are often weaned from the bottle at about 3 years of age. It is not unusual to see a Mexican-American preschool child with a bottle or pacifier.

The introduction of solid foods to the infant also varies with cultures. In Mexican-American families, infants are fed on demand. Table foods are introduced when the baby is about 6 months old and may include bean broth, mashed beans, rice, soup, and eggs. In Vietnamese families, solid foods are introduced in a somewhat different order than in American families: fruits, vegetables, meats, and finally cereal. In American families cereal is usually offered as the first food.

Changes in child care within the family are occurring in all cultures. Mothers in Western, more industrialized societies are rediscovering the benefits of breast-feeding, with as many as 75% of American mothers breast-feeding their infants for at least a short period of time. At the same time, mothers in less-industrialized countries are adapting to the convenience of bottle feeding. The use of milk formula and supplemental solid foods could alter the nature of the mother-infant interactions in these countries, as more mothers find that they can leave the nurturing of the infant to others as they seek employment out of the home.

Toileting

In Chinese families, young children are not placed on rigid toilet-training, feeding, or bedtime schedules (Char 1981). Children eat and sleep according to their own needs. The mother learns to recognize the needs of the child and adapts her behavior to the child. She may feed the child several mouthfuls of food when she perceives the child to be hungry. In many homes, no penalties are placed on the child for lapses in toilet training until the child is 4 years old.

Other Variables

Another example of changes in child-care practice in non-Western societies is the abandonment of slings for baby strollers and carriages, high chairs, children's seats, and infant car safety seats. Infants who traditionally were held close to the mother are now separated from the mother. Infants and toddlers, traditionally allowed to freely explore open areas, are now having their activity restricted by playpens. As people from other cultures become more westernized in their child-rearing practices, the nature of the traditional mother-child relationship and thus the role of mother-child interaction in the development of language is likely to change. As the traditional role of women changes in societies in response to increased opportunities outside the home, greater economic pressures, greater educational opportunities, and the entry of women into traditionally male-dominated professions, the system of caring for and interacting with infants is changing.

Research generally indicates that the transmission of culture through maternal speech starts at very early ages and affects the development of communicative competence of young language-learning children. Mother-infant interaction is dependent on the mother's perception of the infant, which is culturally prescribed, her expectations of the child's ability to express his or her needs through verbal communication, and her perception of her role in the development of the cognitive and linguistic skills of the child.

Cross-Cultural Language Development

Child-rearing practices and mother-child interactions show significant cross-cultural differences during the toddler and preschool years. The role of mother-child interactions in child language development has been studied extensively for cross-cultural comparisons. Japanese-American child-rearing practices are discussed here as an example of the many variables that affect child development.

Perhaps because Japanese Americans have been in the United States for many generations, there is more information available on language development in Japanese-American children than other Asian and Pacific island groups. Although it is tempting to generalize the findings across all Asian groups, the vast diversity of the Asian and Pacific groups limits this discussion to the Japanese. Also, because the studies reported were of Japanese Americans, many of whom have been in the United States for several generations, these observations cannot be extended to newly arrived Japanese immigrants. The studies are presented to show that different cultures have different child-rearing practices and to alert the speech-language pathologist to the need to consider carefully the child-rearing practices of all families from the cultural point of view.

Japanese and American mothers share two major characteristics of caregiver-child interaction. First, Japan and the United States are both child-centered societies, in the sense that considerable attention is given to the child and to care giving. Second, mothers in both cultures are usually the primary caregivers and the main source of linguistic input for the children (Fisher 1970; Clancy 1986).

According to Fisher (1970), Japanese caregivers are less likely to talk to their infant children than American middle-class mothers. Japanese mothers emphasize nonverbal communication and control through physical contact, perhaps because nonverbal communication maintains privacy in households in which a large number of family members live together with limited space.

Morikawa and colleagues (1988) compared maternal speech of American and Japanese mothers to their 3-month-old children to show that the transmission of culture through maternal speech starts at the earliest stages of infant development. Extensive ethnographic data collection procedures were used, and the data were analyzed for nationality, infant gaze behavior, and utterance form and function. They found that the Japanese mother's use of multiple syntactic forms and referent categories to prohibit infant actions reflected an indirect speech style. The Japanese mothers also produced more speech directed toward establishing joint activities when the infants were gazing at them and speech aimed at suppressing negative behaviors while the infants were looking away than did the American mothers. American mothers appeared to chat more with or without the intention of affecting their children's activities or conditions; their speech patterns were less constrained by the communicative ability of the infant. They used nonlinguistic forms largely when they focused on the infant's activities, regardless of infant gaze directions, to approximate the utterances of the infant and to control infant behavior.

Cross (1977), Ferguson (1977), Sherrod and colleagues (1978), and Penman and colleagues (1983) also report that Japanese and American mothers used many questions and shortened sentences to communicate with their children and that they produced many utterances that refer to the infant or that have no apparent referent. They reported that mothers were not information-oriented in their verbal behavior toward the 3-month-old infants.

However, several fundamental differences exist between Japanese and American society that affect the caregiver-child interaction and how the mothers perceive their role in the development of the child's language skills. First, the social roles of Japanese children are more socially differentiated than the social roles of adults. Second, Japanese and American societies are distinct from one another in terms of their expectations of the communicative skills of their young children.

Japanese mothers have a different expectation of their role in the development of language by infants. There are differences in the style of maternal speech directed toward Japanese and American infants. According to Fisher (1970) and Caudill (1972), who did extensive work in this area, Japanese caregivers do not discourage speech by their children but are less likely than American mothers to talk to their very young children. From a series of systematic studies involving Japanese, American, and Japanese-American mothers and their infants, Caudill and Weinstein (1978) showed that American mothers chatted more with their babies than Japanese mothers and that American infants had a generally higher level of vocalization and responded with greater amounts of happy vocalization and gross motor activity than Japanese infants. The Japanese mothers did more vocal lulling and rocking of their babies, resulting in babies that were more passive. The Japanese babies had a greater amount of unhappy vocalizations, as their mothers took longer to respond to their signals for attention. Japanese mothers produced speech mainly to soothe their crying or unhappy infants, whereas American mothers talked to their infants when they were happy and alert. The American mothers viewed their babies as separate and autonomous individuals whose cognitive and language development was their responsibility. The Japanese mothers viewed their infants as an extension of themselves, and they therefore considered the child's physical comfort and safety to be their primary responsibility. They responded quickly to cries of physical discomfort, soothing and comforting the child.

Caudill and Weinstein (1978) used these data to support the notion that because of the difference in early care-giving practices between the two societies, when the infants are 3-4 months old, they have already acquired culturally distinctive behaviors. The Japanese infants had developed a pattern of silent togetherness with their mothers, whereas the American babies had learned to interact vocally with their mothers.

Caudill and Frost (1971) and Sengoku (1984) obtained comparable data from third-generation middle-class Japanese-American mothers living in urban areas in the United States. The data showed that, although the

Japanese-American mothers talked less to their infants than the American mothers, their behavior was closer to that of the American mothers than that of the Japanese mothers, indicating changes in child-rearing practices as the families became more acculturated into the American mainstream. This is important, in that it reminds practitioners that child-rearing practices are greatly influenced by acculturation and that one cannot and should not make assumptions about child-rearing or any practice based on ethnicity alone. The amount of acculturation and specific patterns within a family must always be considered.

Japanese mothers socialize their preschool children in the use of language during the preschool years. Social-role distinction is reflected in the more positive and tolerant attitude of the Japanese to the use of the baby talk register and the use of immature speech, which children are permitted to use well into the school years (Sengoku 1984). Japanese mothers believe that children should be treated as children and should be expected to speak like children. Adults do not encourage children to talk like adults but instead allow them to continue to use immature speech as an indication that they are continuing in the role of the child. Japanese adults often use the baby talk register themselves when talking to a child to create a feeling of intimacy with the child. The development of mature linguistic form is of a lesser concern until the child is enrolled in school.

Japanese mothers adjust themselves to the level of the child's communicative development rather than expecting the infant to maintain a high level of communication skills in an adult conversation. The mother's perception of her role in the care of the child is concerned with the child's physical safety and health rather than with the child's cognitive and language development (Slobin 1985).

Cross-Cultural Research on the Role of Families in Child Language Development

Intergenerational Issues in Cross-Cultural Research

With the increase in the number of Mexican Americans in the United States, there has been an increase in the study of speech and language development of Spanish-speaking children and the development of Spanish-English bilingualism. Little has been studied, however, about the role of the parents in the development of language in Mexican Americans. Studying child-rearing patterns of any ethnic group in the United States is difficult because of the need to control for the amount of acculturation of those in the study. Although much attention has been given to bilingual language development among first-generation and newly arrived Mexican immigrants, many Mexican Americans trace their roots to the earliest days of the country, when much of the present Southwest was under Mexican rule. Buriel (1993) compared the child-rearing practices of Mexican-American parents of first-, second-, and third-generation adolescents (i.e., those born in Mexico, those born in the United States of Mexican-born parents, and those born in the United States of United States–born parents). He showed differences across generations for child-rearing practices among the three generations of Mexican-American families. Parents of first- and second-generation adolescents reported a more responsibility-oriented child-rearing style, whereas parents of third-generation adolescents reported a more concern-oriented child-rearing style. The first-generation children grew up in home environments in which Spanish was the primary language spoken between parents and children. In second-generation children, Spanish was spoken in the home until the children entered school. The primary language for the school-aged second-generation children became English, with resulting cultural schisms between Mexican values and newly acquired English values. The third generation is distinguishable from the previous two by the absence of any direct links to Mexico by immigration. Language development, cultural values, and education occurred exclusively in English.

The extent to which a family's immigration history and socialization values are meshed in the semantics and concepts of the home country can influence child rearing. Changes in language use may also be related to changes in child-rearing styles. It is therefore always important to consider the immigration history of families in the conduct of cross-cultural research and in family assessment and intervention.

Family Relationships in Language-Development Research

Much of the study of family patterns in child rearing has focused on the mother-child dyad in white middle-class families. Most of the research that has been published regarding the relation between families and language development has been guilty of one or both of the following errors: (1) Middle-class families serve as the control subjects or the standard against which working-class families are judged and compared, and (2) socioeconomic status and ethnicity or race are intermingled—for example, working-class African American families are compared with middle-class white families. The conclusions drawn are often erroneous in that differences found are attributed to race rather than to socioeconomic status.

Limited nonbiased ethnographic research has been conducted investigating the influence of socioeconomic status on language development. In ethnographic research, the researcher observes and describes communication in naturalistic settings without holding one group as the norm or standard for comparison with another. Ethnographic examinations of the diversity across families as they interact with young children who are learning language are important in that they examine differences in communication in natural family environments. They are based on the principle that each family has its own cultural norm of behavior in child rearing, which influences the normal development of language. Although usually small in sample size, ethnographic studies present interesting differences in the language behaviors of families who differ socioculturally. They describe variations in child-adult interactions that occur within the normal language acquisition process with the variables of ethnicity and socioeconomic status being separated. In addition, they introduce the question of the influence of gender on parent-child interaction and communicative behaviors.

Research that is ethnographic in its theoretical framework and design has the potential to contribute a great deal to our knowledge of language development because the researcher observes and describes communication in naturalistic settings. It eliminates the bias of comparing groups of subjects with a control group that is considered the standard. Ethnographic research therefore reduces the tendency to compare communication behaviors within families from culturally diverse backgrounds with those from traditionally mainstream populations that serve as the norm.

The communication environment is an important variable in the development of child language. Across cultures, two primary types of interaction environments can be distinguished, namely, dyadic and multiparty. Children learning language are primarily involved in one environment or the other. In dyadic environments, such as middle-class families, children are exposed to and participate in primarily dyadic verbal interchanges. The emphasis on dyadic communicative units is reflected in the literature on language development, which analyzes communication based on dyadic units, such as mother-child, father-child, or child-child (Schieffelin and Ochs 1986). In some societies, however, such as Mexican American, Samoan, Kwara'ae, Basotho, and Kalili societies, children are immersed in multiparty exchanges. Children in these configurations understand that communication can involve three or more people (Farran 1982). Several communication partners, instead of a single partner, may respond to the child's utterances. The communication interaction of three-party or multiparty systems differs from that in dyadic interaction, yet multiparty interaction has not been the subject of much study in child language.

Farran (1982) studied the way the social interaction of children in infancy enables them to learn the form and function of language or language socialization. White and African American families of differing income levels were studied as they interacted with children learning language. Middle-class mothers were considered to be the prime communicant of the child, communicating with the child during routine nurturing and caring functions, and thus were the prime agents for transmitting cultural norms and linguistic behaviors to the child. The child in middle-class homes was often in a series of dyadic subgroups—mother-child, father-child, child-child, or caregiver-child. These dyadic relationships have been the focus of research on language development in infancy.

Farran's working-class mothers were not the sole nurturant of the young child. Socialization and child-rearing responsibilities were shared by a number of adults and older siblings. The child was often in a multiparty system, in which conversations were held among three or more people. Verbalizations during nurturing and caring functions were not addressed to the child but rather to other adults in the room.

Farran's study also showed that the type of talk addressed to young children and their expectant roles as a conversationalist differed across families. In the middle-class homes, the conversation was child-centered—that is, it focused on and adapted to the needs of the children. Mothers simplified their language during nurturing routines, talked of the here and now, and shared physical interactions. The children learned protoconversational skills during dyadic exchanges; focused attention on objects, events, and attributes; and were expected to respond to questions for information to confirm their knowledge to improve labeling ability. The children in the middle-class homes were encouraged to talk about what they had done, to explain themselves, to give directions, and to give accurate accounts of activities in which they had participated. The children were involved in preliteracy skills, such as storytelling and retelling, at an early age.

In working-class families, conversations were situation-centered—that is, they focused on the situation or social context. The children were expected to adapt to the social situation. The mothers did not use simplified syntax. They did not address the children directly or develop joint attention to objects, but rather commented on situations generally for all present. Questions were asked for information rather than to encourage problem solving or labeling.

Farran (1982) and Heath (1983) showed that there are differences across families with regard to their perceived role in emergent literacy. The middle-class homes studied had many children's storybooks. Infants were often given books as gifts, which were cared for and prized in the family. Children were frequently read to and understood at early ages the functions of print, books, and fiction storytelling. In the working-class homes, books for literature were not in evidence. Rather, telephone books, magazines, and newspapers were the sources of print in the homes. Children were rarely read to or involved in activities that involved print. Rarely were children involved in storytelling and retelling. Stories that were told were oral recounts of family history rather than fiction or fantasy. Physical development, health, and safety were the primary concerns of the family: Cognitive development and language development were viewed as being as natural as learning to walk and not subject to instruction or nurturing.

The middle-class families perceived their role to be that of the prime agent in rearing children and in developing children's language skills. The working-class families saw children's language as the child's responsibility and left the children to their own devices in developing their potential.

Social interaction between children enables them to learn the content, form, and functions of language. A number of studies have compared mother-infant interactions in poor and middle-class families. These studies have shown little difference in mother-child interaction and the amount of vocalization directed toward infants in the first year of life between these groups, which differed by education, income, or race. The data on the vocalization rate of mothers to their infants are inconclusive. Some studies show middle-class mothers vocalizing more, some show low-income mothers vocalizing more, and some studies show no difference between the two groups. The amount and type of stimulation provided by mothers in the child's first year may be a matter of personal preference (Feagans and Farran 1982).

In a longitudinal study, Farran (1982) videotaped and rated the interaction patterns of 50 low-income mothers and their 6-month-old babies. She found that the mothers' behavior at home when the infants were 6 months old was unrelated to the children's cognitive development at 18 months. However, 4-year-old children whose mothers had shown minimal maternal involvement at 18 months of age scored 10 points lower than their counterparts on an intelligence test. The patterns of play between the two groups were similar at 6 months. The patterns of play showed divergence at 20–36 months and again became similar at 60 months. The middle-class mothers played with their children more than twice as much as the working-class mothers, and each playing session lasted twice as long. The middle-class mothers played until each task was complete, whereas the working-class mothers provided structure and then pulled back and watched. Significant differences were observed in the amount of time in the interaction but not always in the nature of the interaction.

Similar interaction patterns involving poor families have been reported by Feagans and Farran (1982). From observations of mothers and their infants at 12, 18, 24, and 30 months of age, they found that middle-class mothers increased their involvement with their children when the children were between 6 and 20 months old, whereas low-income mothers decreased their involvement during the same period. These differences in involvement were reflected in differences in scores on the Reynell Developmental Language Scale at 30 months.

These findings may derive from different expectations of low-income parents of the competence of young children. When children from low-income homes are able to walk, they are viewed as competent and able to play alone. When children from middle-class families can walk and have begun to talk, their mothers view them as budding conversational partners and increasingly engage in verbal interaction routines such as peek-a-boo, naming games (What's this?), games of naming body parts (Where's your nose?), and animal games (How does a doggy go?).

Heath (1986) studied child-rearing practices in middle-class and working-class African American families and their impact on the development of conversational competence in three children—a middle-class white girl, a working-class white girl, and a working-class African American boy. Conversations that the children had with their parents when the children were 16–24 months old and again when they were 40–48 months old were analyzed. At both age levels, there was a significant difference in the amount of sustained discourse between child and adults and in the nature of narratives used by the children. At both time periods, the middle-class white girl had more extended conversations with her parents than either the working-class white girl or the working-class African American boy had with their parents. The middle-class white girl had 1,522 conversational interactions at 3 years of age, whereas each of the working-class children had only 60 such interactions. In addition, diversity regarding parent-child interaction and the nature of the role of the children in the interactions was observed. The middle-class parents frequently framed invitations to the child to perform narratives. They challenged the child's accounts and asked her for clarification and explanation when the message was unclear. During all interactions, the child was encouraged to event cast and provide accounts of activities. The working-class white girl was frequently asked to give an account of her activities but was rarely challenged or questioned by her parents. Elaboration of detail was not encouraged. Activities were rarely verbalized while they were going on. The working-class African American boy engaged in sustained narratives more frequently with peers and family members than with other adults. Most sustained talk directed at him came from peers and family members in the form of teasing and challenges.

In a similar ethnographic study of working-class African American and white families, Heath (1983) described verbal interactions between children and adults. She found that, in the community that was studied, children in working-class homes were not excluded from adult conversations; however, language input was not specifically modified for them, topics were not addressed to them, and adults did not ask the children questions to engage them in conversation. Adults instead asked questions that were requests for information (e.g., Where is your brother?).

Similar findings were found in a study of poor rural African American families in a Louisiana community. Ward (1982) described how the adults interacted differently with infants than with older children. The adults interacted verbally with their very young children who had not yet begun to talk. The parents attended to the young "lap" babies for longer periods of time than to older talking toddlers. Children were not expected to initiate conversations. When a conversation was initiated by an adult, children were expected to make a minimal response. Children were not expected to direct topic selection in conversations with adults. Rather than expand the children's utterances, the adult caregivers expanded their own utterances, which tended to be imperatives or information-seeking questions. Like the children in Heath's study, the children in Ward's study were expected to listen and to follow instructions rather than to initiate conversations, select topics, or expand their utterances. Such conversational behavior reflected the adage that children are to be seen and not heard; they are to speak only when spoken to.

A similar expectation of silence in the presence of adults has been described in other cultures (Basso 1972; Harkness and Super 1977). Silence is a sign of deference and respect, reflecting the subordinate relationship between children and adults within societies such as the Kipsigis (Blount 1977), Lou in Kenya (Scollon and Scollon 1981), and the Athabaskan Indians (Porter and Samover 1976). In these cultures, the child's silence in adult-child interactions indicates that they are learning to act as a child—that is, learning when and when not to talk to adults. The Kipsigis' mothers socialize their children to silence by infrequently using question forms that require a verbal response (Blount 1977). The Athabaskan Indians believe that parents and teachers should speak and that children should listen. Verbal expression is not considered to be necessary to language learning. Within the Lou culture in Kenya, children are permitted only to greet adults, then they must retreat in silence. Mealtimes could be a primary source of interaction with adults, but children also eat in silence (Scollon and Scollon 1981).

Several studies have investigated the role of African American families in the development of language in their young children. The studies have reinforced the idea that the distribution and use of language by African

American children has a socioeconomic orientation. Children learn language through the social systems of their cultures, including the values, expectations, roles, and rules for social interaction that are transmitted to them through the primary caretaker, usually the mother. These daily interactions influence the numbers and types of communication functions that develop. Hall and colleagues (1984) audio-recorded the speech of preschool children from middle-class and working-class homes talking with their parents in several different contexts. Although not specified, because of the disproportionate number of African American families living below the poverty level, it can be assumed that Hall, et al. included many African American families. Hart and Risley (1995) compared the amount of speech directed toward infants and toddlers in well-functioning African American professional, working-class, and welfare homes. In both studies, there were significant differences in the amount of words per hour directed toward the children as a function of socioeconomic status of the family. In addition, there was a significant difference in the amount of positive feedback and encouragement provided to the children across the three groups in Hart and Risley's study. The children from professional families received an average of 32 affirmatives and five prohibitions per hour, whereas the children from working-class families received 12 affirmatives and seven prohibitions per hour. Children from the welfare homes received only five affirmatives and as many as 11 prohibitives per hour. The children's language experiences at home were strong predictors of the children's vocabulary growth, vocabulary use, and IQ at age 3 and beyond. The most significant predictors identified by Hart and Risley were the number of different words the child hears; the number of affirmative feedback responses the child receives in relation to the number of prohibitives; the parents' use of prompts and questions rather than commands; the proportion of parent talk with nouns, modifiers, and past tenses; language functions focusing on naming, qualifying, and remembering experiences; and the amount of parent talk in response to the child's social behavior.

An analysis of the language experiences and the interaction of the children with their caretakers led both researchers to conclude that the significant features of parent-child interaction were among strong indicators of children's vocabulary growth, vocabulary use, and cognitive development at age 3 years and later.

Tolson (1995) and Hinton, et al. (1995) studied the effect of the structure of the family on the development of language in African American children. They reported that the amount of speech and conversational interactions within the families was affected by the internal structure of the family. Children from dual-parent homes used significantly more speech and mature sentence types than did children from single-parent homes or homes in which there were more adults than the two parents.

Rosier and Corsaro (1993) examined the values and concerns of working-class African American mothers regarding their children's education. They disagree with the perception that African American mothers do not motivate their children to high educational achievement. The mothers in the study encouraged independent thinking and autonomy in their children's lives. They used highly stylized and frequently eloquent bits of wisdom filled with figurative speech and rich vocabulary. As the children progressed through their preschool years, they were able to adequately use vocabulary words for social, interpersonal, and communicative purposes.

Blake (1993) conducted a 9-month longitudinal study to examine the language development of three African American children from working-class families in mother-child dyads. Analysis of the development of the mean length of utterance and 11 semantic-syntactic relations revealed that the children's productions were similar to those of middle-class white children as reported in Bloom and Lahey (1978) and Miller (1981). Thus, despite differences in the three sociocultural environments, the African American children developed the same linguistic and cognitive structures as white middle-class and white working-class children.

Blake (1994) also examined the development of language use by analyzing the occurrence of eight language functions: (1) interpersonal expressive, (2) effective, (3) objective, (4) directive, (5) self-expressive, (6) self-expressive nonsocial, (7) attentive, and (8) participative functions. For all three subjects, the interpersonal functions (i.e., interpersonal expressive and effective) were the most frequently occurring. More than half of the children's total utterances served social-emotional functions. It is notable that a significant portion of the mother's utterances also were interpersonal expressive. The mothers often restructured, repeated, and interjected utterances with content about interpersonal roles, appropriate behavior, and the children's internal states. A comparison of Blake's subjects with those of Bloom and colleagues (1975) reveals that the social-emotions topics of conversation did not appear to be a cultural emphasis among the white subjects. In contrast, the cultural emphasis among the white subjects was a factive, objective orientation. These finding are extremely significant in pointing out the differences in cultural orientation in the mother-child interaction through which children learn language.

Mount-Weitz (1996) also reported that the vocabulary development of African American preschool children could be traced to cultural differences in the use of language. She found that the vocabulary words used by the young children were for social, interpersonal, and communicative purposes.

The children experienced problems when they had to meet the monocultural demands of the traditional educational system.

It appears, then, that the nature of the verbal and social interaction between mother and child has a significant impact on the child's language development. It remains to be seen whether the differences in language development across cultures affect the course of language development in children from different cultures. There is need for further research in the patterns of language development in cultures where child-rearing patterns are significantly different from those of the cultures in which language development has been studied.

Assessment and Intervention Considerations

The assessment of the needs of a family to provide services for children and adults with disabilities has become an important function for speech-language pathologists. IDEA focuses on the role of the family in fostering the development of infants and toddlers with disabilities. The law requires an IFSP that includes a statement of the family's strengths and needs related to enhancing the development of the infant or toddler. The IFSP also must include a statement of the major goals for the infant or toddler and the family and a statement of the specific early intervention services needed to meet the unique needs of the infant or toddler and the family. Each family is unique, with individual needs, goals, and expectations. When cultural variables are added to the unique needs, the importance of understanding the family within the context of the culture becomes critical to the delivery of clinical services. As has been shown by the rigid and flexible boundaries of families, not all families are willing to be involved in the assessment and intervention of their family member's needs. The willingness to be involved varies from culture to culture. For some families contributing information, staying informed on progress, and getting the child to treatment may be the extent of possible involvement allowable for the family. Although the family may be concerned about the family member's welfare, they may expect the highly educated clinician and professionals to take control of the assessment and intervention process. They may not expect to provide input or to participate in any way. It is therefore imperative, in the assessment and treatment of clients with disabilities, for the family to be viewed as a unique system with unique subsystems of individuals acting and reacting within the boundaries of interactions allowable by the culture. The boundaries define and redefine who is involved and to what extent family members are involved in the client's care and treatment. Each family is unique and in need of a thorough understanding within the context of its culture to provide culturally appropriate clinical services.

Conclusion

The study of language development in various cultures shows that child-rearing practices and socioeconomic status affect the development of language in young children. Each family has its own culture, set of beliefs, values, and behaviors. Just as there are differences across cultures related to the development of language, there are differences across families, some of which may be related to culture. There is considerable variability within families within cultures. The speech-language pathologist must look at each family as an individual unit to determine which behavioral patterns operate within the particular family.

Although the research is not plentiful and in many cases confuses the variables that are under investigation, it seems to at least partially justify the following conclusions concerning families, culture, and the development of language. (The term *families* is used here to avoid the possibility of forming stereotypes or generalizations across a particular culture.)

1. Although in some families mothers are the prime communicant with the children, especially during nurturing and caring, in other families mothers may not be the prime communicant, particularly after the first year.

2. In some families infants are in a series of dyads (e.g., mother-child, father-child, child-child), and these dyads are the basis of much of the child's language development. In other families, however, children are often in a multiparty system where conversations are held among three or more people.

3. The type of speech and language addressed to young children and their expectant role as conversationalists differ across families. In some families, conversation is child-centered. In these families, the mother simplifies the language she uses to address the child during nurturing routines, talks of the here and now, and shares physical and verbal interactions. In other families, conversation is situation-centered. The children are expected to adapt to the situation present.

4. In some families literacy is encouraged at an early age. The family considers its role in the development of the cognitive and language skills of the children important. In other families, the focus is on activity rather than on preparation for literacy.

5. Families differ in their expectation of communicative competence. In some families, children are encouraged to talk about what they have done, to give explanations, to give oral directions, and to give accurate accounts of events in which they have participated. In other families, learning occurs by observation and participation in activities. The children are expected to observe until they are able to accomplish a task.

6. Socioeconomic status is more critical to the development of language than race or ethnicity. The factor most related to the socioeconomic status

is the education of the mother. The more educated the mother, regardless of race, the larger the vocabulary that is used, the more abstractions are used, the more declarative speech and questions are used (rather than imperatives), and, most significantly, the more time is spent interacting with the children.

7. Children from stable two-parent low-income households have language skills at school entry equal to those of middle-class children. Family income is not an isolated factor in the development of language, but rather family practices and stability have a significant influence on the language development of children.

8. The status of children in relation to adults has implications for the nature of verbal interactions between children and adults in various families. In some families, children are expected to be seen and not heard. These families see silence or minimal responses as the only appropriate behavior for someone who is deferent and respectful.

9. The types and functions of sentences spoken to children and the expected verbal responses vary across families. In families in which discourse between children and adults is encouraged, children tend to hear many questions that are designed to elicit responses from them, and they are expected to elaborate their responses. In some families, children are not viewed as conversational partners. The language directed toward them tends to be directive with minimal responses, and no initiation of conversation is expected.

10. The language, immigration, acculturation, and socialization history of the family is important in considering the interaction of the child in the family.

11. In assessment and intervention, the structure, systems, and subsystems operating in the family must be considered from the point of view of the family within the culture.

12. All family assessments must be conducted with a family-centered and culture-centered view. One critical professional challenge to speech-language pathologists is the lack of language-assessment procedures that differentiate between different cultures. Such procedures will not be available to the practicing speech-language pathologist soon, because too little developmental research is conducted that carefully controls all of the variables known to affect language development. The family's cultural values, experiences, expectations, child-rearing practices and beliefs, and the child's cognitive style and preference all greatly influence the child's language development. These variables show considerable diversity cross-culturally and must be taken into account in the spirit of the principle of nondiscriminatory assessment for all children.

References

Basso, K.I. (1972). To give up on words: Silence in Western Apache culture. In P. Gigiolo (Ed.), *Language and social context* (pp. 213–230). New York: Penguin.

Blake, I. (1993). The socioemotional orientation of mother-child communication in African-American families. *International Journal of Behavioral Development, 16,* 443–463.

Blake, I. (1994). Language development and socialization in young African-American children. In P.M. Greenfield, & R.R. Cocking (Eds.), *Cross-cultural roots of minority child development* (pp. 167–196). Hillsdale, NJ: Erlbaum.

Bloom, L. & Lahey, M. (1978). *Language development and language disorders.* New York: Wiley.

Bloom, L., Lighthood, P., & Hood, L. (1975). Structures and variations in child language. S*cientific Research in Child Development Monographs, 40,* 2.

Blount, B.G. (1977). Ethnography and caretaker-child interaction. In C. Ferguson, & C. Snow (Eds.), *Talking to children* (pp. 297–308). New York: Cambridge University Press.

Buriel, R. (1993). Child-rearing in Mexican-American families: The influence of generational and sociocultural factors. *Journal of Marriage and Family, 55,* 987–1000.

Caudill, W., & Frost, L. (1971). A comparison of maternal care and infant behavior in Japanese-American, American and Japanese Families. In E. Lebra (Ed.), *Mental health research in Asia and the Pacific (Vol. 2)* (pp. 276–291). Honolulu: East-West Center Press.

Caudill, W., & Weinstein, H. (1978). Maternal care and infant behavior in Japan and America. *Psychiatry, 32,* 12–43.

Caudill, W. (1972). Tiny drama: Vocal communication between mother and infant in Japanese and American families. In W.P. Lebra (Ed.), *Transcultural research in mental health.* Honolulu: The University Press of Hawaii.

Chan, S. (1992). Families with Filipino roots. In E.W. Lynch, & M.S. Hanson (Eds.), *Developing cross-cultural competence: A guide for working with young children and their families* (pp. 259–300). Baltimore: Brookes.

Char, E.L. (1981). The Chinese American. In A.L. Clark (Ed.), *Culture and childrearing* (pp. 47–64). Philadelphia: Davis.

Cheng, L.L. (1991). *Assessing Asian language performance: Guidelines for evaluating limited English proficient students.* Oceanside, CA: Academic Communication Associates.

Clancy, P.M. (1986). The acquisition of Japanese. In D.L. Slobin (Ed.), *The crosslinguistic study of language acquisition* (pp. 373–524). Hillsdale, NJ: Erlbaum.

Crais, E. (1991). Moving from family involvement to family centered services. *American Journal of Speech-Language Pathology, 1,* 5–8.

Cross, T.G. (1977). Mothers' speech adjustments: The contribution of selected child listener variables. In C.E. Snow, & C.A. Ferguson (Eds.), *Talking to children: Language input and acquisition* (pp. 151–180). New York: Cambridge University Press.

Donahue-Kilburg, G. (1992). *Family-centered early intervention for communication disorders.* Gaithersburg, MD: Aspen.

Duvall, E. (1985). *Family development (5th ed.).* Philadelphia: Lippincott.

Ehling, M.B. (1981). The Mexican American. In A.L. Clark (Ed.), *Culture and childrearing* (pp. 65–98). Philadelphia: Davis.

Farran, D.C. (1982). Mother-child interaction, language development and the school performance of poverty children. In L. Feagans, & D.C. Farran (Eds.), *The language of children reared in poverty: Implications for evaluation and intervention* (pp. 19–52). New York: Academic Press.

Feagans, L., & Farran, D.C. (1982). *Language of children reared in poverty: Implications for evaluation and intervention.* New York: Academic Press.

Ferguson, C.A. (1977). Baby talk as a simplified register. In C.E. Snow, & C.A. Ferguson (Eds.), *Talking to children: Language input and acquisition* (pp. 219–238). New York: Cambridge University Press.

Fisher, J.L. (1970). Linguistic socialization: Japan and the United States. In R. Hill, & R. Konig (Eds.), *Families in East and West: Socialization process and kinship ties.* The Hague: Mouton.

Galvin, M., & Brommel, B. (1982). *Family communication: Cohesion and change.* Glenview, IL: Scott Foresman & Co.

Hall, W., Nagy, W., & Linn, R. (1984). *Spoken words: Effects of situation and social groups on oral word usage and frequencies.* Hillsdale, NJ: Erlbaum.

Handy, E.S., & Pukui, M.K. (1977). *The Polynesian family system in Ka'u, Hawaii.* Tokyo: Charles & Tuttle.

Hanson, M.J., Lynch, E.W., & Wayman, K.I. (1990). Honoring the cultural diversity of families when gathering data. *Topics in Early Childhood Special Education, 10,* 112.

Harkness, S., & Super, C.M. (1977). Why African children are so hard to test. *Annals of the New York Academy of Sciences, 285,* 326–331.

Hart, B., & Risley, T. (1995). *Meaningful differences in the everyday experiences of young American children*. Baltimore: Brookes.

Heath, S.B. (1983). *Ways with words: Language, life and work in communities and classrooms*. New York: Cambridge University Press.

Heath, S. (1986). Taking a cross-cultural look at narratives. *Topics in Language Disorders, 7(1)*, 84–89.

Hinton, I.J., Wilson, M.N., & Solomon, H., et al. (1995). Effect of familial composition on parent-child interactions in African American families. In M.N. Wilson (Ed.), *African American family life: Its structural and ecological aspects* (pp. 73–84). San Francisco: Jossey-Bass.

Hofferth, S.L. (1984). Kin networks, race and family structure. *Journal of Marriage and Family, 46*, 791–806.

Joe, J.R., & Malach R.S. (1983). Families with Native American roots. In E.W. Lynch, & M.J. Hanson (Eds.), *Developing cross-cultural competence: A guide for working with young children and their families* (pp. 89–115). Baltimore: Brookes.

Johnson, C.L., & Barer, B.M. (1990). Families and networks among old inner-city blacks. *The Gerontologist, 30*, 726–734.

Kim, S.C. (1985). Family therapy for Asian Americans: A strategic-structural framework. *Psychotherapy, 22*, 342–348.

Lacay, G. (1981). The Puerto Rican in mainland America. In A.L. Clark (Ed.), *Culture and childrearing* (pp. 123–147). Philadelphia: Davis.

Lund, N. (1986). Family events and relationships: Implications for language assessment and intervention. *Seminars in Speech and Language, 7*, 415–432.

Miller, J. (1981). *Assessing language production in children*. Baltimore: University Park Press.

Mokuau, N., & Tauili'ili, P. (1992). Families with native Hawaiian roots and Pacific island roots. In E.W. Lynch, & M.J. Hanson (Eds.), *Developing cross cultural competence: A guide for working with young children and their families* (pp. 301–318). Baltimore: Brookes.

Morikawa, H., Shand, N., & Kosawa, K. (1988). Maternal speech to prelingual infants in Japan and the United States: Relationships among functions, forms and referents. *Journal of Child Language, 15*, 237–256.

Mount-Weitz, J. (1996). Vocabulary development and disorders in African American children. In A.C. Kamhi, A.G. Pollack, & J.L. Harris (Eds.), *Communication development and disorders in African American children: Research, assessment, and intervention* (pp. 189–226). Baltimore: Brookes.

Mutran, E. (1985). Intergenerational family supports among blacks and whites: Response to culture or to socioeconomic influences. *Journal of Gerontology, 40,* 382–389.

Penman, R., Cross, T., Milgrom-Friedman, J., & Meares, R. (1983). Mothers' speech to prelingual infants: A pragmatic analysis. *Journal of Child Language, 10,* 17–34.

Porter, R.E., & Samover, L.A. (1976). Communicating interculturally. In L.A. Samover, & R.E. Porter (Eds.), *Intercultural communication: A reader* (pp. 290–341). Belmont, CA: Wadsworth.

Public Law 107–115 (1997). Individuals with Disabilities Education Act. P.L. 107–115. June 1997. Washington DC: House Congressional Record.

Pukui, M.K., Haertig, E.W., Lee, C., & McDermott, J. (1972) *Nana I ke kumu (Vol. 2).* Honolulu: Hui Hanai.

Red Horse, J. (1983). Indian family values and experiences. In G.J. Powell (Ed.), *The psychological development of minority group children* (pp. 258–274). New York: Brunner/Mazel.

Roberts, R.N. (1990). *Developing culturally competent programs for families of children with special needs (2nd ed.).* Washington, DC: Georgetown University Child Development Center.

Roberts, J.E., Medley, L.P., Swartzfager, J.L., & Neebe, E.C. (1997). Assessing the communication of African American one-year-olds using the Communication and Symbolic Behavior Scales. *American Journal of Speech-Language Pathology, 6(2),* 59–65.

Rosier, K.B., & Corsaro, W.A. (1993). Competent parents, complex lives: Managing parenthood in poverty. *Journal of Contemporary Ethnography, 22,* 171–204.

Satir, V. (1972). *Peoplemaking.* Palo Alto, CA: Science and Behavioral Books.

Schieffelin, B.B., & Ochs, E. (1986). Language socialization. *Annual Review of Anthropology, 15,* 163–191.

Scollon, R., & Scollon, S.B.K. (1981). The literate two-year-old: The fictionalization of self. In R.O. Freedle (Ed.), *Narrative, literacy and face in interethnic communication (Vol. 7). Advances in Discourse Processes.* Norwood, NH: Ablex.

Sengoku, T. (1984). *Itsu Nihonjin Ni Naru Ka.* Tokyo: Shogakukan.

Sharifzadeh, V. (1992). Families with Middle Eastern roots. In E.W. Lynch, & M.J. Hanson (Eds.), *Developing cross-cultural competence: A guide for working with young children and their families* (pp. 319–351). Baltimore: Brookes.

Shelton, T.L., Jeppson, E.S., & Johnson, B.H. (1989). *Family-centered care for children with special health care needs.* Washington, DC: Association for the Care of Children's Health.

Sherrod, K.B., Crawley, S., Peterson, B., & Bennett, P. (1978). Maternal language to prelinguistic infants: Semantic aspects. *Infant Behavior and Development, 10,* 335–345.

Slobin, D. (1985). *The crosslinguistic study of language acquisition: The data (Vol. 1).* Hillsdale, NJ: Erlbaum.

Taylor, R.J. (1985). The extended family as a source of support in elderly blacks. *The Gerontologist, 25,* 488–495.

Tolson, T.F.J., Wilson, M.N., Hinton, I.D., et al. (1995). An analysis of adult-child conversation patterns in diverse African-American families. In M.N. Wilson (Ed.), *African-American family life: Its structural and ecological aspects* (pp. 59–71). San Francisco: Jossey-Bass.

Turnbull, A., & Turnbull, H. (1986). *Families, professionals, and exceptionality: A special partnership.* Columbus, OH: Merrill, 1986.

U.S. Bureau of the Census (1995). *Statistical abstract of the United States: 1995 (115th ed.).* Washington, DC: U.S. Bureau of the Census.

Ward, M.C. (1982). *Them children: A study in language learning.* New York: Irving Press.

Westby C. (in press). Cultural differences in caregiver-child interactions: Implications for assessment and intervention. In L. Cole, & V. Deal (Eds.), *Communication disorders in multicultural populations.* Rockville, MD: American Speech-Language-Hearing Association.

Whiting, J.W.M., & Whiting, B.B. (1960). Contributions of anthropology to the methods of studying child-rearing. In P. Mussen (Ed.), *Handbook of research methods in child development* (pp. 918–944). New York: Wiley.

Whiting, J.W.M., Kluckholm, E., & Anthony, A.S. (1958). The function of male initiation ceremonies on puberty. In E.E. Maccoby, & T. Newcomb (Ed.), *Readings in social psychology* (pp. 359–370). New York: Holt.

Additional Resources

Donahue-Kilburg, G. (1992). *Family centered early intervention for communication disorders.* Gaithersburg, MD: Aspen.

Lynch, E.W., & Hansen, M.J. (1992). *Developing cross-cultural competence: A guide for working with young children and their families.* Baltimore, MD: Brookes.

8

□ □ □
□ □ □
□ □ □
□ □ □

Multicultural Considerations in the Assessment and Treatment of Stuttering

Eugene B. Cooper and Crystal S. Cooper

Cultural considerations in the assessment and treatment of stuttering are not new. Primarily because distinctive features of stuttering vary significantly in relation to the individual's cognitive and affective states, stuttering is the only speech disorder that historically has been viewed, by a significant portion of those writing about it, from the perspective of individuals and their cultural milieu. From the time of Freud's (1920) report of his analysis of a stuttering client through Johnson's (1944) diagnosogenic-based interest in the presence, or lack thereof, of stuttering or a word for *stuttering* among American Indians, to the recent and continuing focus on ethnographic research (Maxwell 1990; Conrad, in press; Watson and Tepner 1996), stuttering has consistently been viewed as a culturally dependent phenomenon. Despite that focus, there are relatively little data concerning cross-cultural variations in the stutterer's affective, behavioral, and cognitive components. In addition, much of the data available are of dubious value in identifying significant cultural variations in stuttering.

Brutten and Miller (1988) and Shames (1989) suggested, as do many others, that the lack of research into cultural variations with respect to stuttering may be primarily the unfortunate result of the attempt by conscientious investigators to isolate independent variables by keeping research populations as homogeneous as possible. By doing so, investigators, for the most noble of reasons, have excluded minority group members from their research; therefore, fluency-related data on members of minority groups are scarce, and data on differences between culturally divergent populations are even more scarce. Fortunately, in recent years, the increased awareness of and sensitivity to the significance of multicultural issues has resulted in a noticeable increase in studies of stuttering in minority populations. For example, Bebout and Arthur (1992) studied the attitudes and beliefs of five cultural groups toward cleft palate, dysfluency, hearing impairment, and articulation disorders. A questionnaire was administered to 166 university students in California and Ontario from Chinese, Hispanic, Vietnamese, and Japanese backgrounds, as well as English-speaking North Americans. The authors found significant differences across the groups in their perceptions of the emotional health of people with speech disorders.

The threat of fostering the development of potentially detrimental stereotypes by focusing on the identification of differences between cultures is ever present. It is particularly so with the problem of stuttering. The fact that individuals with fluency disorders are subject to stereotyping is well documented. The attitudes of members of a variety of groups toward stuttering and stutterers have been studied extensively. Among the groups studied are parents (Crowe and Cooper 1977; Fowlie and Cooper 1978), teachers (Crowe and Walton 1981; Yeakle and Cooper 1986), students (St. Louis and Lass 1981; Turnbaugh, et al. 1981), store clerks (McDonald and Frick 1954), vocational rehabilitation counselors (Hurst and Cooper 1983a), employers (Hurst and Cooper 1983b), and residents from three small rural communities in Newfoundland (Doody, et al. 1993). The attitudes of speech-language pathologists have been the subject of several studies (Woods and Williams 1971, 1976; Yairi and Williams 1970; Cooper 1975; Turnbaugh, et al. 1979; Cooper and Cooper 1982, 1985a, 1996a; Cooper and Rustin 1985). The identification of a recurring pattern of negative stereotyping with respect to the problem of stuttering and to those identified as stutterers is one of the primary results of these studies. Vigilance is required if speech-language pathologists are to avoid creating new stereotypes as they strive to identify culture-dependent influences on the assessment and treatment of stuttering.

In addition to the lack of data pertaining to cultural variations in the nature of fluency disorders, available data on cultures other than the white English-speaking Western cultures are of dubious value for more than gross comparative purposes. This is so primarily because of the historical and continuing lack of universally accepted definitions for terms such as *fluency, dysfluency, stuttering, cluttering,* and *stammering.* Comparisons of the incidence and prevalence of stuttering reported by different investigators within the same culture, for example, are highly suspect because definitions of the *stuttering* studied are frequently either too vague or nonexistent.

The purposes of this chapter, in addition to reviewing the literature concerning the incidence and prevalence of stuttering syndromes in various cultures, are (1) to provide a definition of stuttering that focuses on the essential features of the complex disorder, thereby facilitating the identification of significant cross-cultural differences in its assessment and treatment; (2) to discuss cultural variations in attitudes toward stuttering; and (3) to describe cultural considerations in its assessment and treatment.

Stuttering Defined

Fluency disorders is popularly used as an umbrella term to refer to speech, rate, rhythm, and prosodic abnormalities of any origin. Fluency disorders are observed in the speech of individuals having experienced cerebral vascular accidents; those with Tourette's syndrome; and individuals experiencing such conditions as dysarthria, dyspraxia, cluttering, spasmodic dysphonia, palilalia, and, of course, the most commonly thought of disorder when fluency disorders are mentioned, stuttering. In recent years, more circumspection appears to be justified in using the single term *stuttering* in writing or discussing clinical assessment or intervention strategies for those who stutter. In addition to there being no universally accepted definition of stuttering, researchers are still unable to distinguish between isolated fluency failures of normally fluent speakers and the isolated dysfluencies of chronic stutterers. There is also an increasing understanding of the relationships between dysfluencies and a host of diagnosable diseases, syndromes, and disorders. For these reasons, in place of the term *stuttering*, the terms *fluency, dysfluency, fluency failures,* and *fluency disorders* are suggested as appropriate semantically unburdened and descriptive umbrella terms. Herein, *stuttering* is used as a diagnostic label referring to a clinical syndrome characterized by abnormal and persistent dysfluencies in speech accompanied by characteristic affective, behavioral, and cognitive patterns (Cooper 1990a, b, 1997). The assumption is made that stuttering syndromes result from the interactions of multiple coexisting physiologic, psychological, and environmental factors. No single causative factor leads to the development of stuttering syndrome. Three major stuttering syndromes have been identified: developmental, remediable, and perseverative (Cooper and Cooper 1991, 1995; Cooper 1993a, b, 1997).

Developmental Stuttering

Two of every five children younger than age 7 years who stutter experience the developmental stuttering syndrome (Cooper 1993a). Typically, without significant professional help but with knowledgeable and supportive parental assistance, these children achieve normal fluency control by age 7 years. Few of these children, in subsequent years, can recall their early difficulty with fluency, and virtually none of them, as adults, remember stuttering.

Remediable Stuttering

Two of every three individuals who stutter after age 7 years experience the remediable stuttering syndrome (Cooper 1993a). Typically these individuals, with professional assistance and a supportive home environment, are able to learn and successfully apply techniques that change the way they speak, feel, or think to achieve normal fluency. In adulthood, they typically can recall their struggle with stuttering but generally do not think of themselves as still stuttering.

Chronic Perseverative Stuttering

One of every five individuals who are said to stutter because of fluency problems beyond normal developmental dysfluencies experience the chronic perseverative stuttering syndrome (Cooper 1987). For these individuals, maintaining an acceptable level of fluency is a lifelong challenge. Although no known cure for chronic perseverative stuttering exists, the outlook is not bleak. With professional assistance, most, if not all, of these individuals are able to maintain an acceptable level of fluency. The abundant number of professionally and personally successful individuals who are chronically dysfluent supports an optimistic outlook for those experiencing the chronic perseverative stuttering syndrome.

The ABCs of Stuttering

Because stuttering is a multidimensional disorder consisting of characteristic *affective*, *behavioral*, and *cognitive* patterns (the ABCs of stuttering), it is immediately apparent that cultural factors play a significant, if not dominant, role in determining the course of a stuttering syndrome in an individual's life. Considerations of cultural influences on the progression of a stuttering syndrome, to be complete, include assessments of feelings and attitudes as well as dysfluencies. The study of differences in the ABCs of stuttering from one culture to another is critical to our understanding of fluency disorders.

Universality, Incidence, and Prevalence of Stuttering

The Universality of Stuttering

The universality of stuttering syndromes in ethnic and cultural groups throughout the world is beyond question. Van Riper's (1982) review and discussion of the evidence of stuttering's universality is compelling in its completeness. He traces the evidence for stuttering's universality from references to it on clay tablets in early Mesopotamia to its current existence in small and relatively isolated cultures in such disparate locales as the Arctic Circle and South Africa.

Van Riper (1982) and Bloodstein (1995) both reviewed in detail the series of events that led to the interesting, thought-provoking, and illuminating controversy regarding the presence of stuttering among various American and Canadian Indian tribes. The controversy is summarized here because it alerts speech-language pathologists in the search for understanding of multi- and intercultural issues having an impact on the assessment and treatment of fluency disorders to the danger of being hung by their frameworks. Johnson (1944), who proposed the still influential but unsubstantiated and discounted theory that a primary cause of stuttering is its diagnosis by parents overconcerned and anxious about their child's normal dysfluencies, reported that in certain American Indian tribes, which had no word for stuttering, stuttering did not exist. Substantiation of Johnson's observations about the lack of stuttering among American Indian tribes appeared to be presented in subsequent research publications. Bullen (1945) compared the prevalence of stuttering among several nonwhite populations, including the Navajos, to that of the white population in the United States through questionnaires mailed to sociologists living among the various tribes Bullen studied. She found stuttering to be almost nonexistent in the nonwhite cultures, and the onset of the rare cases that were found were related to the child entering a white school system. Snidecor (1947), Johnson's former student, after interviewing informants purportedly familiar with the Shoshone and Bannock American Indian tribes, noted that no stuttering was reported. He related the lack of stuttering, in part, to the nonexistence of a word for stuttering in the languages and to the lack of a significant relationship in the cultures between social adjustment and the ability to speak. Stewart (1959), also Johnson's former student, compared 30 American Indian families of the Ute tribe with 30 Cowichan

(Vancouver Island) Indian families and reported no stuttering among the Utes; however, Van Riper (1982) noted that Stewart's protocols indicated that two mothers had reported that their children stuttered.

The controversy as to whether American Indian tribes had words for stuttering and whether the prevalence of stuttering was markedly different for American Indians and American whites began soon after Johnson's 1944 article. Lemert (1953), a social anthropologist, reported finding numerous stutterers among the Salish, Kwakiutl, and Nootka tribes of British Columbia and Vancouver Island. He reported that some Indians stuttered but did not challenge directly the suggestion that some Indian tribes have no word for it and have no stuttering. Clifford and colleagues (1965) reported finding 32 stutterers among 1,799 children in several South Dakota Indian schools but attributed the incidence in this population to the fact that the children were raised under the influences of a white culture. According to Van Riper (1982), the controversy generated by these reports became public with the Liljeblad (1967) presentation to the Nevada State Speech Association titled *The Indians Have a Word for It.* With the publication of a report by Zimmerman and colleagues (1983) that included data gathered by Liljeblad, Frank, and Cleeland between 1937 and 1968, it became evident that, in fact, stuttering existed among the Bannock and Shoshone tribes and that there are several phrases, if not words, in the tribal languages to describe stuttering behaviors.

Zimmermann and colleagues (1983) suggested that discrepancies between initial reports and more recent studies reflected an increasing sophistication in intercultural research, with the objectivity of the researcher being a key factor. In addition, the early studies were based on second-hand reporting and not on controlled surveys. The questions posed by the surveyors and the manner in which they were asked may have caused informants to "protect" the tribes by denying problems. Zimmerman, et al. noted that the investigators' unfamiliarity with the tribes' native languages may have also interfered with the informants identifying words and phrases used by the investigators for stuttering as well as in their ability to identify individuals who stuttered.

The "Indians have no words for it" controversy can be viewed as a valuable learning experience for all who undertake cross-cultural research.

Incidence and Prevalence of Stuttering

Having determined that fluency disorders are common to all cultures, the question arises whether incidence and prevalence vary from among cultures. Apparently they do in some cases. As noted previously, however, universally accepted definitions do not exist regarding what constitutes the fluency disorders that the English terms *stuttering* and *stammering* and their equivalents in other languages have come to encompass and symbolize. In addition, with methodologies varying between investigators and any number of sources of error possible, it is difficult, if not impossible, to compare with any degree of certainty the results of incidence and prevalence studies conducted by different investigators in differing cultures. Nevertheless, assuming there have been more similarities than critical differences in the definitions and methodologies employed in the significant number of incidence and prevalence studies reported on populations throughout the world, their review provides helpful insights.

General American Populations

After extensive reviews of incidence and prevalence studies, Van Riper (1982) and Bloodstein (1995) concluded that for the general American population, the prevalence of stuttering is about 0.8%, whereas the incidence of the problem over the lifetime of that population is somewhere between 5% and 10%, depending primarily on how developmental dysfluencies are defined and whether children experiencing them are included in the stuttering count.

African American Populations

Van Riper (1982) cited three early studies suggesting the prevalence of stuttering to be higher among African Americans than among the general population and one study suggesting no difference. Van Riper noted that Waddle (1934) tested 1,582 children in segregated schools in Topeka, KS, and found a ratio of 1.7 to 1, with African Americans in the majority. Carson and Kantner (1945) reported the prevalence of stuttering among African American children in Baton Rouge, LA, schools to be 60% higher than white children. Pritchett (1966) reported a ratio of 1.3 to 1.0 black to white stuttering children in East St. Louis schools. Van Riper (1982), however, noted that Neeley (1960) carefully studied children in the New Orleans parochial elementary schools and found no significant difference in the prevalence of stuttering between African American children and white children.

Two additional studies add to the evidence that stuttering is more prevalent among African Americans than in the general population. Gillespie and Cooper (1973) studied the prevalence of speech problems in junior and senior high schools in Tuscaloosa, AL. Between March and June 1971, 5,054 junior and senior high-school students were interviewed individually regarding their speech by a graduate student in communicative disorders from the University of Alabama. The subjects included 2,380 African American students (1,351 in the junior high and 1,029 in the senior high) and 2,674 white students (1,483 in the junior high and 1,191 in the senior high). Stuttering was found to be almost four times more prevalent among the African American children (2.8%) than among the white children (0.7%).

Conrad (1980) screened 1,271 adult African American students ranging in age from 17 to 70 years in a Chicago community college. She found the prevalence of stuttering to be 2.7%, or more than three times higher than the 0.8% prevalence generally accepted for the total population. On the basis of the data currently available, it appears that the prevalence of stuttering is higher in the African American population than in the general population.

Another difference with respect to the prevalence of stuttering in the African American and in the general populations may be the male-to-female ratio of stutterers in the two populations. Goldman (1967) surveyed 694 school children in Tennessee. He found a male-to-female ratio of 2.4 to 1.0 among African American children and a 4.9 to 1.0 male-to-female ratio among white children. Conrad (1980) studied 1,271 adult African American students. She found a male-to-female ratio of 2 to 1. Both the Goldman and the Conrad data indicate that, although twice as many African American males stutter than African American females, the prevalence of stuttering in African American females is almost twice as high as the prevalence of stuttering in white females.

African Populations

Investigations concerning the prevalence of stuttering in black populations in Africa also suggest a higher prevalence of stuttering among African Americans. Bloodstein (1995) summarized Morgenstern's (1953, 1956) reports of a high prevalence of stuttering among the Ibo and Idoma tribes of West Africa. Stuttering was reported in 2.67% of 5,618 Ibo school children. Aron (1962) studied 6,581 Bantu school children in Johannesburg, South Africa, and judged the prevalence of stuttering to be 1.26%, which she found to be similar to prevalence data reported in Europe. Kirk (1977) reported a high incidence of a dysfluent speech pattern in Ghana among speakers of Ga, many of whom considered the dysfluencies as nonpathologic. Goodall and Brobby (1982), also cited in Bloodstein (1995), noted a 5.5% prevalence of stuttering in Dakar school children and a 3.5% prevalence in the Accra district of the Gold Coast.

Citing those reports along with Goodall and Brobby (1982) and personal communication with R. Armstrong (1983), Nwokah (1988) concluded that the incidence of stuttering in Nigerians and West Africans may be the highest in the world. Nwokah also cited personal communication with L. Rustin (1988), of the Bloombury, Hampstead, and Islington Health Authorities in London, in reporting that the number of Nigerian children referred for or receiving therapy in London is high compared with other ethnic groups. On the basis of these reports, it appears that the prevalence of stuttering in at least some black populations in Africa is higher than it is among general populations in the United States and Europe.

Caribbean Populations

In their report on the prevalence of stuttering among school-children in Nassau, Bahamas, Leith and Gibson (1991) cited McCartney's (1971) observation that the incidence of stuttering appears unusually high in the Bahamas. They also report the results of eight stuttering prevalence surveys conducted on schoolchildren in Nassau between 1972 and 1977, citing the Ministry of Education and Culture, Nassau, Bahamas. The prevalence of stuttering ranged in the eight surveys from a low of 1.07% to a high of 4.46%, giving support to McCartney's observation of a high stuttering prevalence among Bahamians. Ralston (1981), who used stuttering as an index of cultural stress in a study of cultural stress in the Caribbean, reported stuttering prevalence to be 4.7% in a school population of 1,999 children. Leith and Gibson (1991) employed six speech-language pathologists who had received training to determine the presence of stuttering and its severity to examine 1,217 children in the public schools in Nassau. They reported a stuttering prevalence of 3.6%. On the basis of these reports and data, it appears that the prevalence of stuttering in the Caribbean is higher than it is in the general U.S. population and similar to the prevalence figures reported for some African American populations.

Hispanic Populations

Leavitt (1974), comparing the prevalence of stuttering among Puerto Ricans in New York City and in San Juan, found the prevalence of stuttering in 10,445 New York City Puerto Ricans to be 0.84% and in 10,499 Puerto Ricans in San Juan to be 1.50%. Ardila and colleagues (1994) surveyed 1,879 Spanish-speaking university students from Bogota, Colombia, to determine the prevalence of stuttering and its relation to other disorders, including depression symptoms, central nervous system risk factors, and associated disorders (e.g., dyslexia, smoking, allergies). Stuttering was found to occur in 2% of the population.

Asian Populations

Van Riper (1982) cited Toyoda (1959) and Ozawa (1960), who reported a 0.82% stuttering prevalence in a population of 140,000 Japanese school children and a 0.90% stuttering prevalence in a population of 7,600 Japanese school children, respectively. These reports suggest that the prevalence of stuttering in Japan is similar to that observed in the United States. Of note, Lemert (1962), an anthropologist who relied on informants for his prevalence data, reported his impression that there were more stutterers among the Japanese than among Polynesians.

As of this writing, no data are available with respect to the prevalence of fluency disorders in Asian-American populations.

Summarizing Prevalence Studies

On the basis of the data available, it appears that the prevalence of fluency disorders varies among the cultures of the world, with some indications that the prevalence of fluency disorders or stuttering is higher among African American, black African, and Caribbean populations than white or Asian populations.

Speculations as to why the prevalence of fluency disorders varies from one culture to another can be found in many of the studies reported above. Leith (1986) provides a provocative discussion of the impact of "easy" cultures and "tough" cultures on the prevalence of stuttering. Citing the works of Arsenian and Arsenian (1948), Gordon (1964), and Leavitt (1974), all of whom promulgated the concept of easy and tough cultures, Leith suggested that one would expect to find more stuttering occurring in the industrialized cultures of Europe and America than in the more rural and presumably less anxious or stressful cultures of the American Indians and South Sea islanders.

As fetchingly simplistic and patently plausible as these recurrent speculations might appear, neither the prevalence data nor any significant body of data pertaining to the etiology of stuttering supports them. In addition to there being a serious question as to the usefulness of conceptualizing the world into two types of societies, the saga of the search to determine if "the American Indians had a word for it" should alert speech-language pathologists to the danger of allowing notions about stuttering to limit interpretations of clinical observations. Perhaps the most that can be concluded from a review of the studies of the incidence and prevalence of stuttering is that the frequency of fluency disorders varies from one culture to another and that the universality of stuttering indicates that stuttering is not simply the result of cultural variations.

Bilingualism and Stuttering

Most Americans speak only one language. One could guess, however, that most of those same Americans would not be surprised when reminded that most of the world's population is bilingual, if not multilingual, and that bilingualism in the United States is increasing at an accelerating rate. As Watson and Kayser (1994) observed, given such developments speech-language pathologists are increasingly called on to serve fluency-disordered bilingual and multilingual clients.

The literature is replete with definitions of bilingualism that range from complete or functional mastery of all aspects of two languages to functional mastery of at least one aspect of the second or least-mastered language (Beatens-Beardsmore 1986). Watson and Kayser (1994) state that "bilingualism is a dynamic, evolving condition that reflects varying levels of language proficiency which should not be equated with language preference." This definition is used as the basis for the discussion of bilingualism and its relationship to stuttering that follows.

As Dale (1977) observed in describing factors related to dysfluent speech in bilingual Cuban-American adolescents, dysfluencies observed solely in the second language or even in the first language may be related to the acquisition of two languages rather than stuttering. Rom and Alpern (1994) described their attempts to differentiate dysfluencies observed in language-learning disabled monolingual and bilingual high-school students. Noting the paucity of data differentiating dysfluency types observed in bilingual stutterers from those observed in monolingual stutterers, Rom and Alpern, citing Bernstein-Ratner and Benitez (1985), suggested that similar syntactic constraints determine the locus of stuttering when differences in the syntactic structures of the two languages are taken into account. Although Rom and Alpern's results do not address the issue directly, their categories of dysfluency types and their data analysis procedures are instructive for researchers wishing to identify differences between bilingual stutterers and monolingual stutterers with respect to dysfluency types. As one might predict, Rom and Alpern concluded their ambitious and enlightening report by stating that differential diagnosis of language disorders in bilingual students remains a difficult task and further research is warranted.

Karniol (1992) reported the case of a bilingual child (English and Hebrew) who began stuttering at age 25 months. The parents reportedly allowed the child to drop the nondominant language. As the child became a monolingual speaker, he ceased stuttering. Karniol described the child's linguistic behaviors up to the age of 39 months and suggested the possibility that the child's stuttering may have been a function of syntactic overload. In another single-subject study, Jankelowitz and Bortz (1996) reported observing dysfluency type, expectancy, adaptation, and consistency of dysfluencies in a bilingual stutterer. Noting the caution with which one must interpret the results of single-subject studies, they concluded that it is the clinician's responsibility to assess and treat bilingual individuals who stutter in the language in which they are proficient.

Due in large part to the basic research concerning the nature and loci of dysfluencies that began in the 1930s (see, for example, Brown 1945), it is possible to conclude that certain types of dysfluencies (e.g., voiced and unvoiced sound prolongations and part-word repetitions) are suggestive of stuttering, whereas other dysfluencies (e.g., whole-word and phrase repetitions) are suggestive of language-acquisition behaviors. Enough is known about stuttering syndromes and their development, however, to enable clinicians to differentiate stuttering from language-acquisition behavior with far more than the type of the dysfluencies observed. Although the type and frequency of speech dysfluencies are significant factors in arriving at the diagnosis of stuttering, clinical experience indicates that the universal characteristic affective and cognitive components of stuttering syndromes are frequently more useful than dysfluency types in arriving at a differential diagnosis between stuttering and dysfluencies related to second-language acquisition. Simply stated, the clients' thoughts and feelings about his or her speech are far more significant in arriving at a differential diagnosis than the types of dysfluencies in the speech.

The ABCs of Stuttering by Culture

Only a few investigators have specifically addressed cultural differences in the affective, behavioral, and cognitive components of stuttering.

Affective Differences

The feelings of those who stutter are the subject of countless studies throughout the world, and an even greater number of autobiographic, biographic, historical, analytical, anecdotal, and speculative reports that appear monthly, if not weekly, in newspapers, magazines, books, and the popular media. It is universally acknowledged that the feelings of loss of control, fear, embarrassment, and even shame are integral parts of the stuttering syndrome. The extent to which such feelings affect an individual's ability to cope with the stuttering syndrome appears to vary from culture to culture as such feelings vary from individual to individual. What does not appear to vary from culture to culture is the fact that individuals who stutter find their fluency-related feelings typically are paramount in any consideration of what constitutes a stuttering syndrome. Unfortunately, there are insufficient data regarding the effect of cultural differences on the feelings and attitudes of those who stutter to provide much insight into the dynamics of a stuttering syndrome's interactive causative factors. However, there are data sufficient to sensitize speech-language pathologists to the need for being aware of cultural factors when assessing and treating the affective and cognitive aspects of a stuttering syndrome. For example, Ralston (1981) studied stress factors in relation to fluency problems observed in Caribbean classrooms. In addition, results of DiLollo and Crowe's (1996) study of the communication attitudes of African American and white elementary-school children affect our understanding of fluency-disordered children in those groups.

Despite differences that undoubtedly have significant ramifications on the development of efficient and effective intervention strategies, there is also evidence of the universality among cultures of characteristic affective and cognitive components of the stuttering syndrome. The professional as well as the popular literature concerning stuttering abound in evidence as to the universality of certain feelings and attitudes as central components in the definition of stuttering syndromes. Cross-cultural studies of clinician attitudes toward stuttering, such as those reported by Cooper and Cooper (1982) and Cooper and Rustin (1985), indicate differences between the cultures studied. Such studies also provide compelling data as to the universality of critical affective and cognitive components of the stuttering syndrome.

Behavioral Differences

Conrad (in press) reports that Nathanson (1969) studied the types of dysfluencies exhibited by normally speaking African American and white 6- and 7-year-old children in Chicago parochial schools and found that African American children produced a greater number of part-word repetitions and prolongations than did their white counterparts. Jayaram (1983) studied 10 monolingual and 10 bilingual (English and Kannada, a language of India) stutterers reading aloud a list of 16 words (eight in each language for the bilingual stutterers). No differences in either the pattern or the distribution of stuttering on various sound groups were found in the two languages of the bilingual stutterer. Bernstein-Ratner and Benitez (1985) studied the loci of stuttering in a bilingual (English and Spanish) subject and observed a greater frequency of dysfluencies in Spanish, which the authors related to the greater frequency of occurrence of vowel-initiated words in the Spanish sample. Conrad interpreted this study, as well as that of Jayaram, as indicating that differences in the structures of language may influence both the loci and frequency of stuttering.

Leith and Mims (1975) contrasted the dysfluencies and stuttering-related behaviors of 25 African American and 25 white adolescent and young-adult stutterers. They found that although African American stutterers tended to exhibit fewer sound prolongations and repetitions than white stutterers, they exhibited more stuttering-related behaviors, such as eye blinks, head movements, facial contortions, and other behaviors that the authors attributed to attempts at avoiding, terminating, or masking stuttering.

In recent years, a few studies have been reported describing dysfluencies in specific cultural populations. Conrad (in press) cites Anderson's (1981) study of the speech of 40 nonstuttering African American children with respect to the frequency and types of dysfluencies exhibited as a function of age as being the kind of research that is needed. Conrad (1985) compared the interactions of 10 African American mother-child dyads in which the children were stutterers with 10 African American mother-child dyads in which the children were normally fluent. She found that differences existed between the interaction of African American mothers and their stuttering children and African American mothers and their nonstuttering children. Children who stuttered produced longer utterances and took longer turns. Mothers of children who stuttered produced fewer expressives than did mothers of children who did not stutter.

In discussing the kinds of normative studies needed with respect to dysfluencies in Hispanic groups, Conrad (in press) cited Tint (1984) and Wakefield (1985). Tint evaluated the rate of speech and types of dysfluencies in thirteen 4- to 5-year-old Spanish-speaking children and found that filled pauses were the most frequently observed dysfluency type with whole and part-word repetitions being second in frequency. Wakefield studied the rate of speech and dysfluencies in 30 normally speaking 18- to 40-year-old Spanish speakers of Puerto Rican descent. Their rates of speech were found to be lower than those reported for English speakers, and interjections were the most frequently observed dysfluency type, with whole-word repetitions being second in frequency. Brutten and Miller (1988) studied the dysfluencies of 20 first-grade African American boys and girls and found that they displayed interjections most frequently, with all other types of dysfluencies being equally displayed.

Robinson and Crowe (1987) studied speech dysfluencies in nonstuttering African American and white college athletes. Ninety-two male college athletes were screened in the areas of articulation, voice, fluency, and hearing. The African American subjects exhibited significantly more total dysfluencies in reading and displayed significantly more word and phrase repetitions than did the white subjects. In conversation, however, no significant differences were found between the subject groups, although the white subjects displayed significantly more hesitations. Grammatically, both subject groups were most dysfluent when using pronouns, nouns, adverbs, verbs, and adjectives, which is consistent with most, if not all, previous findings on the loci of speech dysfluencies. Robinson (1992) subsequently studied speech fluency skills in African American preschool children and found that all of the subjects experienced significantly more dysfluencies during narrative discourse than during conversation.

Although the above-noted studies that identify cultural differences in the behavioral aspects of normal fluency and stuttering are few and cannot be considered as a body of research on which to base conclusions, a few tentative observations are warranted. Sound repetitions and voiced and unvoiced sound prolongations are the universal behavioral components of the stuttering syndrome, and concomitant stuttering behaviors, such as eye blinks and extraneous facial, limb, and body movements, are universally observed. It is also apparent that the loci of dysfluencies vary between languages and cultures because of the infinite variety of articulatory, phonatory, prosodic (melody), and rhythmic (beat) features that characterize the world's spoken languages.

Cognitive Differences

It is useful to differentiate between the terms *affect* (feelings) and *cognition* (thinking) as they are used in this discussion. *Affect* refers to autonomic nervous system responses to internal (e.g., thinking) or external (e.g., observing an accident) stimuli that may or may not be congruent with the thinking of the individual. *Cognition* refers to the cerebrally based activity of thinking. The term *attitude*, for this discussion, refers to a cognitively determined, rather than affectively determined, perception.

As noted, an individual's feelings and attitudes may or may not be congruent. For example, individuals may think they should feel good about something but feel miserable. The distinction between feelings and attitudes and their congruence, or lack thereof, are useful constructs in understanding their interactions in those coping with a stuttering syndrome.

The feeling of loss of control appears to be the most significant universal affective response of individuals who have chronic perseverative stuttering syndrome (Cooper 1965, 1968, 1987, 1997; Manning and Shrum 1973; Cooper and Cooper 1976, 1985b; Perkins 1990). In fact, the presence or absence of the loss-of-control feeling during dysfluent episodes may be the single most important clue in determining whether a young child is experiencing the developmental stuttering syndrome rather than either the remediable or chronic perseverative stuttering syndromes (Cooper 1990a, b, 1993a). The concept also appears to be a helpful construct in discriminating between cluttering and stuttering. Nevertheless, the feeling of loss of control during moments of dysfluency is universally characteristic of the chronic stutterer. Unfortunately, other than observing changes in vital signs resulting from autonomic nervous system responses, the objective differentiation, identification, and measurement of feelings remain difficult.

Nevertheless, on the basis of countless identical descriptions of the dysfluent moment by chronic stutterers and Cooper and Cooper's clinical experiences, the observation of the universality of the loss-of-control feeling during episodes of dysfluency among chronic stutterers appears justified.

Clinical experience, as well as the literature concerning stuttering, suggests that feelings such as fear, shame, and embarrassment are far more difficult to define than the feeling of control or the loss thereof. Feelings such as fear and embarrassment, however, are not universally observed in chronic stutterers and do not appear to be as central to the disorder as does the feeling of loss of control. It is with respect to feelings such as shame and embarrassment that cultural differences are frequently reported (Leith and Mims 1975; Ralston 1981; Leith 1986).

Attempts to Identify Affective, Behavioral, and Cognitive Differences

In an attempt to gather examples of culture-specific affective, behavioral, and cognitive characteristics of stuttering, as well as examples of how stuttering is perceived and treated differently in specific cultures, Cooper and White (1991) interviewed 54 nationally bilingual-certified speech-language pathologists and audiologists. Each participant in the study was asked to identify the nongeneral American culture with which they were familiar. Eleven cultures were identified: Eastern European, Asian, Eastern Indian, Hispanic American, French, Greek, Filipino, German, Swedish, Italian, and Japanese. Twenty-eight percent of the respondents perceived differences in the incidence and prevalence of stuttering between the general American culture and the second culture with which they were familiar. Thirty-three percent perceived no difference. Only 4% of the respondents reported that treatment programs for stutterers were not available in the non-American culture with which they were familiar. Only 13% of the respondents believed that the American stuttering therapy goals and techniques with which they were familiar were inappropriate in the second culture. Although a few specific examples of potential areas of conflict with respect to stuttering therapy goals were reported, no respondent suggested that stuttering in the non-American culture with which they were familiar was significantly different, or that the American treatment goals and techniques with which they were familiar would present major difficulties for clinicians. As would be expected, several respondents expressed the hope that clinicians, not knowledgeable of cultures other than their own, would be sensitive and responsive to general variables such as family member roles, gender roles, caregiver roles, belief systems, and customs. Cooper and White concluded that the data received from

54 bilingual and nationally certified speech-language pathologists supported previous observations of the universality of the nature of stuttering as well as of the universality in the appropriateness of the typical goals and techniques used in American stuttering treatment programs.

Following is a list of specific culture-dependent factors that have been suggested by various authors as being particularly relevant to the assessment and treatment of fluency disorders. The list is presented primarily to illustrate the kinds of fluency disorder–related factors to which speech-language pathologists should be sensitive when treating individuals from a different culture. The validity of these observations is subject to question. Generalizations concerning the feelings, attitudes, and behaviors of members of a culture are seldom, if ever, helpful to speech-language pathologists. Such lists are helpful only to the extent that they sensitize speech-language pathologists to the infinite heterogeneity of the human condition. To the extent that they establish or reinforce stereotypes, they are detrimental. The list is intended to be instructive, not destructive, and intended to be representative, not exhaustive:

- Therapy involving touching is frowned on in some Arab and Lithuanian cultures (Leith 1986; Cooper and White 1991).
- Eye contact has negative implications in some American-Hispanic cultures (Leith 1986).
- Clinical assignments to be completed outside of the clinical situation are viewed skeptically in some Chinese cultures (Cooper and White 1991).
- Parents are hesitant to verbalize openly during parental conferences in some Hispanic populations (Leith 1986).
- Play activities, no matter how therapeutically oriented, are questioned by some Japanese societies (Leith 1986).
- Group-play therapy is effective in some Japanese cultures (Wakaba 1983).
- A fluency disorder in a multilingual speaker needs to be assessed in each language spoken (Nwokah 1988).
- Languages such as Spanish and German contain sound patterns that interfere with the use of some fluency-eliciting vocal adjustments commonly used in America (Cooper and White 1991).
- Frequently occurring sounds in spoken French interfere with the use of gentle or easy onset of phonation (Cooper and White 1991).
- Discussions of feelings about stuttering may be frowned upon in certain Lithuanian cultures (Cooper and White 1991).
- The encouragement of client expressions of negative feelings toward the clinician or the therapy process to foster the development of an open and honest relationship between client and clinician is frowned on in certain British cultures (Cooper and White 1991).

- Treatment programs encouraging overt stuttering for control purposes are frowned upon in some urban African American cultures (Cooper and Rustin 1985).

Ethnography and the Assessment and Treatment of Stuttering

The assessment and treatment of fluency disorders histori- cally have been viewed from the perspective of the individual and the indi- vidual's milieu. Ethnography, a research style developed in the field of anthropology, focuses on an individual's sociocultural context in seeking understanding of an individual's or a culture's affective, behavioral, and cognitive responses (Agar 1986; Maxwell 1990). The development of ethnography and its application to the discipline of human communica- tion sciences and disorders obviously is in response to the rapid increase in the multicultural nature of the American society and to the accompanying increased awareness of the significance of culture in understanding human behavior. Ethnography and the history of the assessment and treatment of stuttering have much in common. They share the same roots in semantics (Korzybski 1941), field theory (Lewin 1935), interpersonal theory (Sullivan 1947), and phenomenology (Rogers 1950; Combs and Snygg 1959).

Johnson, a student of Korzybski, focused attention on the significance of language in creating the milieu in which fluency disorders occur (Johnson 1944). Pragmatics pioneer Backus (1951, 1952), citing the works of Sullivan (1947), Lewin (1935), and Rogers (1950), focused on creating the growth- facilitating milieu. The principles of ethnography (Maxwell 1990), as well as its practices for the communicative disorders practitioner (Paganos and Bliss 1990; Westby 1990; Cheng 1990; Maxwell 1990), complement and signifi- cantly advance the work of pioneers in understanding and responding to individual differences in varying sociocultural contexts.

The following discussions of fluency assessment and treatment proce- dures are directed toward enhancing awareness of, and sensitivity to, cul- tural differences. The principles of phenomenology and ethnology underlie the procedures prescribed.

Cultural Considerations in the Assessment of Stuttering

A comprehensive assessment of a fluency disorder addresses the affective, behavioral, and cognitive components of the problem in the context of the individual's life situation. Obviously, complications can arise when the individual, whose fluency disorder is being assessed, is a member of a culture unfamiliar to the examiner. This brief discussion focuses on the kinds of information necessary for an adequate fluency assessment and a frequently observed error committed in assessing fluency disorders.

A common error in assessing fluency disorders is an excessive, if not obsessive, focus on dysfluency frequency counts. Unfortunately, this practice may increase as cultural differences between clinician and client become more frequent and the assessment of client attitudes and feelings become even more challenging. The focus on frequency counts in the assessment of fluency disorders has been labeled the *frequency fallacy* (Cooper and Cooper 1976, 1985b). The frequency fallacy is the belief that the single most reliable and valid measure of stuttering severity is dysfluency frequency counts. In an overzealous attempt to arrive at numbers on which to base clinical decisions, clinicians and researchers overlook the unreliability and the meaninglessness of dysfluency frequency counts obtained in clinical situations. Unfortunately, therapy program developers have gone so far as to design progressions of therapeutic activities based on dysfluency frequency counts.

Effective culture-independent stuttering syndrome assessment instruments are constructed with an awareness of the frequency fallacy and of the syndrome's more critical elements: the types of dysfluencies; the physiologic correlates of dysfluencies; the consistency of dysfluencies; the variability of dysfluency types; the semantic, syntactic, and pragmatic features of the fluency failures; and, most important, the individual's dysfluency-related affective and cognitive responses. In addition, instruments facilitating the assessment of the attitudes and feelings of significant others provide information as to the individual's sociocultural milieu. Fortunately for the fluency clinician, in recent years there has been a proliferation of commercially available fluency disorders assessment instruments. In many instances these instruments are modifiable to account for cultural differences and designed to assess the ABCs of the stuttering syndromes. For example, the Cooper Assessment for Stuttering Syndromes programmed protocols (Cooper and Cooper 1996b, c), which were created for adolescents and adults (CASS-A) and children (CASS-C), were developed to assess the affective, behavioral, and cognitive components of stuttering syndromes in as culturally unbiased a manner as is possible given the current level of understanding of the stuttering syndromes.

Cultural Considerations in the Treatment of Stuttering

Crowe and colleagues (1996) suggested that effective fluency intervention is structured within the context of each client's "cultural system" and "cultural environment." They noted that the cultural system "includes values, attitudes, perceptions, myths, and so on, and to a large extent determines the reality within which clients exist." They describe a client's cultural environment as comprising all aspects of the client's environment, including the client's "phenomenal field, access to experience, semantic environment, significant other relationships, and language environment."

The Culturally Independent Universal Fluency Therapy Goal: The Feeling of Control

The feeling of fluency control, as the end-goal of fluency therapy, is a culturally independent construct. The term *feeling of control* is not meant to be abstract. Rather, it is meant to refer to a response-specific visceral reaction universally experienced, whether it be in typing class, shooting baskets in basketball, or having successfully survived a day on a diet. The feeling of control that fluency-disordered individuals are encouraged to develop is perceived as a concrete experience rather than a hypothetical construct. Typically, once a chronically fluency-disordered individual has experienced the feeling of control and has learned to maintain it, even for brief periods, less psychic energy is required on subsequent occasions to earn and sustain an acceptable level of fluency. Fluency, for the chronically dysfluent, can be viewed as a by-product of the feeling of fluency control.

Unfortunately, as is too commonly the practice today, an arbitrarily selected frequency-of-dysfluency rate may be set as the end goal of therapy. In addition to being impossible to assess, such goals focus the individual's attention on a variable that has little relation to the complex syndrome of attitudes, behaviors, and feelings that constitute fluency disorders. Fortunately, the feeling of control is a universally recognizable construct that generally can be communicated easily despite cultural barriers.

A Culturally Sensitive Stuttering Therapy Process

Cooper and Cooper's (1985b, 1991) Personalized Fluency Control Therapy–Revised program's STAR therapy process was developed to be consistent with phenomenologic principles and thus to be culturally sensitive and adaptable. A brief summary of the four stages follows:

1. Structuring stage. The clinician assists the client in identifying behaviors occurring during moments of dysfluency and behaviors adopted as a result of the dysfluencies. The clinician informs the client of the procedures to be followed in the therapy process in as much depth and detail as is

appropriate for the client's age and understanding. With older clients, the clinician discusses the rationale for focusing in the client-clinician relationship to assist the client in enhancing fluency-facilitating feelings, attitudes, and behavior.

2. Targeting stage. The clinician asks the client to modify behaviors identified in the first stage of therapy. The clinician observes the client's affective, behavioral, and cognitive response patterns. Having targeted patterns that facilitate therapy, the clinician assists the client in becoming aware of them and in planning strategies to modify the impeding patterns and enhance the facilitating patterns.

3. Adjusting stage. The clinician reinforces appropriate and enhancing verbalizations of feelings and attitudes as well as fluency-facilitating behavioral modifications. The clinician instructs the client in self-reinforcement procedures and in fluency initiating gestures (FIGs). The stage is brought to a close when both clinician and client agree that the client has made sufficient adjustments with respect to fluency-related attitudes, feelings, and behaviors to enable the client to begin to strive for the feeling of fluency control in situations outside of the therapy and home environment.

4. Regulating stage. The clinician guides the client in the use of FIGs in life situations with the goal of earning and maintaining the feeling of fluency control.

Culturally Independent Universal Fluency Initiating Gestures

There are six FIGs, which are referred to as *universal* because they can be used to enhance fluency in most speakers whether abnormally or normally dysfluent. They are defined as follows:

Slow FIG	A reduction in the rate of speech typically involving the equalized prolongation of syllables
Easy FIG	A gentle superimposition of phonation on a gentle exhalation
Deep FIG	A consciously controlled inhalation before the initiation of phonation
Smooth FIG	Continuous phonation in conjunction with the use of light articulatory contacts modifying plosives and affricates to resemble fricatives
Loud FIG	A conscious and sustained effort in varying vocal intensity

Beat FIG   Altering the prosody (melody) and rhythm (beat) of the speech

The FIGs have been found to be easily communicated to culturally diverse populations and adaptable in languages with significantly different phonologic, prosodic, and rhythmic characteristics. The set of six FIGs enables the speaker to shift the "locus of focus" from one area of the speech production system to another when one FIG fails to initiate fluency. FIG switching is taught to enhance the client's maintenance of the feeling of fluency control. For use with young children, the FIGs have been cartoonized into the super-hero SuperFIG and six FIG friends, each with its own personality.

References

Agar, M. (1986). *Speaking of ethnography: Qualitative research methods (Vol. 2)*. Beverly Hills, CA: Sage.

Anderson, B. (1981). *An analysis of the relationship of age and sex to type and frequency of dysfluencies in lower socioeconomic preschool black children*. Ph.D. dissertation, Northwestern University.

Ardila, A., Bateman, J.R., Nino, C.R., et al. (1994). An epidemiologic study of stuttering. *Journal of Communication Disorders, 27*, 37–48.

Aron, M. (1962). The nature and incidence of stuttering among a Bantu group of school going children. *Journal of Speech and Hearing Disorders, 27*, 116–148.

Arsenian, J., & Arsenian, J. (1948). Tough and easy cultures. *Psychiatry, 11*, 377–385.

Backus, O. (1951). Personality structure in relation to speech therapy. *Quarterly Journal of Speech, 36*, 51–56.

Backus, O. (1952). The use of group structure in speech therapy. *Journal of Speech and Hearing Disorders, 17*, 116–122.

Beatens-Beardsmore, H. (1986). *Bilingualism: Basic principles (2nd ed.)*. San Diego: College Hill.

Bebout, L., & Arthur, B. (1992). Cross-cultural attitudes toward speech disorders. *Journal of Speech and Hearing Research, 35*, 45–52.

Bernstein-Ratner, N., & Benitez, M. (1985). Linguistic analysis of a bilingual stutterer. *Journal of Fluency Disorders, 10*, 211–219.

Bloodstein, O. (1995). *A handbook on stuttering (5th ed.)*. San Diego: Singular.

Brown, F. (1945) The loci of stuttering in the speech sequence. *Journal of Speech and Hearing Disorders, 10*, 181–192.

Brutten, G., & Miller, R. (1988). The dysfluencies of normally fluent black first graders. *Journal of Fluency Disorders, 13*, 291–299.

Bullen, A.K. (1945). A cross cultural approach to the problem of stuttering. *Child Development, 16*, 1–88.

Carson, C., & Kantner, C.E. (1945). Incidence of stuttering among white and colored school children. *Southern Speech Journal, 10*, 57–59.

Cheng, LL. (1990). The identification of communicative disorders in Asian-Pacific students. *Journal of Childhood Communication Disorders, 13(1)*, 113–119.

Clifford, S., Twitchell, M., & Hull, R. (1965). Stuttering in South Dakota Indians. *Central States Speech Journal, 16*, 59–60.

Combs, A., & Snygg, D. (1959). *Individual behavior: A perceptual approach to behavior*. New York: Harper.

Conrad, C. (1980). *An incidence study of stuttering among black adults.* Unpublished research project, Northwestern University.

Conrad, C. (1985). *A conversational act analysis of black mother-child dyads including stuttering and nonstuttering children.* Ph.D. thesis, Northwestern University.

Conrad, C. (in press). Fluency in multicultural populations. In L. Cole, & V. Deal (Eds.), *Communication disorders in multicultural populations.* Rockville, MD: American Speech-Language-Hearing Association.

Cooper, E.B. (1965). An inquiry into the use of interpersonal communications as a source for therapy. In D. Barbara (Ed.), *New directions in stuttering* (pp. 78–105). Springfield, IL: Thomas.

Cooper, E.B. (1968). A therapy process for the adult stutterer. *Journal of Speech and Hearing Disorders, 33*, 246–260.

Cooper, E.B. (1975, November). *Clinician attitudes toward stutterers: A study of bigotry?* Presented at the annual meeting of the American Speech-Language-Hearing Association, Washington, DC.

Cooper, E.B. (1987). The chronic perseverative stuttering syndrome: Incurable stuttering. *Journal of Fluency Disorders, 12*, 381–388.

Cooper, E.B. (1990a). Stuttering nuggets from a perennially perplexed but persevering prospector. *The Clinical Connection, 4(1)*, 1–4.

Cooper, E.B. (1990b). *Understanding stuttering: Information for parents.* Chicago: National Easter Seal Society.

Cooper, E.B. (1993a). Chronic perseverative stuttering syndrome: A harmful or helpful construct? *American Journal of Speech-Language Pathology, 3*, 11–22.

Cooper, E.B. (1993b). Red herrings, dead horses, straw men, and blind alleys: Escaping the stuttering conundrum. *Journal of Fluency Disorders, 18*, 375–387.

Cooper, E.B. (1997). Fluency disorders. In T.A. Crowe (Ed.), *Applications of counseling in speech-language pathology and audiology* (pp. 145–166). Baltimore: Williams & Wilkins.

Cooper, E.B., & Cooper, C.S. (1976). *Personalized fluency control therapy: An integrated behavior and relationship therapy.* Austin, TX: Learning Concepts.

Cooper, C.S., & Cooper, E.B. (1982). Clinician attitudes toward stuttering in the United States and Europe. *Journal of the Speech and Hearing Association of Alabama, 11(2),* 11–19.

Cooper, E.B., & Cooper, C.S. (1985a). Clinician attitudes towards stuttering: A decade of change. *Journal of Fluency Disorders, 10,* 19–33.

Cooper, E.B., & Cooper, C.S. (1985b). *Cooper personalized fluency control therapy—revised.* Austin, TX: PRO-ED.

Cooper, E.B., & Cooper, C.S. (1991). A fluency disorders prevention program for preschoolers and children in the primary grades. *American Journal of Speech-Language Pathology, 1,* 28–31.

Cooper, E.B., & Cooper, C.S. (1996a). Clinician attitudes towards stuttering: Two decades of change. *Journal of Fluency Disorders, 21,* 119–135.

Cooper, E.B., & Cooper, C.S. (1996b). *Cooper assessment for stuttering syndromes—adolescent and adult version (CASS-A).* San Antonio, TX: The Psychological Corporation.

Cooper, E.B., & Cooper, C.S. (1996c). *Cooper assessment for stuttering syndromes—children's version (CASS-C).* San Antonio, TX: The Psychological Corporation.

Cooper, E.B., & Cooper, C.S. (1995). Treating fluency disordered adolescents. *Journal of Communication Disorders, 28,* 125–142.

Cooper, E.B., & Rustin, L. (1985). Clinician attitudes toward stuttering in the United States and Great Britain: A cross cultural study. *Journal of Fluency Disorders, 10,* 1–17.

Cooper, E.B., & White, J. (1991). *Bilingual speech-language pathologists and audiologists' perceptions of multicultural considerations in the assessment and treatment of stuttering.* Unpublished study. The University of Alabama.

Crowe, T.A., & Cooper, E.B. (1977). Parental attitudes toward stuttering. *Journal of Communication Disorders, 10,* 343–357.

Crowe, T.A., Robinson, T.L., & DiLollo, A. (1996). A multicultural framework for evaluation and treatment of fluency disorders. *American Speech-Language-Hearing Association Special Interest Division #14 Newsletter, 2(4),* 3–5.

Crowe, T.A., & Walton, J.H. (1981). Teacher attitudes toward stuttering. *Journal of Fluency Disorders, 6,* 163–174.

Dale, P. (1977). Factors related to disfluent speech in bilingual Cuban-American adolescents. *Journal of Fluency Disorders, 2,* 311–314.

DiLollo, A., & Crowe, T.A. (1996). *Communication attitudes of African-American and white elementary school children.* Presented at the

Memphis research symposium: Communication in African American children and youth, Memphis, TN: University of Memphis.

Doody, I., Kalinowski, J., Armson, J., & Start, A. (1993). Stereotypes of stutterers and nonstutterers in three rural communities in Newfoundland. *Journal of Fluency Disorder, 18,* 363–373.

Fowlie, G.M., & Cooper, E.B. (1978). Traits attributed to stuttering and nonstuttering children by their mothers. *Journal of Fluency Disorders, 3,* 233–246.

Freud, S. (1920). *A general introduction to psychoanalysis.* New York: Liveright.

Gillespie, S.K., & Cooper, E.B. (1973). Prevalence of speech problems in junior and senior high schools. *Journal of Speech and Hearing Research, 16(4),* 739–743.

Goldman, R. (1967). Cultural influences on the sex ratio in the incidence of stuttering. *American Anthropologist, 69,* 78–81.

Goodall, H.B., & Brobby, G.W. (1982). Stuttering, sickling, and cerebral malaria: A possible organic basis for stuttering. *Lancet, 8284,* 1279–1281.

Gordon, M.M. (1964). *Assimilation in American life.* New York: Oxford University.

Hurst, M., & Cooper, E.B. (1983a). Vocational rehabilitation counselors' attitudes toward stuttering. *Journal of Fluency Disorders, 8,* 13–27.

Hurst, M., & Cooper, E.B. (1983b). Employer attitudes toward stuttering. *Journal of Fluency Disorders, 8,* 1–12.

Jankelowitz, D.L., & Bortz, M.A. (1996). The interaction of bilingualism and stuttering in an adult. *Journal of Communication Disorders, 29,* 223–234.

Jayaram, M. (1983). Phonetic influences on stuttering in monolingual and bilingual stutterers. *Journal of Communication Disorders, 16,* 287–297.

Johnson, W. (1944). The Indians have no word for it. I. Stuttering in children. *Quarterly Journal of Speech, 30,* 330–337.

Karniol, R. (1992). Stuttering out of bilingualism. *First Language, 12,* 255–283.

Kirk, L. (1977). Stuttering and quasi-stuttering. *Georgia Journal of Communication Disorders, 10,* 109–126.

Korzybski, A. (1941). *Science and sanity: An introduction to non-Aristotelian systems and general semantics.* New York: Non-Aristotelian Library, 1941.

Leavitt, R.R. (1974). *The Puerto Ricans: Cultural change and language deviance.* Tucson, AZ: University of Arizona Press.

Leith, W.R. (1986). Treating the stutterer with atypical cultural influences. In K.O. St. Louis (Ed.), *The atypical stutterer* (p. 9). New York: Academic.

Leith, W.R., & Gibson, A. (1991). *The prevalence of stuttering among school children in Nassau, the Bahamas.* Unpublished manuscript, Wayne State University.

Leith, W.R., & Mims, H.A. (1975). Cultural influences in the development and treatment of stuttering: A preliminary report on the black stutterer. *Journal of Speech and Hearing Disorders, 40(4),* 459–466.

Lemert, E.M. (1953). Some Indians who stutter. *Journal of Speech and Hearing Disorders, 18,* 168–174.

Lemert, E.M. (1962). Stuttering and social structure in two Pacific societies. *Journal of Speech and Hearing Disorders, 27,* 3–10.

Lewin, K. (1935). *Dynamic theory of personality.* New York: Harper.

Liljeblad, S. (1967, November). *The Indians have a word for it.* Presented at the annual meeting of the Nevada State Speech Association.

Manning, W.H., & Shrum, W. (1973). The concept of control in stuttering therapy: A reappraisal. *Division for Children with Communication Disorders Bulletin IX, 9,* 32–34.

Maxwell, M.M. (1990). The authenticity of ethnographic research. *Journal of Childhood Communication, 13,* 1–12.

McCartney, T.O. (1971). *Neurosis in the sun.* Nassau, Bahamas: Executive Ideas of the Bahamas.

McDonald, E.T., & Frick, J.V. (1954). Store clerk's reaction to stuttering. *Journal of Speech and Hearing Disorders, 19,* 306–311.

Morgenstern. J.J. (1953). *Psychological and social factors in children's stammering.* Ph.D. dissertation, University of Edinburgh.

Morgenstern, J.J. (1956). Socioeconomic factors in stuttering. *Journal of Speech and Hearing Disorders, 21,* 25–53.

Nathanson, S. (1969). *A study of the influence of race, socioeconomic status and sex on the speech fluency of 200 nonstuttering fifth graders.* Ph.D. dissertation, Northwestern University.

Neeley, M.M. (1960). *An investigation of the incidence of stuttering among elementary school children in the parochial schools of Orleans Parish.* Master's thesis, Tulane University.

Nwokah, E.E. (1988). The imbalance of stuttering behavior in bilingual speakers. *Journal of Fluency Disorders, 13,* 357–373.

Ozawa, Y. (1960). Studies of misarticulation in Wakayama district. *Journal of Medicine, University of Osaka, 5,* 319.

Paganos, J.M., & Bliss, L.S. (1990). Presuppositions for speech therapy lessons. *Journal of Childhood Communication Disorders, 13(1),* 19–38.

Perkins, W.H. (1990). What is stuttering? *Journal of Speech and Hearing Disorders, 55(2),* 370–382.

Pritchett, M. (1966, November). *The role of the East St. Louis Schools: A study of the effectiveness of the multi-approach in stuttering therapy.* Proceedings of the Annual Meeting of the Illinois Speech Association, Chicago.

Ralston, L. (1981). Stammering: A stress index in Caribbean classrooms. *Journal of Fluency Disorders, 6,* 119–133.

Robinson, T. (1992). *An investigation of speech fluency skills in African-American preschool children during narrative discourse.* Ph.D. dissertation, Howard University.

Robinson, T.L., & Crowe, T.A. (1987). A comparative study of speech dysfluencies in nonstuttering black and white college athletes. *Journal of Fluency Disorders, 12,* 147–156.

Rogers, C.R. (1950). *Client-centered therapy.* Boston: Houghton-Mifflin.

Rom, A., & Alpern, C. (1994). Dysfluencies in language-learning disabled monolingual and bilingual high school students. *HEARSAY, 9,* 2.

Shames, G.H. (1989). Stuttering: An RFP for a cultural perspective. *Journal of Fluency Disorders, 14,* 66–77.

Snidecor, J. (1947). Why the Indian does not stutter. *Quarterly Journal of Speech, 33,* 493–495.

St. Louis, K.O., & Lass, N.J. (1981). A survey of communicative disorders students' attitudes toward stuttering. *Journal of Fluency Disorders, 6,* 49–80.

Stewart, J. (1959). Problem of stuttering in certain North American Indian societies. *Journal of Speech and Hearing Disorders, 24(Suppl 6),* 1–87.

Sullivan, H.S. (1947). *Conceptions of modern psychiatry.* Washington, DC: William Alanson White Psychiatric Foundation.

Tint, D. (1984). *Rate assessment and dysfluent behaviors in normal Spanish-speaking children.* Unpublished manuscript, Temple University.

Toyoda, B. (1959). A statistical report. *Clinical Paediatrics, 12,* 788.

Turnbaugh, K.R., Guitar, B.E, & Hoffman, P.R. (1979). Speech clinician's attributions of personality as a function of stuttering severity. *Journal of Speech and Hearing Research, 22,* 37–45.

Turnbaugh, K.R., Guitar, B.E., & Hoffman, P.R. (1981). The attribution of personality traits: The stutterer and nonstutterer. *Journal of Speech and Hearing Research, 24,* 288–291.

Van Riper, C. (1982). *The nature of stuttering.* New York: Prentice-Hall.

Waddle, P. (1934). *A comparison of speech defectives among colored and white children.* Master's thesis, University of Iowa.

Wakaba, Y. (1983). Group therapy for Japanese children who stutter. *Journal of Fluency Disorders, 8,* 93–118.

Wakefield, L. (1985). *Non-fluent behaviors in normal Spanish-speaking adults.* Unpublished manuscript, Temple University.

Watson, J.B., & Kayser, H. (1994). Assessment of bilingual/bicultural children and adults who stutter. *Seminars in Speech and Language, 15(2),* 149–163.

Watson, J.B, & Tepner, L.D. (1996). Stuttering in multicultural populations: Clinical research highlights. *American Speech-Language-Hearing Association Special Interest Division Newsletter #14, 2(4),* 10–12.

Westby, C.E. (1990). Ethnographic interviewing: Asking the right questions to the right people in the right ways. *Journal of Childhood Communication Disorders, 13,* 101–111.

Woods, C.L., & Williams, D.E. (1971). Speech clinicians conceptions of boys and men who stutter. *Journal of Speech and Hearing Disorders, 36,* 225–234.

Woods, C.L., & Williams, D.E. (1976). Traits attributed to stuttering and normally fluent males. *Journal of Speech and Hearing Research, 19,* 267–278.

Yairi, E., & Williams, D.E. (1970). Speech clinicians' stereotypes of elementary school boys who stutter. *Journal of Communication Disorders, 3,* 161–170.

Yeakle, M.K., & Cooper, E.B. (1986). Teacher perceptions of stuttering. *Journal of Fluency Disorders, 11,* 345–359.

Zimmermann, G.N., Liljeblad, S., Frank, A., & Cleeland, C. (1983). The Indians have many terms for it: Stuttering among the Bannock-Shoshoni. *Journal of Speech and Hearing Research, 26,* 315–318.

Additional Resources

American Speech-Language-Hearing Association. (1996). *Issues in assessing and treating speech fluency behaviors.* Rockville, MD: American Speech-Language-Hearing Association.

Cooper, E.B. (1997). Fluency disorders. In T.A. Crowe (Ed.), *Applications of counseling in speech-language pathology and audiology* (pp. 145–166). Baltimore: Williams & Wilkins.

http://doombox.mankato.msus.edu/dept/comdis/Kuster/stutter.html

McCallien, C. (1956). Problems of speech defect in the Accra district. *Speech, 20,* 15–19.

Stut-HLP@BGU.EDU (listserv for those who stutter and their families)

Stutt-L@VM.Temple.edu (listserv open to all)

Stutt-X@ASUVM.INRE.ASU.EDU (listserv for academicians and students)

Watson, J.B., & Kayser, H. (1994). Assessment of bilingual/bicultural children and adults who stutter. *Seminars in Speech and Hearing, 15(2),* 149–163.

Wright, L., & Sherrard, C. (1994). Stuttering therapy with British-Asian children. I: A survey of service delivery in the United Kingdom. *European Journal of Disorders of Communication, 29,* 307–324.

Wright, L., & Sherrard, C. (1994). Stuttering therapy with British-Asian children. II: Speech and language therapists' perceptions of their effectiveness. *European Journal of Disorders of Communication, 29,* 325–337.

9

Voice and
Voice Disorders

Glenda DeJarnette and
R. Wayne Holland

Voice reflects the health status of the body through its connection with neurologic and endocrinologic systems. Moreover, the health status of subglottal and supraglottal systems is often reflected in the voice. To both the trained and untrained ear, the voice suggests a person's age, sex, and emotional state. Speech-language pathologists are trained to consider these traditional aspects of the voice in clients. As of this writing, clinical protocols do not presuppose that racial, ethnic, or cultural factors contribute to the quality of voice. In fact, few acoustic and physiologic data exist that compare laryngeal structure and function across racial, ethnic, and cultural groups. A few perceptual studies exist that allude to the fact that culturally determined linguistic patterns both color the tone of voice of speakers and influence the listener's perception of voice tone.

The perception of the voice is not restricted to the phonatory apparatus and its functioning. Indeed, the perceived aerodynamic and torque interactions of the phonatory system with respiratory and resonatory systems provide the greatest appreciation of voice. Thus, a full examination of multicultural issues affecting normal and abnormal voice function ultimately must consider the variables that affect these combined systems to generate the vocal product. Throughout this chapter, information is shared that pertains to the respiratory system, laryngeal system, and supralaryngeal resonatory systems because it is believed that quality assessment of voice disorders and intervention must consider the interactions of these systems.

There is a paucity of information on the impact of multicultural variables on the production of normal and abnormal voice. This chapter presents the information that is available regarding voice in culturally diverse groups.

Specifically, the chapter examines (1) incidence of voice-related pathologies in minority groups in the United States; (2) health issues related to voice dysfunction; (3) racial and ethnographic factors related to voice; and (4) the role of the speech-language pathologist in prevention, assessment, and intervention. The reader is cautioned that the categorization of minority groups is an artificial contrivance in that several groups (e.g., Asian and Hispanic groups) have racially, ethnically, or culturally distinct subgroups.

Incidence of Voice-Related Pathologies in Minority Groups in the United States

A review of the literature concerning the epidemiology of voice-related pathologies in minority groups yields insufficient data on the national distribution of all disorders. In some instances, the incidence reports extend beyond the United States to suggest racial distributions. Subsequently, studies of the incidence of the various voice-related pathologies among minority groups in the United States await epidemiologic investigation on a national scale. The available literature scans a few of the pathologies related to the vocal cords and the nasal and oropharyngeal ports. This literature is reviewed in "Incidence of Oral and Nasopharyngeal Pathologies" and is followed by an examination of health information that reiterates the need for increased research of voice-related pathologies in culturally diverse populations in the United States.

Incidence of Vocal Cord Pathologies

Incidence of all vocal cord disorders among minority groups in the United States is difficult to ascertain because no studies currently exist that are cross-sectional for race or ethnicity. This section discusses a recent report of the incidence of laryngeal cancer in the United States, with a focus on black and white adults. A second report is presented that examines the incidence of laryngeal pathologies in Asian, black, and white children.

Yang and colleagues (1989) reported the incidence of laryngeal cancer by subsite for adult blacks and whites across sex, with ages ranging from younger than 29 to 79 years. Blacks constituted 10% of the subject pool. Medical records for 1973–1982 were used to report the data. Subjects were identified through the National Cancer Institute's Surveillance, Epidemiology, and End Results (SEER) program. Comparative ratios for incidence of squamous cell carcinoma revealed that both black and white men exhibited a higher incidence than women for all subsites. The rate ratios were largest between the sexes for the glottis subsite as compared with the supraglottis and subglottis. The investigators indicated that anatomic and physiologic differences between the sexes may have accounted for the disparity in the incidence rates. Although Yang and colleagues did not comment on the differences in incidence between the races, the data reflect that, compared with white men, black men had a higher incidence of all subsite laryngeal cancers, most notably cancer of the glottis. Likewise, compared with white women, black women had a higher incidence of all subsite laryngeal cancers, except for the glottis.

The incidence of laryngeal pathologies in children was investigated by Dobres and colleagues (1990), who used medical chart inspection as the method of data collection. A portion of the medical charts were marked for race. Asian children constituted 0.02% of the subjects; black children constituted 5%; and white children constituted 79%. Thirty laryngeal pathologies were noted in the data. Overall, the incidence of laryngeal pathologies was greater among males than females, and subglottic stenosis showed the highest incidence. The investigators suggested that the distribution of laryngeal pathologies across the races mirrored the overall finding for the total sample. Asians had the greatest male-to-female incidence ratio (4.3 to 1.0), whites had the second greatest (1.8 to 1.0), and blacks had the lowest (1.4 to 1.0). It is unclear if the results for age-related incidence in the total sample is the same across the races because the age breakdown for race was not shared. Moreover, visual inspection of the data suggests that there might be proportional differences in the distribution of the pathologies as well as some sex-related differences across race groups. For all groups, the occurrence of subglottic stenosis was the highest. Subsequent pathologies, however, showed patterns for minority groups that differed from that of the white children. Although vocal nodules were clearly more prevalent in white males as compared with white females, vocal nodules were only slightly more prevalent in Asian males compared with Asian females. Among the black children, the females showed a higher incidence of vocal nodules as compared with males.

In the case of laryngomalacia, a pattern difference occurred as well in that neither the Asian nor the black children followed the sex ratio distribution that was observed in the white children (Dobres, et al. 1990). The incidence of laryngomalacia was higher among white males than among white females; however, the pattern among blacks was the reverse. The incidence was higher among black females. Laryngomalacia was equally disbursed among Asian males and females. Only five of the 30 pathologies (i.e., subglottic stenosis, vocal nodules, laryngomalacia, dysphonia [normal larynx], and vocal fold paralysis) were clearly evidenced across all groups. Of course, as Dobres and colleagues (1990) suggested, the minority sample sizes were small, making definitive comparisons difficult.

Incidence of Oral and Nasopharyngeal Pathologies

Other than cleft palate, the incidence of oral and nasopharyngeal pathologies in minority groups has not been investigated. The most accurate method of reporting the incidence and prevalence of a cleft palate is not perfected in reporting practices, according to Sayetta and colleagues (1989). Methodologic difficulties include varied methods of case selection (e.g., through birth or death certificates, professional reports, or hospital records), semantic confusion over incidence versus prevalence in data reports, inaccuracies in cleft classifications, and exclusion of stillbirths and aborted fetuses from incidence data. Despite these methodologic encumbrances, investigators have provided evidence of differing distributions of cleft palate occurrence across racial groupings (Vanderas 1987). Vanderas (1987) examined the literature on epidemiologic studies of cleft lip, cleft palate, and cleft lip and palate across racial groupings and provided a picture of the incidence of a cleft palate in blacks, American Indians, Chinese, and Japanese. Some of the data were extracted from international studies, as well as from studies on the incidence in the United States. For the minority groups on which Vanderas focused, the incidence of cleft palate in the United States per 1,000 population was highest for Chinese (4.04), second highest for American Indians (0.79–3.62), third highest for Japanese (0.82–2.41), and fourth highest for blacks (0.80–1.67). Vanderas looked at one study from multiple sources to report incidence in Chinese, whereas multiple sources were used to report incidences for other groups. Incidence reports for Filipinos and Hispanics were shared from a more limited pool of studies (Vanderas 1987). For Filipino births in Hawaii, the incidence was 2.45 per 1,000 population. An international focus on Puerto Ricans and Mexicans showed incidence ranging from 0.42 to 2.27, with Puerto Ricans showing slightly greater incidence than Mexicans per 100,000 population (Vanderas 1987).

Vanderas (1987) also reported on incidence trends of the different kinds of conditions (i.e., cleft lip, cleft palate, and cleft lip and palate). Among blacks, the incidence of cleft palate tended to be greater than that of cleft lip with cleft palate, which in turn was greater than that of cleft lip alone. For American Indians, the incidence of cleft lip with palate tended to be greater than the incidence of cleft lip alone or cleft palate alone. For Chinese, the incidence of cleft lip with cleft palate tended to be greater than that of cleft lip or cleft palate alone in some studies. In other studies, the incidence of cleft lip with cleft palate tended to be equal to that of cleft palate, although the incidence of both was greater than that of cleft lip alone. For Japanese, the incidence of cleft lip with cleft palate was greater than that of cleft lip alone, which was greater than the incidence of cleft palate alone.

The sex ratios for each racial group revealed that, for the most part, males tend to have a higher incidence of cleft palate than females. Specifically, for each group and each cleft classification the following was noted:

- Black males showed a greater incidence for all cleft types than black females.
- American Indian males showed a greater incidence for cleft lip with palate and cleft palate alone than American Indian females. Both showed an equal incidence of cleft lip alone.
- Chinese showed an unclear ratio on sex differences for cleft lip with cleft palate, but males showed a greater incidence of cleft palate alone than females.
- Japanese males showed a greater incidence of cleft lip with palate, but females showed a greater incidence of cleft palate alone. It was unclear which sex dominated the ratio for cleft lip alone.

In summary, it appears that except for blacks, minority groups follow the incidence trend of the general population—that is, a cleft lip with cleft palate occurs more often than a cleft palate alone (Shaw, et al. 1991). Among blacks, a cleft palate occurs more often. The sex ratio is less clear for minority groups and may not follow the trend found in the general population (i.e., that females are more likely to be born with a cleft palate alone than males) (Shaw, et al. 1991). American Indians and Japanese followed this trend; however, it is not followed by Chinese (females equal males in the incidence of cleft palate alone) or blacks (male incidence of cleft palate is greater than that of females).

Health Issues Related to Voice Dysfunction

To adequately address voice disorders in multicultural groups, the health-related conditions that predispose and precipitate voice disorders must be considered. This section therefore examines health problems that have either a direct or an indirect effect on the voice production system. The data-base material was taken from the 1988–1992 SEER program (Miller, et al. 1996). The SEER program collected data on the incidence of cancer in the general population. SEER data for 1988–1992 represented 14% of the total United States population. The areas that supplied the SEER database for 1988–1992 were Connecticut; Hawaii; Iowa; New Mexico; Utah; Atlanta; Detroit; Los Angeles, San Francisco, Oakland, San Jose, and Monterey, CA;

Seattle and Puget Sound; and areas identified by the Alaska Area Native Health Service.

Carcinomas with Direct or Indirect Effect on Voice

According to the National Cancer Institute (1996), overall cancer incidence rates were higher in males than females for regions included in the SEER database. SEER data showed trends that affected racial groupings. Racial groupings reported in the SEER data included black, American Indian, Alaska Native, Chinese, Filipino, Hawaiian, Hispanic (nonwhite), Hispanic (white), Japanese, Korean, non-Hispanic white, Vietnamese, and white. For males, the average annual rate of cancer per 100,000 population from highest to lowest incidence by racial and ethnic group is as follows:

Black (560)
Non-Hispanic white (481)
White (469)
Alaska native (372)
Hawaiian (340)
Hispanic (white) (336)
Vietnamese (326)
Japanese (322)
Hispanic (nonwhite) (319)
Chinese (282)
Filipino (274)
Korean (266)
American Indian (New Mexico) (196)

For females, the "average annual" rate of cancer per 100,000 population from highest to lowest incidence by racial and ethnic group is as follows:

Black (319)
Hawaiian (239)
Alaska Native (225)
Non-Hispanic white (217)
White (213)
Chinese (139)
Hispanic (white) (134)
Japanese (133)
Hispanic (nonwhite) (129)

American Indian (New Mexico) (123)
Filipino (105)
Korean (N/A)
Vietnamese (N/A)

Predispositions to Cancers That Affect Voice

Genetic Factors

The genetic predisposition for cancer is unclear, despite the fact that research on skin cancer tentatively shows genetic differences between blacks and whites in the development of cancer. Moreover, the genetic influence on cancers that have environmental causes is even less clear. Certain teratogens and health practices put people at risk for cancer. Known risk factors include tobacco (including smokeless tobacco), alcohol, certain diet ingredients, and carcinogenic substances in the workplace and environment.

Smoking

Smoking is known to be causally related to cancer of the larynx, oral and pharyngeal cavities, lungs, and esophagus. In 1994, an estimated 48.0 million adults (men and women) were smokers. A 1996 Centers for Disease Control report states that "[r]acial/ethnic group-specific prevalence was highest for American Indians/Alaskan Natives...and lowest for Asians/Pacific Islanders...With the exception of persons with 0–8 years of education, smoking prevalence varied inversely with level of education and was highest among persons with 9–11 years of education...Smoking prevalence was higher among persons living below the poverty level...than among those living at or above poverty" (Centers for Disease Control 1996). Miller et al. (1996) reported the following smoking rates for men and women in the United States:

	Men	Women
American Indians and Alaskan Natives	53.7%	33.1%
Blacks	33.9 %	21.8%
Whites	28%	24.7%
Hispanics	24.3%	15.2%
Asian and Pacific islanders	20.4%	7.5%

Alcohol

Alcohol is known to increase the risk for cancer of the oral cavity, pharynx, larynx, and esophagus. The percentage of use across minority groups is difficult to ascertain because of small sample sizes within the large national studies. However, existing data suggest that alcohol consumption patterns vary across racial groupings (Page and Asire 1985). The occurrence of cirrhosis of the liver has been used as an indicator of alcohol consumption patterns, although caution is exercised because confounding socioeconomic variables have an impact on health care provision and can inflate incidence rates among minorities. The cirrhosis data, however, reveal that the death rate for those with cirrhosis of the liver is highest for American Indians (males, 43.7%; females, 29.9%), second highest for blacks (males, 29.4%; females, 13.5%), and lowest for Asians and Pacific Americans (Page and Asire 1985). The death rate for Hispanics was not available.

Nutrition

Nutritional factors tend to combine with other risk factors to affect the cancers that have an impact on voice-related concerns. Exposure to teratogenic agents combined with a reduced nutritional intake probably increases the risk of cancer. Indeed, it is suggested that salt-cured, smoked, and nitrite-cured foods are linked to cancer of the esophagus. Although no data exist that implicate nutritional factors in the development of cancers that have an effect on vocal systems, it has been suggested that dietary habits influence disease incidence (Baquet, et al. 1991). Dietary ingredients implicated in cancer control include carotenoid (found in dark vegetables, fruits, and carrots), vitamin A (found in liver, milk, cheese, butter, and egg yolks), fiber (found in fruits, vegetables, beans, peas, and whole-grain cereals), vitamin E, and selenium. Dietary ingredients known to cause cancer include fats ingested at high levels and molds and fungi produced in foods that use curing agents. Culturally rooted dietary habits, often reinforced by conditions of poverty or low socioeconomic potential, can put minority groups at risk for cancer (Baquet, et al. 1991). For example, Hargreaves and colleagues (1989) reviewed the nutritional habits of African Americans and found that African American food tended to be high in protein, fat, and carbohydrates and low in fiber, thiamine, riboflavin, vitamins A and C, and iron.

Environmental and Chemical Factors

Exposure to carcinogenic substances in the workplace puts individuals at risk for cancers that affect the vocal production systems (Parnes 1990). No studies exist that show correlations between cancer and occupational trends among minority populations. However, low-paying, high-risk jobs have historically been the employment avenues for minorities in the United States (National Center for Health Statistics 1991). As such, these groups have been exposed to industrial processes and chemicals that increase the risk of cancer. The National Cancer Institute has identified exposure to chemicals in the workplace as an environmental risk (Page and Asire 1985). Among the industries with a high risk of exposure are furniture manufacturing, boot and shoe manufacturing and shoe and boot repair, auramine manufacturing, rubber manufacturing, mining (with exposure to radon), isopropyl alcohol manufacturing, and nickel refining. Among the carcinogenic chemicals to which workers are exposed are 4-aminobiphenyl, arsenic and arsenic compounds, asbestos, benzene, benzidine, Bis(2-chloroethyl)-2-naphthylamine (chlornaphazine), Bis(chloromethyl)ether and technical-grade chloromethyl methyl ether, chromium and certain chromium compounds, 2-naphthylamine, soot, tars, oils, and vinyl chloride.

Incidence of Cancers in Minority Groups

Laryngeal Cancer
    The annual incidence of laryngeal cancer in the United States is most often reported for whites and blacks. According to SEER data for 1988–1992, black males had a higher incidence than white males and both black and white females (Miller, et al. 1996). Black males showed an incidence of 12.7 cases per 100,000 population as compared with 7.5 per 100,000 for white males. Black females showed an incidence of 2.5 cases per 100,000 population as compared with 1.5 per 100,000 for white females (Miller, et al. 1996). Of all minority groups, blacks had the highest incidence of laryngeal cancer (Miller, et al. 1996). Several minority groups had less than 25 cases of laryngeal cancer per 100,000 population, and calculations were not conducted for them. Groups affected by the low incidence were Alaska Native, American Indian (New Mexico), Hawaiian, Korean, and Vietnamese.

Esophageal Cancer
    SEER data for 1988–1992 on the incidence of esophageal cancer show that blacks (both men and women) have a higher incidence of this cancer than whites and other minority groups (Miller, et al. 1996). This report states that "[t]he incidence rate for black men is 60% higher than that for Hawaiians and more than 2.7 times greater than the rate for non-Hispanic white men. The rates for Chinese, Japanese, and non-Hispanic white men are similar to each other (within the range of 5.2 to 5.6 per 100,000 men) and are

modestly higher than the rate for white Hispanic men." Limited data were available for women with only black, white, and Hispanic groups represented. Hispanic and non-Hispanic white females had lower incidences of esophageal cancer than black females.

Lung Cancer

SEER data for 1988–1992 on the incidence of lung and bronchus cancer show that, "[a]mong men...lung cancer incidence rates (per 100,000) range from a low of about 14 among American Indians to a high of 117 among blacks, an eightfold difference. Between these two extremes, rates fall into two groups ranging from 42 to 53 for Hispanics, Japanese, Chinese, Filipinos, and Koreans and from 71 to 89 for Vietnamese, whites, Alaskan Natives and Hawaiians. The range among women is much narrower, from a rate of about 15 among Japanese to nearly 51 among Alaska Natives...Rates for the remaining female populations fall roughly into two groups with low rates of 16 to 25 for Korean, Filipino, Hispanic, and Chinese women and rates of 31 to 44 among Vietnamese, white, Hawaiian, and black women" (Miller, et al. 1996).

Nasopharyngeal Cancer

The Chinese are suspected to have a genetic predisposition to nasopharyngeal cancer (Hung-Dhiu Ho 1982). Mortality rates among Chinese are as high as 11.5 for females and 13.5 for males in population-specific regions of the United States (Rice and Yu 1982). According to SEER reports for 1988–1992, the highest incidence rates of nasopharyngeal cancer were among the Chinese (Miller, et al. 1996). Rates were also high in Vietnamese and Filipino males. Black, white, and Hispanic males and white females showed low incidences compared with males and female Chinese, Filipinos, and Vietnamese.

Oral Cavity Cancer

SEER data for 1988–1992 indicate that for males, oral cavity cancer is highest in blacks, followed by whites, Vietnamese, and native Hawaiians. For females, high rates occur in non-Hispanic whites, blacks, and Filipinos (Miller, et al. 1996).

Thyroid Cancer

SEER data for 1988–1992 show that thyroid cancer affects females more than males. The highest rates for thyroid cancer were among Filipino females, Vietnamese females, and Hawaiian females. The lowest were among black females (Miller, et al. 1996).

Thyroid Disease with Direct or Indirect Effects on Voice

The incidence of endocrinologic diseases among minority populations has been researched very little. Williams (1975) identified some of the disorders among blacks based on international and national cases. Thyrotoxicosis, often symptomatic of Graves' disease, was listed among the diseases affecting blacks. It is known to produce conditions of hyperthyroidism and toxic nodular goiters. The incidence of Graves' disease among black Africans has been studied, and it is suggested that toxic nodular goiter does not often accompany the disease, although some degree of hyperthyroidism is evidenced (Kalk and Kalk 1989). The Chinese have also shown a susceptibility to thyrotoxicosis (Blum 1982; Gee 1982). In a study that investigated the incidence of thyroid dysfunction in adults 55 years of age and older, differences in the incidence rates for blacks and whites were observed as well (Bagchi, et al. 1990). The incidence of hypothyroidism and hyperthyroidism was lower in blacks compared with whites. The study contained more women than men, which may have affected the results; however, both black and white women showed a greater proportional incidence than black and white men (Bagchi, et al. 1990).

Respiratory Disease with Direct or Indirect Effects on Voice

Upper and lower respiratory tract bacterial and viral infections need to be researched relative to their distribution among the races. Current data-reporting and management systems do not appear to track the allergens and infectious causes of respiratory distress across racial groups. Chronic and persistent cough has been noted in the Chinese population and indicates a variety of respiratory difficulties including postnasal drip, chronic bronchitis, bronchial asthma, and pulmonary tuberculosis (Chen 1982). According to the Centers for Disease Control, tuberculosis showed an increase of 9.4 cases per 100,000 population between 1989 and 1990 and 2.3 cases per 100,000 population between 1990 and 1991. The incidence figures for 1990 showed that minorities account for the greatest incidence of tuberculosis. The cases per 100,000 population were 41.6 Asian and Pacific Americans, 33.0 blacks, 18.9 American Indians, 21.4 Hispanics, and 4.2 whites (Centers for Disease Control 1991). It has been noted that some races have less resistance to tuberculosis, which suggests a genetic predisposition to the disease (Williams 1975). Other reasons for the increase in tuberculosis infections may be the virus that causes acquired immunodeficiency syndrome, homelessness, drug use, and the influx of immigrants who are at high risk for tuberculosis.

Cerebrovascular Disease with Direct or Indirect Effects on Voice

It is known that conditions of neuromotor compromise often result in dysarthric conditions and can affect the system of voice production. Age-adjusted death rates for cerebrovascular disease for 1988 were higher for black men (57.8) and women (46.6) per 100,000 population than for white men (30.0) and women (25.5) (National Center for Health Statistics 1991). Across minority groups, the 1988 death count due to cerebrovascular disease was 8,098 for black men, 10,381 for black women, 791 for Asian and Pacific-American men, 789 for Asian and Pacific-American women, 171 for American Indian men, and 200 for American Indian women (National Center for Health Statistics 1991).

Racial and Ethnographic Factors Related to Voice

Current knowledge about the anatomic, physiologic, acoustic, and perceptual parameters related to the normal voice of minority populations in the United States is almost nonexistent. The few existing studies focus on the voice characteristics of African Americans, and these are shared in this section. Specifically, this section mentions literature that suggests anatomic, physiologic, acoustical, and perceptual differences between African Americans and the majority population. At the end of this section is a discussion of how the voice is used in the cultural-linguistic patterns of African American English to perpetuate the oral tradition of the culture. It is probable that other minority groups use parameters of voice to maintain cultural connection as well; however, existing literature has best identified this phenomenon in African Americans.

Anatomic Factors

In examining the larynges of blacks in South Africa, Boshoff (1945) found that the larynges of black cadavers were larger than those of white cadavers. It has been suggested that blacks have shorter trunks and longer limbs, which contributes to respiratory differences (Williams 1975). Cole (1980) reviewed the orofacial characteristics of blacks that must be considered in the health and professional service to cleft palate patients. Among the structural traits were a short columella, obtuse nasal arch, wide nasal tripod, septal cartilage producing a rounded nasal tip relative to the bridge of the nose, fullness of the vermilion border of the lips, propensity to develop keloids, and depigmentation or hypopigmentation when scarring of the skin occurs.

Physiologic Factors

Williams (1975) reviewed research of pulmonary function in blacks. This research suggested that black males of all ages have smaller vital capacities than those of whites of the same age, height, and weight. Black females also demonstrated smaller vital capacities than white females. Additionally, total lung capacity and residual volume were found to be smaller in blacks compared with whites.

Acoustic Factors Across Age Groups

The fundamental frequency characteristics of black children, preadolescents, adolescents, young adults, and elderly have undergone some investigation. For all age groups, the fundamental frequency of blacks is reportedly lower than that of whites, even when this lower frequency level does not appear to be statistically significant (Awan and Mueller 1996; Wheat and Hudson 1988; Hollien and Malcik 1962; Hudson and Holbrook 1981; Ducote 1983). The following review of the literature moves chronologically across the age span to illuminate racial differences that may be present and observable through acoustical analysis.

Awan and Mueller (1996) compared speaking fundamentals of black, Hispanic, and white kindergartners (ages 5 years to 6 years and 3 months). Visual inspection of the mean speaking fundamental measures taken from this study revealed that the fundamental frequencies of white and Hispanic females and males were closer in range to each other than were the fundamental frequencies of female and male black children. The mean values for females and males, respectively, were 243.35 Hz and 240.07 Hz for whites, 248.04 Hz and 248.99 Hz for Hispanics, and 231.48 Hz and 241.31 Hz for blacks. The mean speaking fundamental for black females was lower than any other group (males and females). Black female's standard deviation (14.99 Hz) was near to the lowest noted in the study, with deviation ranging from 14.45 (Hispanic females) to 22.17 Hz (white females). Despite this observable sex difference in the data, statistical analysis suggested that there was no significant difference between the groups for sex. Moreover, Awan and Mueller (1996) found no statistically significant difference in fundamental frequency variability (i.e., pitch sigma for sex or across racial grouping). One statistically significant finding in this study was that male and female black kindergarten children exhibited a lower mean speaking fundamental frequency compared with Hispanics (236.40 Hz and 248.51 Hz, respectively). No statistically significant difference was found between the mean speaking fundamental frequencies of white kindergarten children (241.71 Hz) and either black (236.40 Hz) or Hispanic (248.51 Hz) groups. A finding in the study was that the speaking range (in semitones) was more reduced for the Hispanic kindergartners than for either the black or white groups. Awan and Mueller (1996) interpreted their findings to suggest that applying normative mean speaking fundamental frequency measures from one racial grouping to another may not be appropriate.

Studies that precede that of Awan and Mueller also indicate that for young children, racial differences can be traced in the acoustic properties of voice output. Wheat and Hudson (1988) conducted a study with children ranging in age from 6 years to 6 years and 11 months. The fundamental frequencies were 219.5 Hz for black males and 211.3 Hz for black females. These pitch levels are lower than those determined for whites, who had a range of 280–365 Hz for males and 270–395 Hz for females (Wilson 1979). No significant difference was found for sex in the fundamental frequencies of 6-year-old blacks (Wheat and Hudson 1988).

Racial differences can be detected acoustically in preadolescent and adolescent youths. Hollien and Malcik (1962) measured the fundamental frequency of preadolescent and adolescent black males. Mean fundamental frequency values were 210 Hz at 10 years old, 158 Hz at 14 years old, and 121 Hz at 18 years old (Hollien and Malcik 1962), as compared with the majority norms of 235 Hz, 190 Hz, and 125 Hz for the respective ages (Wilson 1979).

Hudson and Holbrook (1981) measured the fundamental frequency of young adult black men and women from 18 to 29 years of age and compared their findings with data gathered for young adult white men and women (Fitch and Holbrook 1970). Both black men and women showed mean fundamental frequency ranges that were greater than those of their white counterparts. The mean modal fundamental frequency for black men was 110.15 Hz (Hudson and Holbrook 1981) as compared with 116.65 Hz for white men (Fitch and Holbrook 1970). The fundamental frequency for black women was 193.10 Hz (Hudson and Holbrook 1981), as compared with 217.00 Hz for white women (Fitch and Holbrook 1970). Hudson and Holbrook (1981) noted that the variability of frequency in blacks was double that of whites and that blacks tended to have greater flexibility above their mean modal frequencies. Findings for whites were just the opposite. Whites showed a greater range below their mean modal frequency. Hudson and Holbrook (1981) suggested that the lower modal frequency and degree of change above the modal frequency are factors that lead to racial identification through the voice.

Ducote (1983) measured the fundamental frequency of black men and women ages 50–79 years. This study examined fundamental frequencies while the subjects were reading and speaking. The reading fundamentals showed significant differences between the younger male speakers (50–60 years old) and the older group; female speakers showed no differences. For black men, the mean fundamental frequencies for speaking across the age groups were 118.13 Hz (50–60 years old), 113.33 Hz (60–70 years old), and 116.33 (70–79 years old). These measures are below the fundamental frequency as reported for the majority male population within this age span, which is 162 Hz (Hon and Isshiki 1980). For black women, the mean fundamental frequencies for speaking across the age groups were 168.22 Hz (50–60 years old), 163.26 (60–70 years old), and 150.46 Hz (70–79 years old) (Ducote 1983). These measures are below the fundamental frequency as reported for the majority female population within this age span, which is 177 Hz (Hon and Isshiki 1980).

As these data suggest, the fundamental frequencies for black males and females tend to be lower than those of white males and females. In some instances the differences between fundamental frequency in blacks and whites appear to be significant (e.g., for 6-, 10-, 14-, and 50- to 79-year-old males and for 6-, 18- to 29-, and 60- to 79-year-old females). In all instances, the actual measures are different and must be taken into account as levels of normal production are considered. It appears that the fundamental frequency for speaking for aged black men falls close to the range for the 18- to 29-year-old group (Hudson and Holbrook 1981). If this holds true with additional research, the general population trend, which indicates an increase in fundamental frequency as men age, should be revisited as data on minority groups are added to the reference tables for norms.

To further support the need for revised norms to reflect racial variation, research of voice onset time differences across races is emerging. In a preliminary study of differences in voice onset time between blacks and whites, Ryalls, et al. (1997) found that there is significantly more prevoicing during voiced consonant production in blacks than in whites.

Perceptual Variables

Since 1962, perceptual studies of the speech and voice of blacks have been conducted (Dickens and Sawyer 1962; Irwin 1977; Lass, et al. 1978, 1979, 1982; Baker 1982; Saniga, et al. 1984; Wright, et al. 1976; Larimer, et al. 1988; Walton and Orlikoff 1994). Paradigms have included panelist judgment of (1) unaltered recorded samples of black speakers (Dickens and Sawyer 1962; Irwin 1977; Lass, et al. 1979; Baker 1982; Saniga, et al. 1984; Walton and Orlikoff 1994), (2) altered recorded samples to determine whether or not temporal features affect perception of race in the speech and voice (Lass, et al. 1978; Wright, et al. 1976), and (3) samples of vocally disguised speech wherein white speakers disguise their speech and voices to feign black native production (Lass, et al. 1982).

Under the unaltered-recorded-samples paradigm, judges correctly identified the speaker's race or racial attributes, which implies a differentiation between the races (speakers were black or white). This occurred regardless of whether the judges were black or white. One attribute noted in a study of the use of vocal fry register in black and white speech was that black speakers were perceived to use vocal fry vocalization more often than white speakers (Saniga, et al. 1984). A second attribute alluding to racial differentiation is the tendency for older blacks to be perceived as younger than their age more frequently than whites (Baker 1982). Although studies using the unaltered-speech paradigm suggest that racial differences are perceivable in the speech and voice, factors often affect perception, particularly when the judge is not a member of the racial group targeted for study.

In a study of personality as portrayed through speech and voice (Larimer, et al. 1988), social class status affected the judgment of white panelists. White judges tended to rate low-income blacks lower on the scaled items than they rated middle-class black and white speakers. White judges did not rate middle-class black and white speakers with significant difference. On the other hand, black judges rated black speakers equally regardless of social class.

Under the altered-recorded-samples paradigm, judges tended to have difficulty and performed at the chance level in identifying the race of the speaker. One study reported a bit greater than chance performance among judges who identified white and black male speakers based on prolonged vowel productions (Walton and Orlikoff 1984). When the unaltered recorded sample and the altered sample appeared in the same study, however, judges clearly identified race with significant degrees of accuracy under the unaltered speech or voice condition (Wright, et al. 1976). The distortions used to alter the speech and voice parameters appear to interfere with listener judgment. Indeed, these paradigms attempt to determine the aspects of the speech and voice act as perceptual clues to racial identity. Thus far the examination of timing alterations seems to suggest that timing is a critical parameter for perception of racial differences. That is, listeners lose their capability to identify the speaker's race when timing is distorted or when timing is isolated as the only cue to the speaker's racial identity (Lass, et al 1978; Wright, et al. 1976) In addition to timing, judges appear to note a characteristic of noise in the voice of black speakers as compared with white speakers (Walton and Orlikoff 1994).

Under the vocal-disguise paradigm, judges were able to distinguish race when speakers used their native speech characteristics and when they attempted to disguise the speech to sound like black speakers. Because only white speakers and white judges were the subjects of the disguise study, it is difficult to determine the veracity of the paradigm in identifying racial perceptions (Lass, et al. 1982).

Cultural and Linguistic Variables

It is known that speech and voice interact in the production of linguistic suprasegmentals and that speakers are recognized by their pitch contours (Atal 1968; Atkinson 1973; van Dommelen 1987). These features of the voice appear to play a pivotal role in speaker identification (van Dommelen 1987; Pittam and Gallois 1986; Pittam 1987), ethnic background (Lass, et al. 1978, 1979, 1982; Baker 1982; Saniga, et al. 1984; Wright, et al. 1976; Larimer, et al. 1988), and cultural-linguistic heritage (Vandepitte 1989; Tarone 1973; Smitherman 1975; Pitts 1989). The oral traditions of blacks are used to illustrate the point that cultural-linguistic inheritance is portrayed in the speaker's use of voice.

Discourse analysis of communication and of miscommunication in speaker-listener dyads has suggested that intonation and the use of tone serve pragmatic functions (Vandepitte 1989). The use of intonation contours and tone is said to indicate the speaker's assumptions about the background knowledge of the listener as well as to suggest the speaker's illocutionary force or commitment to the relevance of information being shared (Vandepitte 1989; Tarone 1973). Tarone (1973) provided the following anecdotal account of how voice can be misinterpreted by those outside the relevant cultural sphere and experience. A white police officer arrested several African American youths when he mistook their lively verbal jousts to be indications of hostility and threats of violence. The African American youths were demonstrating their commitment to the verbal game, but their illocutionary force was misinterpreted by the officer who did not share their background and was not aware of the intent of the verbal exchange (Tarone 1973).

Acquired oral traditions of cultures probably bespeak the function of the voice and speech production systems as much as do genetically inherited racial, anatomic, or physiologic traits. As noted above, acoustic findings have suggested that African American speakers have low fundamental frequencies and flexible ranges and tend to use the higher end of the range more flexibly than the lower end (Wheat and Hudson 1988; Hollien and Malcik 1962; Hudson and Holbrook 1981; Ducote 1983). These findings seem to be corroborated by studies of the oral traditions used by African American speakers (Tarone 1973; Smitherman 1975; Pitts 1989). Intonation features of speakers of African American English include (1) the use of a wide range of pitches that frequently shift to falsetto register when points of emphasis are being made, (2) frequent use of level and rising final pitch contours on all sentence types, (3) use of falling pitch contours (demanding format) in formal and threatening contexts to express yes-and-no questions (which in Standard English requires a rising intonation), and (4) use of nonfinal intonation contours to express conditionality in a sentence (Tarone 1973).

The oral traditions that affect the use of voice in African American English have been identified in the linguistic literature (Smitherman 1975; Pitts 1989). Smitherman (1975) discussed sacred and secular discourse modes used in African American English. Both types of discourse capture the vocal habits of speakers of African American English and are vestiges of African cultural-linguistic styles. The speech patterns that are found in secular and sacred discourse have accompanying vocal traits. Among them are the low moaning and groaning ("mm...hmm") vocal postures that are used in the call-and-response pattern and the loud whispered and raspy affirmation ("yessuh") in the same pattern. Other examples are rhythmic, loud, and sometimes shrieking falsetto that is used in the "songified" pattern and vocal strain from the loud, rapid, and quickly varying vocal tones in the more secular styles of the playing the dozens, signifyin', or the toast (Smitherman 1975).

Pitts (1989) verifies these vocal traits in his observations of West African poetics in the style of preaching used by African American ministers. He suggests that the voice as used by African American preachers has a West African heritage. The preacher's style includes use of vocal harshness; varying speech rate, from rapid to slowed and chanting; use of loud falsetto shrieks; rushing many syllables into a single breath group; loud gasping inhalations; and inhalatory stridors (Pitts 1989). Both secular and sacred oral traditions of African Americans preserve the cultural-linguistic heritage. The examination of African American English suggests that the voice is used as a cultural-linguistic device, and that the voice plays a role in cultural transmission.

Obviously, the oral traditions of other minority groups should be examined as well. For instance, it is interesting to observe the vestiges of tonality in Asian groups and how this affects the use of the voice and voice production.

Research Needs

The literature reviewed in this chapter indicates that anatomic, acoustic, physiologic, and perceptible differences exist for the speech and voice of blacks and whites. It is unclear exactly which parameters within each of these studies make the differences and whether a combination of these parameters is critical to racial or ethnic identification in speech and voice. It is clear that laryngeal dynamics are affected by the subglottic and supraglottic systems (Zajac 1990) and that these systems work synergistically to produce a voice that is unique to individuals and their group affinity. Research of the anatomic support for racial differences should review more than the weight of the larynges. It should also consider the body type configurations that affect voice, including weight, height, thoracic cavity, and oropharyngeal and nasopharyngeal cavity construction. These areas of study indicate how the vocal source is structured to coordinate with the subglottal and supraglottal systems. Physiologic research needs to examine the pulmonary functions to determine how racial differences in volumes and capacities affect the voice production system. Additionally, physiologic studies of the supralaryngeal systems as they couple with the subglottic and glottic systems should be conducted to determine any differences between the races. Research of the acoustic support for racial differences needs to examine fundamental frequency across all age groups to determine which ranges fall within or outside the norm. Moreover, acoustic research needs to examine the concept of pitch contouring, as habitually used by differing racial and ethnic groups. Such examination would provide insight to the source and filter characteristics that coordinate to make the voice identifiable to a racial or ethnic group. Research of the perceptual support for racial differences needs to examine intraracial and interracial factors (e.g., cultural-linguistic biases) that affect the listener's perception of speech and voice. Moreover, perceptual research needs to examine how perceptions of rate, rhythm, stress, prosody, and intonation influence judgment of racial or ethnic affinity of a speaker. Obviously, all these research efforts need to be conducted across all minority groups in the United States and internationally.

The Role of the Speech-Language Pathologist in Prevention and Assessment

Prevention

The projected changes in the composition of the American population in the next few decades require that speech-language pathologists join other health care professionals in rethinking their assumptions about the consumers of health services. To assist in this effort, the literature reviewed in this chapter attempts to identify evidence of real and probable service needs of minority populations in the United States as related to voice and its disorders. The incidence, mortality, and survival information suggests that disease and hereditary conditions that affect the voice and its functioning are variously found among the minority groups. Moreover, it appears that disease susceptibility may have a racial basis, which is evidenced by the incidence of nasopharyngeal cancer among certain groups in the Asian population. The ethnographic information suggests that different ethnic groups may have anatomic, physiologic, and acquired cultural traits that work singularly or interactively to affect the use of the voice. It is the speech-language pathologist's task to be knowledgeable about the predisposition to voice disorders for these groups. Furthermore, the speech-language pathologist must be prepared to join other health care professionals in prevention programs for racially, ethnically, and culturally diverse populations. Marge (1984) discusses three levels of prevention and defines them as follows:

1. "Primary prevention is the elimination or inhibition of the onset and development of a communicative disorder by altering susceptibility or reducing exposure for susceptible persons."
2. "Secondary prevention is the early detection and treatment of communicative disorders. Early detection may lead to the elimination of the disorder or the retardation of the disorder's progress."
3. "Tertiary prevention is the reduction of a disability by attempting to restore effective functioning. The major approach is rehabilitation of the disabled individual who has realized some residual problem as a result of the disorder."

These prevention roles have been adopted by the American Speech-Language-Hearing Association as best-practice procedures for professionals (Marge 1984). Moreover, the American Speech-Language-Hearing Association indicated that taking on the professional role of preventionist means (1) playing a "significant role in the development and application of prevention strategies...(2) expand[ing] research into the causes of communication disorders and variables which influence the development and maintenance of communication abilities...[, and] (3) educating colleagues and the general public relative to personal wellness strategies as they relate to prevention" (ASHA 1988).

Predisposers and precipitants of voice pathology that are preventable include vocal abuse, upper respiratory infections, allergies, airborne irritants, smoking, trauma and injury, faulty respiration (due to allergies, infections, and emphysema), substance abuse, and some genetic disorders (Marge 1984). Clearly, a need exists for additional epidemiologic data to determine whether certain minority groups are more susceptible than others to predisposing and precipitating conditions affecting voice. Moreover, a need exists for information on the incidence (rate of new occurrences) and prevalence (total proportion of cases in the population at any one time) of vocal pathologies within the minority groups.

Despite the need for additional research, the speech-language pathologist must use the information that is currently available to develop prevention strategies that are culturally sensitive and relevant. Several prevention strategies are already used by health professionals and can be adapted for multicultural groups presenting voice-related disorders (Marge 1984). They include the following:

- Prenatal care (as related to cleft palate especially)
- Genetic counseling (as related to cleft palate)
- Mass screenings and early identification (across the ages for any voice related concern)
- Early intervention (as related to vocal abuse)
- Public education about vocal hygiene and voice-related disorders (across the ages)
- Advocacy and political action on all issues related to health care that affect the voice and its functioning (including environmental quality control and government programs to ensure that minority groups have the resources to effectively prevent and reduce debilitating conditions that lead to voice disorders)

Critical to the success of these prevention strategies is their employment in a culturally sensitive manner. It must be remembered that each cultural minority group is heterogeneous and that subgroupings exist within each basic group. Thus, it behooves the speech-language pathologist to be always cognizant that the clientele within these groups do not "look alike" nor are they "all the same." The speech-language pathologist needs to engage in community-based prevention programs, which means distributing materials to targeted groups through community organizations (e.g., churches, public and private community schools, and social groups). The language used in all public awareness programs must be appropriate to the targeted population (ASHA 1985). The speech-language pathologist must be sensitive to the cultural traits (e.g., thoughts, beliefs, traditions, mores, teachings) that affect the interactions of the various groups with the health professional.

The Secretary's Report on Black and Minority Health attempted to identify "social characteristics" of the minority groups (U.S. Department of Health and Human Services 1985). A recurrent theme across all groups was the strength of family ties. Health beliefs and comfort with health professionals varied among the groups. To some degree all groups showed underuse of health-related services. This underuse appears to have been caused by a preference for non-Western medical treatments and lack of economic access. The preferences for non-Western health care included folk medicine for African Americans; the healing force of family for Hispanics; herbalists, acupuncturists, and traditional non-Western medicine for Asians and Pacific Americans; and medicine men for American Indians. These traditional patterns of health care affect beliefs about the usefulness of health professionals in meeting health care needs.

In addition to beliefs and levels of comfort with health professionals, some members of ethnic or racial minority groups have reduced economic capability, which also acts as a deterrent to health care use. The Institute of Medicine (1989), in its study of allied health professions, noted the following:

- Minorities are more likely than whites to lack health care insurance, and they consistently report greater difficulty than whites in gaining access to medical care.
- Twenty-six percent of Hispanics have no medical coverage compared with 9% of whites and 18% of blacks.

These differences between whites and minorities in access to health care are reflected in health care use rates. Twenty percent of blacks and 19% of Hispanics indicate that they have no usual source of medical care, compared with 13% of whites. Between 1978 and 1980, the percentage of people 4–16 years old who had never received dental care was higher among Mexican Americans (30.7) than among blacks (22.3) or whites (9.7). Similarly, the percentage of individuals with no physician contact was higher among Mexican Americans (33.1) than among other Hispanics (3.9), blacks (23.8), or whites (20.4).

The roles and responsibilities of prevention, in light of addressing the needs of minority groups, present both opportunity and challenge to the profession of speech-language pathology. Speech-language pathologists are encouraged to familiarize themselves with the voice-related health problems of multicultural populations and with the cultural deterrents to health care use. These vital pieces of knowledge make the work of prevention easier.

Assessment

It is important for the speech-language pathologist to understand normal voice functioning before embarking on assessment techniques of the abnormal voice. The voice of humans has often been likened to musical instruments. The organs of the voice are similar to wind instruments. To make pitch adjustments the larynx follows patterns found in string instruments. In many cultures the melodic patterns of voice may be considered music to the ear (e.g., the songified pattern of African American English or the chant of the African American preacher). No one definition of what constitutes a normal voice is accepted by all. In this chapter, voice is considered as unique as a person's eyebrow pattern, fingerprint, or smile. It is influenced by race, sex, age, socioeconomic standing, emotional swings, and situational moments. Normal voice is also defined as that which is accepted by the listener and the native speaking environment. Physiologically, the normal voice can be affected by viral infections, benign or malignant tumors, neurologic impairments, and psychological factors. Currently, we have little guidance from research to direct our efforts to address the factors that affect normalcy judgments as made by various racial or ethnic groups (DeJarnette 1996). The speech-language pathologist must therefore interview the patient to determine what is aesthetically pleasing. In doing so, he or she should use questions such as the following (DeJarnette 1996):

- What voice pitch do you believe would best represent you to family, everyday community, religious community, and work community?
- What loudness level (soft or loud) do you believe would work best for your voice with family, everyday community, religious community, and work community?
- What vocal tone (smooth, breathy, or harsh and rough) do you believe would work best for your voice with family, everyday community, religious community, and work community?
- What degree of versatility do you believe would work best for your voice with family, everyday community, religious community, and work community?

Responses to these questions allow the speech-language pathologist to search for a culturally appropriate voice that fits with the client's best voice production capability. Moreover, these questions can provide important insight as the speech-language pathologist tries to identify and decrease abuse and misuse vocal behaviors. Having the client identify cultural models of voice can enhance the clinical relationship and provide a sense of ownership and commitment to the therapeutic process.

When assessing voice disorders among multicultural populations, the speech-language pathologist should first consider the patient's point of view. Many minority groups, if they accept professional intervention at all, approach clinical diagnosis and intervention cautiously. Some are hesitant to trust professionals who have a cultural perspective that differs from their own; this may be based on past experience or the perception that mainstream cultural values are used to judge capability and progress. Others may trust only certain professionals, such as doctors, believing that all others are pseudoprofessionals. Therefore, the speech-language pathologist should be prepared for the patient who approaches the diagnostic appointment with reticence. If the patient is a child, the speech-language pathologist should consider the anxiety level of the changes and parents. In all cases, the speech-language pathologist must be aware that the patient's attitudes can be influenced by age, source of the referral, family status, occupation, and understanding of his or her own voice. The clinician should remember that before clinical intervention begins, medical clearance is warranted. Achieving medical clearance can be affected by the client's experience or lack of experience in negotiating medical systems, the client's belief system regarding Euro-American medicine, or both. The speech-language pathologist, therefore, may need to assist the client with negotiating medical systems.

General Outline of Diagnostic Procedures

Before the diagnostic session, the speech-language pathologist needs to get a sense of the client's cultural point of view to know what clinical procedures the client sees as taboo (e.g., physical contact, direct eye contact). The speech-language pathologist uses perceptual and acoustic measures, when possible, to determine the patient's voice characteristics, the severity of the disorder, and the benefit that can be derived from therapy. Much of the data for making these determinations are based on findings from a monocultural source—that is, from mainstream speakers and voices. As noted above, there is a sparse database to inform the speech-language pathologist of multicultural factors to use in determining normal versus deviant voice in multicultural populations. However, a more client-centered approach can fill that knowledge gap at the present time.

A client-centered approach allows the speech pathologist to consider the notion that racial, ethnic, and cultural groups can present more risk for specific types of organic voice disorders (e.g., laryngeal, esophageal, and lung cancer in blacks and nasopharyngeal cancer in Asian populations). Moreover, a client-centered approach allows the speech pathologist to be informed by the patient regarding the cultural influences that affect voice production and voice intervention. Indeed, the diagnostic intake and interview provide opportunities for the speech-language pathologist to be client-centered. Much like the questions listed in "Assessment," above (DeJarnette 1996), the client should be asked to inform the speech-language pathologist of cultural beliefs or practices that might affect evaluation and intervention.

Good clinical practice should be informed by a client-centered approach. An assessment protocol should include at least (1) a description of the patient, including culturally relevant biographical information and observation of the client's physical presentation at the time of the diagnostic session; (2) the history of the disorder, including events in the patient's life that appear to be related to the problem; (3) a description of the speech mechanism and the characteristics of the voice (e.g., measures of fundamental frequency, optimum and habitual pitch, vocal range); (4) an audio or video recording during the interview and spontaneous voice sampling procedures; (5) the results of an indirect examination of the vocal cords; (6) a video fluoroscopic study (when appropriate); and (7) the patient's self-assessment of voice.

Although medical clearance must be ensured before intervention is initiated, the speech-language pathologist must not hesitate to inspect the patient's medical status for voice-related concerns. The speech-pathologist should explain all procedures thoroughly. He or she must secure the client's permission to touch the patient and conduct any physical examination. It is imperative that the speech-language pathologist conduct an examination of the vocal tract (i.e., respiratory tract, larynx, oro- and nasopharynx, and oral peripheral cavity), keeping in mind possible health and environmental conditions that affect various racial and ethnic groups. Knowledge of the vocal tract improves the speech-language pathologist's ability to communicate effectively with medical staff and to understand the patient's physical limitations and conditions. If the client's ethnic or cultural beliefs prohibit such an examination or physical contact, the speech-pathologist should explain the need and invite suggestions from the client about how to conduct the examination. For instance, significant others can be trained to position a client for clinical observation by the speech-pathologist; this should be accepted as a way to conduct the examination.

The diagnostician should exercise caution when using norms that are based on measures of predominantly white subjects because differences between majority and minority populations exist for anatomic, physiologic, acoustic, and perceptual parameters related to voice. As data accrue on these parameters in multicultural populations, these differences will be clarified, and norms will be generated that are more racially or culturally appropriate. It is exceedingly important for speech-language pathologists to keep this in mind as they prepare to provide services to minority populations. Care should be taken to investigate what is considered normal for each group and subgroup.

Examination of the External Vocal Tract

The speech-language pathologist's examination follows the audio or video recording of the patient. It should start with the external observation of the neck area and include palpation of the larynx and neck muscles. Notation should be made of the patient's breathing pattern and the resting position of the lips. The mobility of facial muscles, puckered lips, and protruded tongue should be noted. These procedures reveal general control and symmetry of the face. Clearly, facial muscles are not involved at the glottal level of voice production; however, their asymmetry can signal neurologic concerns. The speech-language pathologist must consider the research on the anatomic differences between races as such observations are made.

Examination of the Oral Pharynx

Attention should next be directed to the oropharynx. The symmetry, color, and condition of teeth should be observed. The protruded tongue and its mobility must be examined. Again, abnormal function could be indicative of neurologic concerns. Standard oral cancer assessment techniques should be followed that include palpation of the oral cavity. Note the coloration of mucosal lining and any edema, as these are important for future medical referrals. Note the movement of the velum when the patient produces the sound /a/ ("ah") or /e/ ("eh"). The soft palate should move upward and backward quickly and symmetrically bilaterally. If not, paralysis is suspected. If scars or any abnormality are observed in this structure, exploratory questions and medical consultation should be sought. The examination continues with viewing the faucial and pharyngeal regions. Scars are observed if tonsils have been removed. If the posterior wall of the pharynx slides laterally when an attempt is made to close the velopharyngeal valve, unilateral paralysis of the pharyngeal constrictor muscle is indicated.

Nasal passages should be observed during the production of a prolonged hum by occluding one ala of the nostril at a time. If partial or complete stoppages are present, attention to denasal voice quality should be noted. The patient should be questioned regarding allergies, colds, and injuries.

Examination of the Interior Larynx

The final phase of the examination is the interior larynx. The authors suggest that experience be gained in using the laryngeal mirror or the telescopic laryngeal scope. Medical staff normally complete fiberoptic, stroboscopic techniques. If the speech-language pathologist is not experienced in these techniques, he or she should at least be present during the medical examination. The function of the vocal cords during examination is pertinent to planning therapeutic techniques.

Observation of vocal cord color and size; movements in adduction and abduction; and the presence of symmetry, nodules, edema, and papillomas should all be noted. Photographs or video recordings can contribute to the rehabilitation plan.

Assessment and Intervention of Voice Disorders

The speech-language pathologist should be sensitive to the fear factor when approaching the assessment and intervention of a culturally diverse client with organic voice disorders. In addition, a thorough educational approach must be followed to ensure that the patient clearly understands the medical implications of the disorder.

It is not uncommon for an African American laryngectomee not to ask the doctor about his or her chances for survival, quality of life, or body hygiene techniques. This is why it is imperative that the speech-language pathologist be knowledgeable about the patient's disorder and be able to disseminate this knowledge at the patient's level of understanding.

The following steps are suggested for assessing vocal disorders such as nodules, polyps, paralysis, and alaryngeal voice:

1. Review all medical records—that is, operative reports, radiologic reports (including viewing of x-rays), pathology reports, and discharge summaries. It is imperative that the speech-language pathologist thoroughly understand all medical interventions. For example, the speech-language pathologist must recognize when a gastric pull-up procedure has been performed in addition to removal of the larynx.
2. Educate the patient about the disorder using graphs and video presentation. Verbal instructions should be accompanied by visual imagery.
3. Time is a critical factor in patient education, counseling, and therapeutic success. Often, the fact that the speech-language pathologist can offer extended time for discussion with the patient allows rapport and trust to develop, thus ensuring a positive therapeutic relationship.

An additional consideration that must be kept in mind is the patient's perception of what constitutes an aesthetically normal voice for his or her cultural community. As a way of determining what the client thinks is the ideal voice, he or she might be asked to provide models or recordings of voices from the cultural community that he or she would like to emulate. Additionally, the speech-pathologist can develop a library of voice recordings from various cultural backgrounds and allow the client to choose among them.

In terms of intervention strategies, the speech-language pathologist must be cognizant that a number of the voice-facilitating techniques can seem awkward, if not culturally inappropriate, to clients from various racial or ethnic backgrounds. For example, "chant talk," with its monotone presentation, may be awkward for the African American speaker who uses pitch and intonation shifts to express meaning and commitment, and it may be equally difficult for speakers of tonal-based languages (Asian-American speakers). Other techniques, such as head positioning, open-mouth approach, tongue protrusion, yawn and sigh, use of artificial laryngeal devices, and so on, can be perceived as obtrusive to cultural styles. Thus, the speech-language pathologist must explain the technique, determine the client's cultural comfort level with using the technique, and be prepared to make adaptations to the technique so that it fits the client's cultural style. Again, the speech-pathologist should check with the client about the usefulness of any intervention strategy in the client's cultural milieu. Moreover, the speech pathologist must be open to suggestions from the client about how to adapt a technique for greater usefulness

Conclusion

This chapter discusses the incidence of voice-related pathologies in minority groups in the United States; health issues related to voice dysfunction; ethnographic and racial factors related to voice; and the role of the speech-language pathologist in prevention, assessment, and intervention. A review of the literature concerning the epidemiology of voice-related pathologies in minority groups illuminates the need for increased research of the incidence and prevalence of causal factors leading to voice disorders and the types of voice disorders found among the minority populations in the United States. The available literature suggests that health risk factors are variously distributed among the minority groups in terms of their incidence and prevalence rates and their sex ratios. Among these risk factors are access to health care (Institute of Medicine 1989), occupational and daily living exposure to teratogens, substance abuse, and possible predispositions to certain disease processes that are the combined effect of biological inheritance and environmental conditions (U.S. Department of Health and Human Services 1985, 1986; National Center for Health Statistics 1991; Baquet, et al. 1991; Hargreaves, et al. 1989; Parnes 1990; Hung-Dhiu Ho 1982; Rice and Yu 1982; Williams 1975; Kalk and Kalk 1989; Blum 1982; Gee 1982). As in the case of carcinoma, the health risks tend to affect the entire vocal tract system and include respiratory and laryngeal and supralaryngeal resonatory systems. Moreover, health risks include disease and trauma effects on the endocrinologic system and on cerebrovascular functioning in as far as these affect voice production (National Center for Health Statistics 1991; Williams 1975; Kalk and Kalk 1989; Blum 1982; Gee 1982). Vocal pathologies can also have different patterns of distribution in terms of proportions and sex ratios across multicultural groups (Dobres, et al. 1990; Sayetta, et al. 1989; Vanderas 1987; Shaw, et al. 1991). Thus, speech-language pathologists need to ascertain the magnitude of the health risks and the incidence and prevalence rates of voice disorders among the various minority groups so that prevention, identification, diagnosis, and intervention can be effectively provided for these groups.

The delivery of appropriate, relevant, and quality voice care to multicultural groups is affected by the speech-language pathologist's knowledge of the racial, ethnographic, and cultural factors that affect voice production and use. This chapter makes the case that ethnographic implications exist for all parameters of study that provide a knowledge base of what voice is across the spectrum of the human continuum (Williams 1975; Boshoff 1945; Cole 1980; Awan and Mueller 1996; Wheat and Hudson 1988; Hollien and Malcik 1962; Hudson and Holbrook 1981; Fitch and Holbrook 1970; Ducote 1983; Hon Jo and Isshiki 1980; Dickens and Sawyer 1962; Irwin 1977; Lass, et al. 1978, 1979; Baker 1982; Saniga, et al. 1984; Walton and Orlikoff 1994). These parameters include anatomic, physiologic, acoustic, perceptual, cultural, and linguistic realms of study. It is suggested that each avenue of study has the potential to expose knowledge about the "differences that make a difference" in the production and perception of voice in racially, ethnically, and culturally differing groups. For the speech-language pathologist, the acquisition of knowledge about the ethnocultural differences between groups is as critical to quality care as is knowledge of the health risks. Developing culturally sensitive, client-centered, and relevant approaches to voice service delivery permits speech-language pathologists to fulfill their roles and responsibilities as preventionists, diagnosticians, and interventionists in working with multicultural groups.

References

ASHA Committee on Prevention of Speech, Language and Hearing Disorders. (1988). Prevention of communication disorders. Position statement. *ASHA, 30(3)*, 90.

ASHA Committee on the Status of Racial Minorities. (1985). Clinical management of communicatively handicapped minority language populations. *ASHA, 27(6)*, 29–32.

Atal, D.S. (1968). *Automatic speaker recognition based on pitch contours.* Ph.D. dissertation, Polytechnic University.

Atkinson, J.E. (1973). *Aspects of intonation in speech: Implications from an experimental study of fundamental frequency.* Ph.D. dissertation, University of Connecticut.

Awan, S.N., & Mueller, P.B. (1996). Speaking fundamental frequency characteristics of white, African American, and Hispanic kindergartners. *Journal of Speech and Hearing Research, 39*, 573–577.

Bagchi, N., Brown, T.R., & Parish, R.F. (1990). Thyroid dysfunction in adults over age 55 years: A study in an urban U.S. community. *Archives of Internal Medicine, 150(4),* 785–787.

Baker, L.L. (1982). *Speech and voice characteristics of aging Afro-American female and male speakers based on listener perceived age estimates.* Ph.D. dissertation, Wichita State University.

Baquet, C.R., Horm, J.W., Gibbs, T., & Grenwald, P. (1991). Socioeconomic factors and cancer incidence among African Americans and whites. *Journal of the National Cancer Institute, 83(8),* 551–557.

Blum, A.S. (1982, May). *Thyrotoxicosis among the Chinese.* Presented at the Conference on Health Problems Related to Chinese in America, San Francisco.

Boshoff, P. (1945). The anatomy of the South African Negro larynges. *South African Journal of Medical Sciences, 10,* 35–50.

Centers for Disease Control. (1991). Surveillance summaries. *Morbidity and Mortality Weekly Report, 40,* 3.

Centers for Disease Control. (1996). Cigarette smoking among adults—United States, 1994. *Morbidity and Mortality Weekly Report, 45,* 588–591.

Chen, H. (1982, May). *Chronic persistent cough in Chinese in America.* Presented at the Conference on Health Problems Related to Chinese in America, San Francisco.

Cole, L. (1980). Blacks with orofacial clefts: The state of the dilemma. *ASHA, 22,* 557–560.

DeJarnette, G. (1996, December). *Multicultural issues in voice care: Focus on the African American voice.* Paper presented at meeting of the American Speech-Language-Hearing Association, Seattle.

Dickens, M., & Sawyer, G.M. (1962). An experimental comparison of vocal quality among mixed groups of whites and Negroes. *Southern Speech Journal, 18,* 178–185.

Dobres, R., Lee, L., Stemple, J.C., et al. (1990). Description of laryngeal pathologies in children evaluated by otolaryngologists. *Journal of Speech and Hearing Disorders, 55(3),* 526–532.

Ducote, C.A. (1983). *A study of the reading and speaking fundamental frequency of aging black adults.* Ph.D. dissertation, Louisiana State University.

Fitch, J.L., & Holbrook, A. (1970). Modal vocal fundamental frequency of young adults. *Archives of Otolaryngology, 92,* 379–382.

Gee, P. (1982, May). *Thyrotoxic periodic paralysis: An unusual presentation of thyrotoxicosis in Oriental men.* Presented at the Conference on Health Problems Related to Chinese in America, San Francisco.

Hargreaves, M.K., Baquet, C., & Gamshadzahi, A. (1989). Diet, nutritional status and cancer risk in American African Americans. *Nutrition and Cancer, 12(1)*, 1–28.

Hollien, H., & Malcik, E. (1962). Adolescent voice change in southern Negro males. *Speech Monographs, 29(1)*, 53–58.

Hon Jo, I., & Isshiki, N. (1980). Laryngoscopic and voice characteristics of aged persons. *Archives of Otolaryngology, 106*, 149–150.

Hudson, A.I., & Holbrook, A. (1981). A study of the reading fundamental vocal frequency of young African American adults. *Journal of Speech and Hearing Research, 24*, 197–201.

Hung-Dhiu Ho, J. (1982, May). *Etiology and control of nasopharyngeal carcinoma (NPC)*. Presented at the Conference on Health Problems Related to the Chinese in America, San Francisco.

Institute of Medicine Committee to Study the Role of Allied Health Personnel. (1989). *Allied health services avoiding crises*. Washington, DC: National Academy Press.

Irwin, R.B. (1977). Judgments of vocal quality, speech fluency and confidence of African American and white speakers. *Language and Speech, 20(3)*, 261–266.

Kalk, W.J., & Kalk, J. (1989). Incidence and causes of hyperthyroidism in African Americans. *South African Medical Journal, 75(3)*, 114–117.

Larimer, G.S., Beatty, E., & Broadus, A.C. (1988). Indirect assessment of interracial prejudices. *Journal of Black Psychology, 14(2)*, 47–56.

Lass, N.J., Mertz, P.J., & Kimmel, K.L. (1978). The effect of temporal speech alterations on speaker race and sex identifications. *Language and Speech, 21*, 279–290.

Lass, N.J., Tecca, J.E., Mancuso, R.A., & Black, W.I. (1979). The effect of phonetic complexity on speaker race and sex identifications. *Journal of Phonetics, 7*, 105–118.

Lass, N.J., Trapp, D.S., Baldwin, M.K., et al. (1982). Effect of vocal disguise on judgments of speakers' sex and race. *Perceptual and Motor Skills, 54(3)*, 1235–1240.

Marge, M. (1984). The prevention of communication disorders. *ASHA, 26*, 35–38.

Miller, B.A., Kolonel, L.N., Bernstein, L., et al. (1996). *Racial/ethnic patterns of cancer in the United States, 1988–1992*. Washington, DC: National Institutes of Health, National Cancer Institute (NIH Pub. No. 96-4104).

National Center for Health Statistics. (1991). *Health United States, 1990*. Washington, DC: U.S. Government Printing Office (Department of Health and Human Services Pub No. PH591-1232).

Page, H.S., & Asire, A.J. (1985). *Cancer rates and risks (3rd ed.).* Washington, DC: National Institute of Health (DHHS Pub No. 85-691).

Parnes, S.M. (1990). Asbestos and cancer of the larynx: Is there a relationship? *Laryngoscope, 100(3),* 254–261.

Pittam, J. (1987). The long-term spectral measurement of voice quality as a social and personality marker: A review. *Language and Speech, 30,* 1–12.

Pittam, J., & Gallois, C. (1986). Predicting impressions of speakers from voice quality: Acoustic and perceptual measures. *Journal of Language and Social Psychology, 5(4),* 233–237.

Pitts, W. (1989). West African poetics in the African American preaching style. *American Speech, 64(2),* 137–149.

Rice, D.P., & Yu, E. (1982, May). *Health of the Chinese in America.* Presented at the Conference on Health Problems Related to the Chinese in America, San Francisco.

Ryalls, J., Zipper, A., & Baldauff, P. (1997). A preliminary investigation of the effects of gender and race on voice onset time. *Journal of Speech, Language, and Hearing Research, 40,* 642.

Saniga, R.D., Carlin, M.F., & Farrell, S.C. (1984). Perception of fry register in African American dialect and standard dialect English speakers. *Perceptual and Motor Skills, 59(3),* 885–886.

Sayetta, R.B., Weinrich, M.C., & Coston, G.N. (1989). Incidence and prevalence of cleft lip and palate: What we think we know. *Cleft Palate Journal, 26(3),* 242–247.

Shaw, G.M., Croen, L.A., & Curry, C.J. (1991). Isolated oral cleft malformations: Associations with maternal and infant characteristics in a California population. *Teratology, 43(3),* 225–228.

Smitherman, G. (1975). *Black language and culture: Sounds of soul.* New York: Harper & Row.

Tarone, E.E. (1973). Aspects of intonation in Black English. *American Speech, 48(1–2),* 29–36.

U.S. Department of Health and Human Services. (1985). *Report of the Secretary's Task Force on Black and Minority Health (Vol. 1.): Executive summary.* Washington, DC: Government Printing Office (Department of Health and Human Services, Pub No. 491-313/44706).

U.S. Department of Health and Human Services. (1986). *Report of the Secretary's Task Force on Black and Minority Health (Vol. 2): Cancer.* Washington, DC: Government Printing Office (Department of Health and Human Services, Pub No. 621-605:00171).

van Dommelen, W.A. (1987). The contribution of speech, rhythm and pitch to speaker recognition. *Language and Speech, 30(4),* 325–338.

Vandepitte, S. (1989). A pragmatic function of intonation: Tone and cognitive environment. *Lingua, 79(4),* 265–297.

Vanderas, A.P. (1987). Incidence of cleft lip, cleft palate, and cleft lip and palate among races: A review. *Cleft Palate Journal, 24(3),* 216–225.

Walton, J.H., & Orlikoff, R.F. (1994). Speaker race identification from acoustic cues in the vocal signal. *Journal of Speech and Hearing Research, 37(4),* 738–745.

Wheat, M.C., & Hudson, A.I. (1988). Spontaneous speaking fundamental of 6-year-old African American children. *Journal of Speech and Hearing Research, 31,* 723–725.

Williams, R.A. (1975). *Textbook of black-related diseases.* New York: McGraw-Hill.

Wilson, D.K. (1979). *Voice problems of children (2nd ed.).* Baltimore: Williams and Wilkins.

Wright, C.R., Motley, M.T., & Phelan, J.G. (1976). Discrimination of dialect from temporal patterns of the speech signal. *Psychology Report, 38(2),* 1059–1067.

Yang, P.C., Thomas, D.B., & Davis, S. (1989). Differences in the sex ratio of laryngeal cancer incidence rates by anatomic subsite. *Journal of Clinical Epidemiology, 42(8),* 755–758.

Zajac, D.J. (1990). *Effects of respiratory effort and induced oronasal coupling on laryngeal aerodynamics and oscillatory behaviors.* Ph.D. dissertation, University of Pittsburgh, 1990.

10

Neurogenic Disorders in Adult and Pediatric Populations

Gloriajean L. Wallace

Neurologically based medical problems can affect anyone, regardless of race or ethnicity. According to the available medical literature, however, certain causes of neurologic impairment affect individuals from minority groups to a greater extent than expected given their overall representation in the population at large. These causes include stroke, acquired immunodeficiency syndrome (AIDS), violent crimes that can result in traumatic brain injury (TBI), substance abuse or exposure to drugs, and lupus. In addition, it has been speculated that dementing disease is prevalent among aging minority groups because of specific dietary and hereditary factors. Prolonged exposure to environmental toxins has also been attributed to dementia in aging populations and to language and learning difficulties in pediatric populations. All of these causes of neurologic impairment are associated with disorders that are of interest to the speech-language pathologist. Because minorities are at high risk for neurologically based impairments, it is imperative for neurogenics specialists to acquire the necessary knowledge base and clinical skills to provide quality care to individuals from culturally and linguistically diverse backgrounds. To that end, this chapter presents information about risk factors for neurogenic communication disorders and dysphagia, factors that can have an impact on rehabilitation and general clinical management issues. These topics are discussed as they relate to culturally and linguistically diverse populations, an area of study that is referred to as multicultural neurogenics (Wallace 1996; Wallace 1997). Multicultural neurogenics is discussed here in the context of the five racial and ethnic groups that are recognized by the U.S. government as the most prominent U.S. minority groups. The information presented in this chapter is applicable to other populations. An additional point to note is that African Americans are currently the largest U.S. minority group. For this reason, there is more information available about health-related issues for African Americans than for any other U.S. minority group. There is a great need for additional research to explore health issues that affect other groups, including migrant workers (Rust 1990) and residents of rural U.S. territories (Wallace 1993).

Principal Causes of Neurologic Impairment

The fact that there are major medical risks for neurologic impairment among minority populations suggests that race and ethnicity influence the distribution of disorders on the clinical caseload. For this reason, clinicians should have an understanding of the types of neurologic disorders that are prevalent among populations within the geographical region of their clinical practice. This is helpful in preparing clinicians for providing rehabilitation services in needed specialty areas, based on problems for which the patients are at greatest risk. Likewise, it is helpful for speech-language pathologists to know about populations most likely to be affected by the disorder(s) within their specialty area(s). This knowledge enables the clinician to prepare for cultural and linguistic issues that can have a unique impact on patient care.

Stroke

The leading cause of neurologic impairment among many individuals from the multicultural community (especially blacks, Hispanics, and certain Asian and Pacific-American groups) is stroke (American Heart Association 1996; Moss 1993; Council on Scientific Affairs, American Medical Association 1991; Report of the Secretary's Task Force on Black and Minority Health 1985; Yatsu 1991; Yano, et al. 1985). Primary risk factors for stroke in these minority groups include hypertension, arteriosclerosis, diabetes, sickle cell anemia, and substance abuse (including smoking).

Hypertension

Hypertension is a leading cause of stroke in minority populations, particularly in black populations. Numerous studies report a prevalence of hypertension among blacks, which has been reported to affect approximately 28% of black adults as compared with 17% of white adults (Caplan, et al. 1986; Berkson, et al. 1980; Hypertension Detection and Follow-up Program Cooperative Group 1977). Advanced hypertension is five times more common in blacks, who develop hypertension at an earlier age than whites (Kenton 1991). Minorities do not receive antihypertensive drug therapy to the same extent as the white population (Kenton 1991). Limited access due to the cost of drugs and lack of continuity of care, early intervention, and education about drug effects and benefits have been cited as reasons for the disparity in drug treatment for hypertension among blacks.

The issue of hypertension is also a significant one for children from the multicultural community. Black, Pacific islander (e.g., Samoan), American Indian, Hispanic, and Asian children have all been shown to be at risk for increased blood pressure at an early age (Berenson 1995; Hohn, et al. 1994; Murphy, et al. 1994; Murphy and McGarvey 1994; Broderick, et al. 1993; Botash, et al. 1992). The early onset of high blood pressure and the fact that hypertension is often undetected in younger minority populations place children at great risk for more serious hypertension-related medical problems later in life.

Hypertension often leads to hemorrhagic stroke because of a combination of factors, including elevated arterial pressure, the concomitant development of microaneurysms, and the arteriosclerotic weakening of blood vessels (Singleton and Johnson 1993). Hypertensive brain hemorrhaging results in blood leakage into the subarachnoid space via the ventricular system. As bleeding progresses, adjacent neural tissue compresses, which can cause additional neurologic impairment. Subsequent compression of brain stem areas that are important for the regulation of heart rate and breathing frequently occurs in this type of stroke, which results in coma and death. High mortality after hemorrhagic stroke can also result from individuals not being hospitalized or seen by specialists after illness. The underuse of health care services by minorities (Sacco, et al. 1991) may contribute to the occurrence of repeated strokes, which can result in severe aphasia or multi-infarct dementia.

In addition to hemorrhagic stroke, hypertension can also result in thrombotic and embolic stroke. This occurs because of the thickening and narrowing of the inner arterial walls, which increase the risk of small blood clot formation.

Arteriosclerosis

Arteriosclerosis, associated with high serum cholesterol levels, is a great contributor to stroke among minorities. The consumption of foods that are high in fat and salt content (e.g., pork as a main dish and pork as a major source of seasoning for vegetables) is perhaps the greatest reason for this problem (McGarry, et al. 1985). Arteriosclerosis causes changes in the elasticity of the inner lining of blood vessels and causes blood-vessel constriction. Arteriosclerosis can result in a full-blown stroke in instances where the blood vessels becomes totally blocked.

Minority children are at risk for high cholesterol levels due to heredi-tary and dietary factors. High cholesterol levels contribute to the develop-ment of arteriosclerosis and therefore increase the likelihood of stroke with advancing age.

Diabetes

Diabetes is another risk factor for stroke that is pervasive in the multicultural community (Wallace 1996). Diabetes is a hereditary disease. Risk factors for diabetes include a positive family history of diabetes, race and ethnicity (especially blacks, Mexican Americans, Native Americans, and Asian Americans), and obesity (American Diabetes Association 1997).

There are two types of diabetes: type I (insulin-dependent diabetes) and type II (non–insulin-dependent diabetes) (Time Life Medical 1996). In dia-betes type I, the body is unable to produce insulin. The food that is eaten is normally broken down into simple sugars, such as glucose, which is the source of energy for the body's cells. In diabetes type I, the body has trouble producing insulin. Insulin facilitates the process of glucose entry from the blood into the body's cells (where it can be stored or changed into energy). If the body does not produce insulin, glucose is unable to enter the body's cells, and the individual is unable to use food to produce energy. Diabetes type I is generally diagnosed in children and young adults.

In diabetes type II, which is the most common type of diabetes among minority populations and is generally diagnosed in adulthood, insulin can be produced in the body. The insulin that is produced, however, is ineffective in facilitating the disbursement of glucose to the body's cells. As a result, in diabetes type II, the body has difficulty using the glucose from food to pro-duce energy for the body. Instead of glucose facilitating the production of energy for the body's cells, in diabetes type II, the glucose remains in the blood and produces an abnormally high blood glucose level. Diabetes is a risk factor for stroke because it causes vascular changes that can lead to stroke. Blacks are 1.6 times more likely to incur type II diabetes than the population at large (American Diabetes Association 1992). More than 2 mil-lion blacks are affected by this disease (nearly 6% of all black men and 8% of all black women) (American Diabetes Association 1992). The prevalence of type II diabetes is also high among Hispanics, who are more than 55% more likely to incur diabetes than the population at large (American Diabetes Association 1992). An estimated 2.5 million Hispanics (or one in every 10) living in the United States have diabetes (American Diabetes Association 1992). The incidence of type II diabetes is also high among the American Indian population, who are 10 times more likely to incur diabetes than the general population (Time Life Medical 1996). Asian Americans are also at risk for diabetes type II (American Diabetes Association 1997). Because of the close association between diabetes type II and family history, minority children and others who are at risk for diabetes should be provided with information about how to reduce the risks for developing diabetes. Reducing the risks for and effects of diabetes in minority populations can be accomplished by implementing healthy lifestyles at an early age, including nutritious diet, proper exercise, and low stress.

Sickle Cell Anemia

Sickle cell anemia is another cause of stroke that disproportionately affects certain segments of the multicultural population (Anson, et al. 1992; Adams, et al. 1988). This is particularly true for people of African and Mediterranean ancestry (Barnhart, et al. 1974; Johnson and El-Hazmi 1984; Platt, et al. 1994; Prohovnik, et al. 1989) and those who unknowingly have traces of this ancestry. In blacks, sickle cell anemia has been reported to affect as many as 190 per 100,000 children younger than 16 years of age (Johnson and El-Hazmi 1984).

Sickle cell anemia is an inherited disease that is caused by a flaw in the structure of the hemoglobin molecule (a complex oxygen-carrying protein in the red blood cells) (Whitten 1973). *Sickle-cell disease* refers to the medical problem that results when an individual is homozygous with the sickle cell gene (meaning that they inherited the sickle cell gene from both parents and are symptomatic). *Sickle cell trait* is used to describe an individual who is heterozygous with the sickle cell gene (meaning he or she inherited the sickle cell gene from only one parent and is likely to be symptom free). Although individuals with sickle cell trait are symptom free, they are carriers of the disease and can pass the gene to their offspring.

For individuals with sickle-cell disease, the structure of the hemoglobin molecules is abnormal, which causes the red blood cells to take on an elongated and sickle-like shape. The sickle shape of the red blood cells makes it difficult for them to pass through small blood vessels. As a result, areas of the brain and other organs that are supplied by small blood vessels do not receive oxygen, which can result in stroke.

Other serious health problems that can occur as a result of sickle cell anemia include (1) physical weakness, (2) poor physical development, (3) pneumonia, (4) paralysis, (5) kidney failure, (6) enlargement of the spleen, (7) abdominal pain, (8) rheumatism, (9) heart failure, and (10) impaired mental functioning. Sickle cell anemia can also cause lowered resistance to infections, which may cause neurologic impairment. Meningitis, for instance, has been reported to occur to a greater extent among individuals with sickle-cell disease than among others (Davies 1989).

Language and learning impairments are often associated with children who have sickle cell anemia. These impairments can be caused by stroke or by the cumulative effects of multiple transient ischemic attacks (Abboud, et al. 1996; Lane 1996; Moser, et al. 1996). In addition, children with sickle-cell disease may miss a significant amount of school because of medically related conditions, which puts them behind academically and further exacerbates the challenges they face with academic achievement.

Cocaine Use

The abuse of "crack" cocaine is a problem of disproportionate magnitude in inner-city areas that are often densely populated by minorities. The prevalence of crack cocaine and other drug abuse within inner-city communities has been attributed to despair poverty and the easy accessibility of drugs in the community. Because crack (the inhaled form of cocaine) is a vasoconstrictor, abuse of this drug places the user at risk for stroke (Brust 1993; Kaku and Lowenstein 1990; Wallach 1989; Levine, et al. 1990; Levine, et al. 1987; Mody, et al. 1988).

The use of crack cocaine by pregnant women places the unborn child at risk for medical problems because the drug can cross the placenta barrier. Prenatal exposure to crack cocaine can cause stroke in utero and, if the fetus survives to birth, can contribute to later communication and learning challenges (Bender, et al. 1995; Eyler and Behnke 1995; Hurt, et al. 1995). Even after birth, children may continue to be at risk for the negative effects of drugs as a result of second-hand smoke exposure from inhaled crack smoke. The effects of abuse, neglect, and an aberrant lifestyle (often associated with illicit drug use) (Black, et al. 1994; Hawley, et al. 1995) are additional risk factors for communication and learning challenges in the pediatric drug-exposed population.

Tobacco Smoking

Smoking is a practice that is prevalent in minority communities. Although smoking is not generally viewed as "substance abuse" by the general public, it is viewed as such by the American Lung Association (American Lung Association 1997). The effects of both direct smoking and second-hand smoke exposure have been documented to cause deleterious effects on health (American Lung Association 1997). Smoking can result in blood vessel changes that lead to cardiovascular disease and stroke.

The prevalence of smoking is highest among American Indians and Alaskan Natives (38.7%), next highest among blacks (26%) and whites (25.4%), and lowest among Asians and Pacific islanders (18.2%). Hispanics are less likely to be smokers (20.4%) than non-Hispanic white and black

Americans (American Lung Association 1997). Minority children who smoke often begin smoking at a very young age. For this reason, the prolonged effects of smoking can have serious negative effects on health by the time they reach adulthood.

Some Afterthoughts About Stroke
It is of interest to note that children from diverse racial and ethnic backgrounds are at risk for incurring stroke at a young age and for developing stroke later in life because of hereditary factors (e.g., sickle cell anemia, hypertension, and diabetes) and because of the early effects of nonhealthy lifestyles (e.g., exposure to cocaine and other drugs, exposure to environmental toxins, consumption of foods high in cholesterol, and smoking). Also of interest is the observation that some researchers have reported differences in components of the vascular system (and ultimately the brain) that are affected by stroke when comparisons are made across nonwhite and white populations (Heyman, et al. 1972; Heyden, et al. 1970; Gorelick, et al. 1984; Gorelick, et al. 1985). These data suggest that there may be important medical and behavioral differences in the characteristics of stroke across diverse populations. The relationship between stroke patterns and patient profiles and prognosis for return to functional lifestyle have not been investigated in minority populations.

Traumatic Brain Injury
Although there are only a few published studies addressing the topic of TBI in minority populations, it is likely that TBI is a significant problem given the high rate of documented homicide and nonfatal violence that occurs in urban areas (U.S. Department of Health and Human Services 1986; Sewell, et al. 1989). Homicide is, in fact, a major cause of premature death in the United States and is recognized as the largest single killer of young (younger than age 18 years) black men (Cornwell, et al. 1995; Laraque, et al. 1995; Centers for Disease Control 1995). Homicide is often preceded by a pattern of nonfatal aggravated assault that entails physical injury, which requires medical treatment beyond first aid and can include TBI.

Although violence is a likely factor relating to the occurrence of TBI in inner-city minority populations, nonviolent causes of TBI occur to an equal extent for white and nonwhite individuals in the middle socioeconomic status categories and above. Some investigators have compared figures for the occurrence and causes of TBI among suburban blacks and whites (Whitman, et al. 1974). In both populations, the most common causes of TBI were motor vehicle accidents for middle age groups (16–44 years of age) and falls for the older groups (older than 44 years of age).

Acquired Immunodeficiency Syndrome

AIDS, first recognized and described in 1981, is typically associated with a homosexual lifestyle in the population at large. In minority communities, however, AIDS is also associated with intravenous drug use, a serious problem in large urban areas (Council on Scientific Affairs, American Medical Association 1991; HIV/AIDS Surveillance Report 1989). Among men in racial and ethnic minority groups, 39% of all AIDS cases are due to exposure from male-male sexual relations, and 38% of all AIDS cases are due to exposure from intravenous drug use (Morbidity and Mortality Weekly Report 1994a). Within the multicultural community, AIDS is so pervasive for many groups (especially blacks and Hispanics) that the number of individuals diagnosed with AIDS far exceeds the expected range based on overall population representation (Hu, et al. 1995).

In 1988, the Center for Disease Control reported that approximately 26% of all people with AIDS (more than 19,000 cases) were African Americans, and 15% (nearly 11,000 cases) were Hispanic (HIV/AIDS Surveillance Report 1989). Approximately 1% of AIDS cases were Asian-Pacific Americans and approximately 1% were American Indians and native Alaskans. In 1994, the Centers for Disease Control (Morbidity and Mortality Weekly Report 1994a) reported on a survey of local, state, and territorial health departments that was conducted in 1993. The purpose of the survey was to determine the number of AIDS cases reported during that time frame. According to results of the survey, a total of 58,538 of all reported cases of AIDS during 1993 occurred among racial and ethnic minorities. These cases represented 55% of the 106,949 AIDS cases reported in the United States during that time. This included 38,544 blacks (66% of all reported cases of minorities), 18,888 Hispanics (32% of all reported cases of minorities), 767 Asian and Pacific Islanders (1% of all reported cases of minorities), and 339 American Indigenous and Alaskan natives (1% of all reported cases of minorities). Future projected figures indicate that the prevalence of AIDS will continue to increase rather than decrease among minority groups (Morbidity and Mortality Weekly Report 1994a).

AIDS is also a serious problem among minority infants and children because the AIDS virus can be transmitted through the placenta. Black children constitute 15% of the total U.S. child population but represent 53% of all childhood AIDS cases. Hispanic children comprise 10% of the U.S. child population but represent 23% of all childhood AIDS cases. Children who are diagnosed with AIDS can have difficulty thriving after birth and can have a myriad of central nervous system abnormalities (Cruz 1988). In addition, pediatric AIDS cases are at a great risk of being abandoned after birth and left to the care of the hospital staff. These boarders of the hospital, or *boarder babies* as they are referred to, remain hospitalized, even in instances when there is no medical need, because they have no other place to go. Foster care or adoptive placement is difficult for children with AIDS because of the fatal nature of the disease.

AIDS can result in AIDS dementia complex, which is characterized by a constellation of neuropsychological and motor deficits, most notable during the later stages of the disease (Brew 1992). Associated deficits of interest to rehabilitation specialists include (1) problems with gait and, eventually, ambulation; (2) motor speech impairments; (3) dysphagia; and, (4) finally, memory loss, impaired concentration, decline in orientation, and reduced performance on complex mental tasks (Flower and Sooy; 1987; Rubinow, et al. 1988; Price, et al. 1988; Petito 1988; Parry 1988). The progression of AIDS dementia complex generally (but not always) follows this order of involvement because of the frequent initial compromise of subcortical structures in the AIDS population. This is different from Alzheimer's disease and other cortical dementias that are characterized by a decline in cognitive performance before changes in motor skills are noted.

Alcohol Abuse

There is a prevalence of alcoholism, particularly among American Indian, black, and Hispanic populations (Christian, et al. 1989). Alcoholism is a serious problem in these groups because the pattern of addiction generally begins during the early or middle teen years. The early onset of alcoholism and the prolonged period of alcohol abuse place these individuals at risk for developing associated neurologic impairments. Associated impairments include Wernicke-Korsakoff syndrome and motor impairments secondary to cerebellar degeneration. Reductions in memory, difficulty processing abstract information, motor impairments, difficulty with visual-spatial integration, and impaired learning are all characteristics of Wernicke–Korsakoff syndrome. It should be noted that alcohol abuse is a major contributor to TBI secondary to motor vehicle accidents and violent crime–related accidents (Lindenbaum, et al. 1989). Alcohol abuse can also exacerbate the severity of impairments caused by TBI.

Alcoholism among pregnant women is a serious problem. Alcohol crosses the placental barrier and exposes the unborn fetus to this toxic drug

(Rhodes, et al. 1994). Populations with the highest alcoholism risk for adults (American Indian and blacks) also have a high rate of fetal alcohol syndrome (Morbidity and Mortality Weekly Report 1993, 1994b, 1995; Egeland, et al. 1995; Abel 1995). Fetal alcohol syndrome, a major cause of fetal and developmental anomalies (Hanson, et al. 1978), occurs 10 times more frequently among American Indians and blacks than in the population at large (Institute of Medicine 1985; Shephard and Shephard 1990). Fetal alcohol syndrome is a problem of serious magnitude, which has been esti-mated to account for up to 5% of all birth defects and ranks as a major cause of mental retardation and developmental disability (Wallace 1992; Centers for Disease Control 1991).

Other Drug Abuse and Exposure to Environmental Toxins

Although drug use is prevalent in all aspects of our society, the prevalence appears to be higher in urban areas than suburban areas. This may be due to the accessibility of drugs to residents of the inner city, which is frequently the hub of illicit drug sales. Because a disproportionate number of minorities reside in urban America, it is likely that minority inner-city residents are affected by the problem of substance abuse to a greater extent than the population at large.

A number of life-threatening consequences can be attributed directly as well as indirectly to drug abuse, including fatal and non-fatal drug overdose, hepatitis B infection, and AIDS. In addition, drug abuse (as with alcohol abuse) can indirectly contribute to the incidence of violent crimes, motor vehicle accidents, and other neurologically related injuries.

The direct effects of drugs can result in a range of neuropsychological alterations, including memory deficits, disorientation, and difficulties with comprehension and reasoning. Illicit drug use can also result in motor speech impairments and dysphagia (Wallace 1992).

Environmental lead exposure from lead paint in deteriorating urban housing (lead in deteriorating paint, soil, dust, and water), heavy traffic, and proximity to manufacturing industry has been cited as one of the "most common and preventable pediatric health problems today" (Centers for Disease Control 1991; Sargent, et al. 1995). Exposure to lead is a significant problem in urban areas that are heavily populated by minority children. Lead exposure can result in developmental delay, lan-guage and learning impairments (Dyer 1993), and, in extreme cases, coma and death (Agency for Toxic Substances and Disease Registry 1988).

Dementing Disease

It has been speculated that dementia due to Alzheimer's disease is a problem among aging individuals from the multicultural community (Baker 1988). This may be due to the association between Alzheimer's disease and environmental toxins in urban areas that are heavily populated by minorities. An increased incidence of TBI among minorities has also been cited as a risk factor associated with the prevalence of dementing disease (Gorelick, et al. 1994), as has the occurrence of frequent strokes (which can result in multi-infarct dementia). Results of investigations into the prevalence of Alzheimer's and other forms of dementia among minority populations must be interpreted with caution because aging minorities generally have less education than whites and may speak a language or dialect other than standard English (Bell, et al. 1976; Williams 1980; Hudson 1976). These factors can confound the results of group investigations to explore dementia in minority aging populations (National Council on the Aging 1981). Among some minority groups (e.g., Asians and Pacific islanders), there are documented disparities in the use of support services after dementia has been diagnosed (Roca, et al. 1984).

Lupus

Systemic lupus erythematosus is an autoimmune disease that affects one in every 2,000 Americans, or nearly 1 million individuals (Braun, et al. 1995). Ninety percent of those diagnosed with lupus are between 15 and 45 years of age, and minority women are affected by this disease more than any other group. Black women, for instance, are affected by lupus three times more often than the population at large (National Lupus Foundation 1994). Hispanic and Asian American women (especially those of Chinese and Thai ancestry) are also affected by this disease to a disproportionate extent.

Lupus is a complex, multisystem disease of the immune system that (much like multiple sclerosis) causes a myriad of health problems that can resemble different illnesses at different times (National Institutes of Health 1994; Moore, et al. 1991; Stevens 1991; Lahita 1992; Panush, et al. 1993). Although the etiology of lupus is unknown, it is suspected that environmental, genetic, or hormonal factors may be responsible for this disease.

Although there is great variability in the disease's clinical presentation, the more common features of lupus include anemia, low white blood cell count, low platelet count, polyarthritis (including the wrist, the knees, and one or more joints), kidney inflammation, sores in the mouth and nose, and butterfly-shaped rashes over the cheeks or other skin areas. Other symptoms

include fatigue, fever, and unusual weight and hair loss. Often those diagnosed with lupus present with peripheral and central nervous system disorders (Moore and McGrory 1991). The central nervous system disorders appear
to occur at a relatively higher frequency than the peripheral nervous system
impairments. Nervous system manifestations include higher cortical dysfunction deficits in neuropsychological, communication, and cognitive communication, and motor speech impairments. Lupus can also damage blood
vessels of the brain, cause reduced brain blood supply, and result in stroke of
both the occlusive and hemorrhagic types (Moore and McGrory 1991).

Clinical Management of Minority Populations

Only 6.59% of the American Speech and Hearing Association
(ASHA)-certified speech-language pathology membership is of nonwhite
ancestry (American Speech-Language and Hearing Association 1996). This
includes 2.77% blacks (non-Hispanic), 2.23% Hispanics, 1.33% Asians and
Pacific islanders, and 0.33% American Indians and Alaskan natives. Only a
small fraction of the 6.59% is composed of bilingual speech-language pathologists (American Speech-Language and Hearing Association 1996). For these
reasons, most of the clinical services to culturally and linguistically diverse
cases are, by necessity, provided by monolingual English and monocultural
(mainstream American) speech-language pathologists.

The Role of the Monolingual Speech-Language Pathologist

The monolingual English speech-language pathologist is
qualified to provide direct services to English-speaking patients from the
mainstream American culture. In addition, if the monolingual English speech-
language pathologist is bicultural (based on personal experience, formally
acquired knowledge and clinical experience, or both), he or she is also able to
provide services to clients who differ in terms of culture but who speak standard English or a dialect of English. Monolingual English speech-language
pathologists who are not familiar with the cultural background of their
patients should obtain information before clinical contact. Ten critical pieces
of information that clinicians should obtain about every patient, including
those from culturally diverse backgrounds, are discussed in this section.

Overall Impression of Culture

It is important to obtain an overview impression of cultural
mores of the patient's racial and ethnic group. Obtaining general information

about the patient's racial and ethnic group helps the clinician understand factors that can have an impact on clinical management but lie outside of the clinician's expected scope of considerations given his or her own cultural background. Although it is an easy (although somewhat time-consuming) task to obtain information about culture and language (this information is readily available in printed form), one must also take the time to validate the appropriateness of information obtained on a patient-by-patient basis. This is important to ensure that the obtained information is applicable to the patient. One should always keep in mind that just as diversity can be found across groups, diversity can also be found within groups. Socioeconomic status, highest level of educational achievement, and area of residence (e.g., rural, suburb, or inner city) are factors that can influence the extent of adherence to specific cultural mores and communication patterns observed across members of specific racial and ethnic groups.

History

It is important to obtain information about the history of the patient's racial and ethnic group and information about the patient's immigration or the immigration of his or her ancestors to the United States. Conditions surrounding immigration to the United States can range from relatively pleasant to harsh. Motives for immigration can range from voluntary pursuit of a more prosperous lifestyle to involuntary flight to avoid political persecution. Particular attention should be given to obtaining information about the patient's history, accessibility, and satisfaction with the U.S. health care system. Because many racial and ethnic groups have a long history of discrimination associated with health care services in the United States, information about this area can provide useful insight into the patient's acceptance of health and rehabilitation services.

Generational Status

Information about generational status provides the clinician with information about the length of the patient's residency in the United States. Length of residency is often associated with level of acculturation to mainstream American culture.

Communication Patterns

The clinician should obtain information about the linguistic and nonverbal pragmatic characteristics of the racial or ethnic group. For patients who are dialect speakers, familiarity with the dialect provides the clinician with information on which to base decisions about designations of communication deviancy attributable to the brain injury (which would require clinical intervention) or language differences (which would not require clinical intervention). When working with adult populations, it is important to keep in mind that the purpose of rehabilitation is not to alter the patient's indigenous language pattern but to, as closely as possible, return the individual to premorbid levels of functioning. In this regard, all responses that are made by the adult patient in the dialect language should be considered acceptable. For pediatric populations with acquired neurogenic impairments, the clinician may wish to develop a strategy for weaving in communication competency in standard English. This should not be considered until after the child has first demonstrated proficiency with premorbid indigenous communication patterns. For children with developmental difficulties, greater attention may be given to initial training in standard English, if it is practical to do so based on the age of the child and the predominant language input that the child receives at home.

For the patient who speaks a language other than standard English or who is bilingual in English and another language, the monolingual speech-language pathologist should obtain the assistance of an interpreter or translator. The reader should refer to Wallace (1997) for an expanded discussion of how to work with interpreters and translators during the provision of clinical services with neurogenics populations.

Social Organization

Minorities are often described as having a group orientation with emphasis on group interdependence. The mainstream American population, on the other hand, is often described as promoting independent functioning. It is important that all supportive family and extended family members be identified so that they can contribute to the habilitation or rehabilitation process. Often family and even extended family members are extremely helpful with assistance during clinical management and home carry over of clinical strategies.

Time Concept

There are two major types of interactional styles, based on emphasis or de-emphasis on time. Individuals with monochronic style view time linearly and tend to focus on interactions and activities one at a time. Individuals with monochronic orientation segment their activities according to the element of time and emphasize promptness. Monochronic individuals are able to terminate an activity when the clock indicates that it is time to do so. Punctuality is a major characteristic of individuals who have a monochronic time orientation. Mainstream American culture has been characterized as monochronic. Many minority cultures, on the other hand, have been described as polychronic, placing less emphasis on punctuality.

Time orientation can have an impact on the way in which treatment sessions are structured and on the way in which service delivery is structured. Home-based rather than clinical-based models for service delivery, for example, can promote regular attendance and prompt arrival for clinical appointments for individuals who tend to function according to the polychronic orientation.

Spiritual Orientation

Religion often influences one's belief about the cause of illness and the appropriateness of attempts to cure an illness or obtain rehabilitation services for a disability. Rehabilitation efforts can be unproductive if the patient firmly believes that the illness or disability is deserved.

Some individuals believe that events are independent of their actions and a result of external forces imposed by God or fate. Others believe that events are contingent on their actions and that they can influence their own destiny. In addition to influencing whether a person is receptive to treatment, this feature (referred to by some as *locus of control*) can influence one's approach to treatment tasks, especially tasks that entail cognitively based judgments.

Health Practices

Concepts of health, illness, and the relevancy of rehabilitation vary across racial and ethnic groups. A clinician who is able to understand these issues from the patient's point of view stands a better chance of obtaining patient cooperation for Western rehabilitation services or a combination of non-Western and Western methods than a clinician that does not have sensitivity in this area.

Food Preferences

It is important to obtain information about the patient's food preferences to maximize the likelihood that the patient will comply with dysphagia management efforts.

Risk Factors for Communication Impairments and Dysphagia

Obtaining information about risk factors for communication impairments and dysphagia facilitates clinician efforts to prevent future medical problems that can exacerbate existing problems being managed by the speech-language pathologist.

General Management Considerations

The following is a list of general considerations for the monolingual speech-language pathologist who is involved with the provision of indirect clinical services to patients who are monolingual non-English and bilingual (Wallace 1996):

1. Obtain information about the patient's culture and language. When working with pediatric populations who have acquired impairments, it is important to obtain as much information as possible about premorbid academic performance and level of language development. One should also be informed about languages spoken in the home. If the individual is of school age, the clinician may find it useful to establish close communication networks with the teacher at an early point in the assessment and rehabilitation process.

2. Become familiar with a few key words and phrases in the patient's native language and be able to pronounce them correctly. This will build a basic rapport with the patient and will demonstrate a level of respect for the patient's culture and language. This applies to non-English, bilingual, and polyglot speakers. It does not apply when working with dialect speakers because generally dialect use is only acceptable during communication exchange among members of the dialect group. Use of dialects by individuals outside of a given cultural group represented by the dialect can be viewed as offensive or inappropriate by members of the group.

3. Obtain a good working knowledge of nonverbal communication patterns that are appropriate for the patient's culture and for interaction with individuals in the patient's age category.

4. Locate, train, and work with an interpreter or translator in preparation for the assessment process.

5. Select culturally and linguistically appropriate standardized assessments (making adaptations, as needed) and design criterion-referenced tasks to obtain comparative information across all languages spoken.

6. Determine the most productive language to target during treatment. For children, this also entails a plan of action for incorporating standard English patterns into the child's repertoire after language skills are on-target in the indigenous language system.

7. Develop culturally appropriate treatment materials and strategies.

8. Develop culturally sensitive methods for incorporating the family into the treatment process. In the case of pediatric populations, it

is imperative that the clinician have an understanding and appreciation of the natural interaction style of the mother, which can vary as a function of culture. This allows the clinician to identify and encourage previously established productive patterns of caregiver-child interaction. These patterns of interaction can be interwoven with therapeutic suggestions for enhancing caregiver-child interaction. It is also important to note that for minority children, often both grandmother and mother serve as primary caregivers (Joslin and Brouard 1995). When this is the case, both individuals should be included as an integral part of the habilitation or rehabilitation plan.

9. Locate, train, and work closely with the interpreter (in conjunction with the family and extended family unit). The interpreter provides the direct rehabilitation services in his or her role as support personnel.

10. Determine whether treatment is efficacious and make ongoing adjustments to treatment goals and strategies as necessary.

For pediatric populations, issues involving developmental disabilities and habilitation are different from the rehabilitation issues that must be considered when working with adult populations. The timing of intervention, the status of the child's development before and at the time of intervention, the accessibility of services as mandated by public law, and the scope of services for culturally and linguistically diverse children available through the school system contribute to a myriad of differences in clinical options and opportunities that must be considered when providing services to pediatric versus adult neurogenics cases.

For an expanded discussion of clinical management issues for culturally and linguistically diverse adult neurogenics populations and case study presentations, the reader should refer to Wallace (1997).

Conclusion

The American Speech-Language-Hearing Association promotes the infusion of multicultural information into the framework of clinical management. In fact, it mandates (according to the specifications of the Action Agenda 2000) that multicultural information be infused throughout all aspects of academic and clinical training (American Speech and Hearing Association Committee on the Status of Racial Minorities 1991). This is an important consideration as speech-language pathologists prepare for professional practice in the twenty-first century, which will involve service provision to a growing minority population. Although the promotion of multicultural issues has moved us in a positive direction as a profession, we have not yet developed specific guidelines for the role that speech-language pathologists must play in the management of diverse populations, and we have not yet developed guidelines regarding the scope of information needed.

This chapter provides a beginning point for the understanding of clinical issues relating to adult and pediatric neurogenics cases from culturally and linguistically diverse backgrounds. Greater attention is needed in this area of multicultural neurogenics to provide training for clinicians and researchers who are prepared to explore and improve service delivery to individuals from the multicultural community. This is important so that speech-language pathologists can provide equal access to services, equal use of services, and equal quality of services (in terms of individualized design of treatment) for people from all segments of our community, including those from diverse cultural and linguistic backgrounds.

References

Abboud, M.R., Jackson, S.M., Barredo, J., et al. (1996). Neurologic complications following bone marrow transplantation for sickle cell disease. *Bone Marrow Transplantation, 17(3)*, 405–407.

Abel, E.L. (1995). An update on incidence of FAS: FAS is not an equal opportunity birth defect. *Neurotoxicology and Teratology, 17(4)*, 437–443.

Adams, R.J., Nichols, F.T., McKie, V., et al. (1988). Cerebral infarction in sickle cell anemia: Mechanisms based on CT and MRI. *Neurology, 38*, 1012–1017.

Agency for Toxic Substances and Disease Registry. (1988). *The nature and extent of lead poisoning in children in the United States: A report to Congress*. Atlanta: U.S. Department of Health and Human Services.

American Diabetes Association. (1992). *Diabetes facts*. Alexandria, VA: ADA National Office.

American Diabetes Association. (1997). *Diabetes fact sheet*. Alexandria, VA: American Diabetes Association.

American Heart Association. (1996). Heart attack and stroke in African Americans. *American Heart Association Newsletter: The BEAT*, Winter issue.

American Lung Association. (1997). *American Lung Association fact sheet*. New York: American Lung Association.

American Speech and Hearing Association Committee on the Status of Racial Minorities. (1991). *A comprehensive affirmative action plan to promote parity within the association and professions.* Rockville, MD: ASHA National Office.

American Speech-Language-Hearing Association. (1996). *Demographic profile of the ASHA membership and affiliation for the period January 1, 1996 through June 30, 1996.* Rockville, MD: Management Information Systems Division, ASHA.

Anson, J.A., Koshy, M., Ferguson, L., & Crowell, R.M. (1992). Subarachnoid hemorrhage in sickle cell disease. *Journal of Neurosurgery, 76,* 726.

Baker, F.M. (1988). Dementing illness and black Americans. In J.S. Jackson (Ed.), *The black American elderly: Research on physical and psychosocial health* (p. 215). New York: Springer-Verlag.

Barnhart, M.I., Henry, R.L., & Lusher, J. (1974). *Sickle cell.* Kalamazoo, MI: Upjohn.

Bell, D., Kasschau, P., & Zellman, G. (1976). *Delivering services to elderly members of minority groups: A critical review of the literature* (pp. 81–103). Santa Monica, CA: Rand.

Bender, S.L., Word, C.O., DiClemente, R.J., et al. (1995). The developmental implications of prenatal and/or postnatal crack cocaine exposure in preschool children: A preliminary report. *Journal of Developmental and Behavioral Pediatrics, 16(6),* 418–424.

Berenson, G.S. (1995). The control of hypertension in African American children: The Bogalusa heart study. *Journal of the National Medical Association, 87,* 614–617.

Berkson, D.M., Brown, M.C., & Stanton, H. (1980). Changing trends in hypertension detection and control: The Chicago experience. *American Journal of Public Health, 70,* 389–393.

Black, M.M., Nair, P., Kight, C., et al. (1994). Parenting and early development among children of drug-abusing women: Effects of home intervention. *Pediatrics, 94,* 440–448.

Botash, A.S., Kavey, R.W., Emm, N., & Jones, D. (1992). Cardiovascular risk factors in Native American children. *New York State Journal of Medicine, 92,* 378–381.

Braun, K.L., Takamura, J.C., Forman, S.M., et al. (1995). Developing and testing outreach materials on Alzheimer's disease for Asian and Pacific Islander Americans. *Gerontologist, 35(1),* 122–126.

Brew, B.J. (1992). Medical management of AIDS patients: Central and peripheral nervous system abnormalities. *Medical Clinics of North America, 76,* 63–81.

Broderick, J., Talbot, G.T., Prenger, E., et al. (1993). Stroke in children within a major metropolitan area: The surprising importance of intracerebral hemorrhage. *Journal of Child Neurology, 8(3),* 250–255.

Brust, J.C. (1993). Clinical, radiological, and pathological aspects of cere-brovascular disease associated with drug abuse. *Stroke, 24(Suppl 12),* I129–135.

Caplan, L.R., Gorelick, P.B., & Hier, D.B. (1986). Race, sex, and occlusive cerebrovascular disease: A review. *Stroke, 17,* 648–655.

Centers for Disease Control. (1991). *Preventing lead poisoning in young children.* Washington, DC: U.S. Department of Health and Human Services.

Centers for Disease Control. (1995). *The psychological impact of violence in underserved communities.* Atlanta: Centers for Disease Control, National Center for Injury Prevention and Control, Division of Violence Prevention.

Christian, C.M., Dufour, M., & Bertolucci, D. (1989). Differential alcohol-related mortality among American Indian tribes in Oklahoma: 1968–1978. *Social Science and Medicine, 28,* 275–284.

Cornwell, E., Jacobs, D., Walker, M., et al. (1995). National Medical Association surgical section position paper on violence prevention (a resolution of trauma surgeons caring for victims of violence). *Journal of the American Medical Association, 372(22),* 1788–1789.

Council on Scientific Affairs, American Medical Association. (1991). Hispanic health in the United States. *Journal of the American Medical Association, 265(2),* 248–252.

Cruz D. (1988). Children with AIDS: Diagnosis, symptoms, care. *Association of Operating Room Nurses Journal, 48,* 893–910.

Davies, P. (1989). Long-term effects of meningitis. *Developmental Medicine and Child Neurology, 31,* 398–406.

Dyer, F. (1993). Clinical presentation of the lead-poisoned child on mental ability tests. *Journal of Clinical Psychology, 49,* 94–101.

Egeland, G.M., Perham-Hester, K.A., & Hook, E.B. (1995). Use of capture-recapture analyses in fetal alcohol syndrome surveillance in Alaska. *American Journal of Epidemiology, 141(4),* 335–341.

Eyler, F.D., & Behnke, M. (1995). Prenatal cocaine exposure, consequences for child and family. *Journal of the Florida Medical Association, 82(9),* 603–606.

Flower, M.W., & Sooy, C.D. (1987). AIDS: An introduction for speech-language pathologists and audiologists. *ASHA, 29,* 25.

Gorelick, P.B., Caplan, L.R., Hier, D.B., et al. (1984). Racial differences in the distribution of anterior circulation occlusive disease. *Neurology, 34,* 54–59.

Gorelick, P.B., Caplan, L.R., Hier, D.B., et al. (1985). Racial differences in the distribution of posterior circulation occlusive disease. *Stroke, 16,* 785–790.

Gorelick, P.B., Freels, S., Harris, Y., et al. (1994). Epidemiology of vascular and Alzheimer's dementia among African Americans in Chicago, Ill: Baseline frequency and comparison of risk factors. *Neurology, 44(8),* 1391–1396.

Hanson, J.W., Streissguth, A.P., & Smith, D.W. (1978). The effects of moderate alcohol consumption during pregnancy on fetal growth and morphogenesis. *Journal of Pediatrics, 92,* 457–471.

Hawley, T.L., Halle, T.G., Drasin, R.E., & Thomas, N.G. (1995). Children of addicted mothers: Effects of the "crack epidemic" on the caregiving environment and the development of preschoolers. *American Journal of Orthopsychiatry, 65(3),* 364–379.

Heyden, S., Heyman, A., & Goree, J.A. (1970). Embolic occlusion of the middle cerebral and carotid arteries: A comparison of the predisposing factors. *Stroke, 1,* 363–369.

Heyman, A., Fields, W.S., & Keating, R.D. (1972). Joint study of extracranial arterial occlusion: VI. Racial differences in hospitalized patients with ischemic stroke. *Journal of the American Medical Association, 222,* 285–289.

HIV/AIDS surveillance report. (1989). Atlanta: Centers for Disease Control.

Hohn, A.R., Dwyer, K.M., & Dwyer, J.H. (1994). Blood pressure in youth from four ethnic groups: The Pasadena prevention project. *Journal of Pediatrics, 125(3),* 368–373.

Hu, D.J., Byers, R., Fleming, P.L., & Ward, J.W. (1995). Characteristics of persons with late AIDS diagnosis in the US. *American Journal of Preventive Medicine, 11(2),* 114–119.

Hudson, G.E. (1976). Some special problems of older Black Americans. *The Crisis, 83(3),* 88–90.

Hurt, H., Brodsky, N.L., Betancourt, L., et al. (1995). Cocaine-exposed children: Follow-up through 30 months. *Journal of Developmental and Behavioral Pediatrics, 16(1),* 29–35.

Hypertension Detection and Follow-Up Program Cooperative Group. (1977). Blood pressure studies in 14 communities. *Journal of the American Medical Association,* 237, 2385–2391.

Institute of Medicine Committee to Study the Prevention of Low Birth Weight, Division of Health Promotion and Disease Prevention. (1985). *Preventing low birth weight.* Washington, DC: National Academy Press.

Johnson, M., & El-Hazmi, M. (1984). *The world and the sickle cell gene: A study in health education.* New York: Trado-Medic Books.

Joslin, D., & Brouard, A. (1995). The prevalence of grandmothers as primary caregivers in a poor pediatric population. *Journal of Community Health, 20,* 383–401.

Kaku, D.A., & Lowenstein, D.H. (1990). Emergence of recreational drug abuse as a major risk factor for stroke in young adults. *Annals of Internal Medicine, 113,* 821–827.

Kenton, E.J. (1991). Access to neurological care for minorities. *Archives of Neurology, 48,* 480–483.

Lahita, R.G. (1992). *Systemic lupus erythematosus.* New York: Churchill Livingstone, 1992.

Lane P.A. (1996). Sickle cell disease. *Pediatric Clinics of North America, 43(3),* 639–664.

Laraque, D., Barlow, B., Durkin, M., et al. (1995). Children who are shot: A 30-year experience. *Journal of Pediatric Surgery, 30(7),* 1072–1075.

Levine, S., Washington, J., Jefferson, M., et al. (1987). "Crack" cocaine associated stroke. *Neurology, 37,* 1849–1853.

Levine, S., Brust, J., Futrell, N., et al. (1990). Cerebrovascular complications of the use of the "crack" form of alkaloidal cocaine. *New England Journal of Medicine, 323(11),* 699–703.

Lindenbaum, G.A., Carroll, S.F., Daskal, I., & Kapusnick, R. (1989). Patterns of alcohol and drug abuse in an urban trauma center: The increasing role of cocaine abuse. *Journal of Trauma, 29(12),* 1654–1658.

McGarry, P., Solberg, L., Guzman, M., & Stron, J. (1985). Cerebral atherosclerosis in New Orleans: Comparison of lesions by age, sex, and race. *Laboratory Investigation, 52(2),* 533–539.

Morbidity and Mortality Weekly Report. (1993). Linking multiple data sources in fetal alcohol syndrome surveillance—Alaska. *Morbidity and Mortality Weekly Report, 42,* 312–314.

Morbidity and Mortality Weekly Report. (1994a). Current trends section: AIDS among racial/ethnic minorities: United States, 1993. *Morbidity and Mortality Weekly Report, 43,* 644.

Morbidity and Mortality Weekly Report. (1994b). Prevalence and characteristics of alcohol consumption and fetal alcohol syndrome awareness— Alaska, 1991 and 1993. *Morbidity and Mortality Weekly Report, 43,* 3–6.

Morbidity and Mortality Weekly Report. (1995). Use of international classification of diseases coding to identify fetal alcohol syndrome—Indian Health Service Facilities, 1981–1992. *Morbidity and Mortality Weekly Report, 44,* 253–255, 261.

Mody, C., Miller, B., McIntyre, H., et al. (1988). Neurologic complications of cocaine abuse. *Neurology, 38,* 1189–1193.

Moore, M.E., McGrory, C.H., & Rosenthal, R.S. (1991). *Learning about lupus: A user friendly guide.* Wayne, PA: Mainline Desktop Publishing.

Moser, F.G., Miller, S.T., Bello, J.A., et al. (1996). The spectrum of brain MR abnormalities in sickle cell disease: A report from the cooperative study of sickle cell disease. *American Journal of Neuroradiology, 17(5),* 965–972.

Moss, S. (1993). Neurogenic communication disorders resulting from stroke. *ASHA 35,* 61–62.

Murphy, J.K., & McGarvey, S.T. (1994). Pressor reactivity in American Samoan children: Comparisons with mainland American children. *Ethnicity and Disease, 4(1),* 47–56.

Murphy, J.K., Alpert, B.S., & Walker, S.S. (1994). Consistency of ethnic differences in children's pressor reactivity: 1987 to 1992. *Hypertension, 23(Suppl),* 152–155.

National Council on the Aging. (1981). *Survey highlights and fact sheet based on aging in the eighties: America in transition.* Washington, DC: National Council on the Aging.

National Institutes of Health. (1994). *What black women should know about lupus.* Bethesda, MD: NIH Public Health Service. (NIH Publication No. 93-3219.)

National Lupus Foundation. (1994). *Lupus fact sheet.* Rockville, MD: National Lupus Foundation.

Panush, R.S., Greer, J.M., & Morshedian, K.K. (1993). What is lupus? What is not lupus? *Rheumatoid Disorder Clinics of North America, 19,* 223–234.

Parry, G.J. (1988). Peripheral neuropathies associated with human immunodeficiency virus infection. *Annals of Neurology, 23(Suppl),* S53–S59.

Petito, C.K. (1988). Review of central nervous system pathology in human immunodeficiency virus infection. *Annals of Neurology, 23(Suppl),* S54–S57.

Platt, U.S., Brambilla, D.J., Rosse, W.F., et al. (1994). Mortality in sickle cell disease: Life expectancy and risk factors for early death. *New England Journal of Medicine, 330,* 1639–1644.

Price, R.W., Sidtis, J., & Rosenblum, M. (1988). The AIDS dementia complex: Some current questions. *Annals of Neurology, 23(Suppl),* S27–S33.

Prohovnik, I., Pavlakis, S.G., Piomelli, S., et al. (1989). Cerebral hyperemia, stroke, and transfusion in sickle cell disease. *Neurology, 39,* 344–348.

Report of the Secretary's Task Force on Black and Minority Health. (1985). *Vol. 1: Executive summary.* Washington DC: U.S. Department of Health and Human Services (Pub. No. 491-313/44706.).

Rhodes, J.E., Gingiss, P.L., & Smith, P.B. (1994). Risk and protective factors for alcohol use among pregnant African-American, Hispanic, and white adolescents: The influence of peers, sexual partners, family members, and mentors. *Addictive Behaviors, 19,* 555–564.

Roca, R.P., Klein, L.E., & Kirby, S.M. (1984). Recognition of dementia among medical patients. *Archives of Internal Medicine, 144,* 73–75.

Rubinow, D.R., Berrettini, C.H., Browers, P., & Lane, H.C. (1988). Neuropsychiatric consequences of AIDS. *Annals of Neurology, 23(Suppl),* S24–S36.

Rust, G.S. (1990). Health status of migrant farm workers: A literature review and commentary. *American Journal of Public Health, 9,* 1118–1224.

Sacco, R.L., Hauser, W.A., Mohr, J.P., & Foulkes, M.A. (1991). One year outcome after cerebral infarction in whites, blacks, and Hispanics. *Stroke, 22(3),* 305–311.

Sargent, J.D., Brown, M.J., Freeman, J.L., et al. (1995). Childhood lead poisoning in Massachusetts communities: Its association with sociodemographic and housing characteristics. *American Journal of Public Health, 85,* 528–533.

Sewell, C.M., Becker, T.M., Wiggins, C.L., et al. (1989). Injury mortality in New Mexico's American Indians, Hispanics, and non-Hispanic whites—1958 to 1982. *Western Journal of Medicine, 150,* 708–713.

Shephard, B.D., & Shephard, C.A. (1990). *The complete guide to women's health.* New York: Plume.

Singleton, L., & Johnson, K. (1993). *The black health library guide to stroke.* New York: Holt.

Stevens, M.B. (1991). The clinical spectrum of SLE. *Maryland Medical Journal, 40,* 875–885.

Time Life Medical. (1996). *Diabetes at time of diagnosis: An educational videotape.* New York: Time Life Medical, 1996.

U.S. Department of Health and Human Services. (1986). *Report of the Secretary's task force on Black and minority health. Vol. 5: Homicide, suicide and unintentional injuries.* Washington, DC: U.S. Department of Health and Human Services.

Wallace, G. (1992). Adult neurogenic disorders. In D. Battle (Ed.), *Multicultural issues and speech-language pathology* (pp. 239–255). North Potomac, MD: Andover.

Wallace, G. (1993). Stroke and traumatic brain injury (Ma'i Ulu) in America Samoa. *Hawaii Medical Journal, 52,* 234–250.

Wallace, G. (1996). Management of aphasic individuals from culturally and linguistically diverse populations. In G. Wallace (Ed.), *Adult aphasia rehabilitation* (pp. 234–250). Boston: Butterworth–Heinemann.

Wallace, G. (1997). *Multicultural neurogenics: A resource for speech-language pathologists providing services to neurologically impaired adults from culturally and linguistically diverse backgrounds.* San Antonio, TX: The Psychological Corporation.

Wallach, S. (1989). Medical complications of the use of cocaine. *Hawaii Medical Journal, 48(11),* 461–462.

Whitman, S., Coonley-Hoganson, R., & DeSai, B.T. (1974). Comparative head trauma experiences in two socioeconomically different Chicago area communities. *American Journal of Epidemiology, 119,* 570–580.

Whitten, C.F. (1973). *Highlights of the sickle cell story.* Detroit, MI: National Association for Sickle Cell Disease, Sickle Cell Detection and Information Center.

Williams, B.S. (1980). *Characteristics of the black elderly.* Washington, DC: Office of Human Development Services, Administration on Aging. (U.S. Department of Health, Education, and Welfare publication No. 80-20057.)

Yano, K., Reed, D.M., & Kagan, A. (1985). Coronary heart disease, hypertension and stroke among Chinese-American men in Hawaii: The Honolulu heart program. *Hawaii Medical Journal, 44,* 297–300.

Yatsu, F.M. (1991). Strokes in Asians and Pacific-Islanders, Hispanics, and Native Americans. *Circulation, 83,* 1471–1472.

11

Multicultural Aspects of Hearing Disorders and Audiology

Diane M. Scott

What does it mean to be an audiologist in today's culturally diverse society? To begin, the population of the United States is changing. As shown in Chapter 1 of this text, data from the U.S. Bureau of the Census clearly delineate the changes in the U.S. population. In 1980, 46 million people, or approximately 20% of the population, were identified as members of racially or ethnically diverse groups (U.S. Bureau of the Census 1990). By 1990, that number had increased to 61 million people, or approximately 24% of the U.S. population (U.S. Bureau of the Census 1990). The majority of immigrants to the United States in recent years have not come from European countries, but from Asian, Pacific Rim, and Latin American countries. People of African descent from countries around the world also are emigrating to the United States in increasing numbers. In addition, birthrates play a role in the Census data. Birthrates for racial and ethnic minority groups are higher than the birthrate for whites. All of this means that the population that audiologists serve is changing and will continue to change well into the twenty-first century (U.S. Bureau of the Census 1990, 1992).

The American Speech-Language Hearing Association estimates that 10% of the U.S. population has a disorder of speech, language, or hearing (American Speech-Language-Hearing Association, Research Division 1994). It is estimated that disorders among members of racially and ethnically diverse groups are also at the 10% level (American Speech-Language-Hearing Association, Research Division 1994). It should be noted that, although racially and ethnically diverse groups have the same types of communication disorders, other contributing factors affect the distribution of the types of disorders across racial and ethnic groups. This can be seen in the distribution of black, as compared with white, Americans with hearing impairment shown in Tables 11-1 and 11-2.

Table 11-1   Number (in Thousands) of People with Hearing Impairment in the United States

Age (in years)	Black	White
<45	642	6,314
45–64	478	6,568
≥65	507	9,197
Total	1,627	22,079

Source: Data from V. Benson & M.A. Morano. (1994). *Current estimates from the National Health Interview Survey, 1993. Vital and health statistics series 10 (190)* (pp. 98). Hyattsville, MD: National Center for Health Statistics.

Table 11-2   Percentage of People in the United States Who Have Difficulty Hearing or Who Are Unable to Hear Normal Conversation

	Black	Hispanic
Have difficulty hearing normal speech	8%	4%
Unable to hear normal speech	11%	6%

Source: Data from U.S. Bureau of the Census. (1992). *Survey of income and program participation estimates for United States, 1991–92. Number of people who have difficulty or are unable to hear normal conversation and whose speech is understood only with difficulty or not at all, by race and Hispanic origin.* Washington, DC: U.S. Bureau of the Census.

In a culturally diverse community, audiologists and the patients and families they serve may not share a common language or world view. Lack of a common language can lead to difficulties in establishing rapport between patient and audiologist and in finding language-appropriate test materials. Seeing the world from the family's view is not always easy or reinforcing for an audiologist. The audiologist's values may not be so highly appreciated by others, yet the audiologist must be culturally sensitive. Anderson and Fenichel (1989) define cultural sensitivity as follows:

> Cultural sensitivity cannot mean knowing everything there is to know about every culture that is represented in a population to be served. At its most basic level, cultural sensitivity implies rather a knowledge that cultural differences as well as similarities exist....[C]ultural sensitivity further means being aware of the cultures represented in one's state or region, learning some of the general parameters of those cultures, and

realizing that cultural diversity will affect families' participation in intervention programs. Cultural knowledge helps a professional to be aware of possibilities and to be ready to respond appropriately.

Audiologists and hearing clinics must strive to become culturally competent. Roberts (1990) asserts that cultural competence refers to the ability to honor and respect those beliefs, interpersonal styles, attitudes, and behaviors both of the families who are patients and of the multicultural staff providing services. Cultural competence incorporates these values at the levels of policy, administration, and practice. Clinical programs that are culturally competent do not become that way by accident. There is commitment at all levels of the organization. The organization reaches out to the community it serves and involves the community in establishing short- and long-range objectives and in determining policy. The program hires staff that mirrors the community it serves and continually educates itself regarding cultural issues.

Cultural Issues in the Practice of Audiology

Case History Information

Cultural sensitivity begins with methods used to obtain case history information. The usual audiologic case history form may not contain all of the questions an audiologist should ask to obtain culturally relevant information (e.g., both race and ethnicity, place of birth as well as year of birth, designation of same-sex parents, natural healing methods as well as medications prescribed and taken, and language in the home). (For more information on modifying the case history form to make it culturally appropriate, see Orque, et al. 1983.)

One in seven U.S. residents speaks a language other than English at home (U.S. Bureau of the Census 1993). At least 31.8 million Americans therefore speak a language other than English at home, up from 23.1 million in 1980. Spanish, spoken by 17.3 million people, is now the most common language other than English in American homes (U.S. Bureau of the Census 1993). The number of at-home native Spanish speakers has increased 50% since 1980 (U.S. Bureau of the Census 1993). Other languages showing a rapid growth in native speakers (a more than 50% increase) include Chinese (1.2 million speakers), Tagalog (0.8 million speakers), Korean (0.6 million speakers), and French Creole (0.2 million speakers) (U.S. Bureau of the Census 1993).

School systems have seen an explosion in the number of native languages spoken by students. As an example, public school children in Kansas in 1994–95 spoke at least 18 native languages other than English, including Spanish, Vietnamese, Lao, Cambodian (Mon Khmer), Ilocano, Mandarin,

Russian, and German (S. Martínez, personal communication, 1995). The U.S. Bureau of the Census (1995) estimates that 14% of school-age children (more than 6.3 million) speak a non-English language at home, and that 4% of school-age children live in households that are "linguistically isolated"— that is, in households in which no member age 14 or older speaks English at least "very well." Most speak Spanish or an Asian language (U.S. Bureau of the Census 1993).

Audiologists who can provide clinical services in a language other than English are in demand. If a program that serves a large non-English speaking population does not have an audiologist who can speak and understand the cultural views of the non–English-speaking population served on staff, the hiring of cultural and linguistic interpreters is strongly recommended. Interpreters should be trained in the necessary clinical issues related to audiologic services, thus ensuring that the interpretations given to the clients and the audiologist are accurate. As stated earlier, being able to communicate with clients in their first language helps establish rapport and develops trust.

Finally, as audiologists read the information obtained from a case history, they need to know if certain auditory disorders (e.g., otitis media, presbycusis, and noise-induced hearing loss) are more common in certain racially and ethnically diverse populations than in others. They then can be on the lookout for these symptoms associated with a given auditory disorder.

Assessment

Cross-Racial Factors

Cultural knowledge is needed at the next step in the audiologic evaluation, the assessment. Research studies have indicated that there are differences in auditory sensitivity between male and female populations and between black and white populations, particularly in those older than 30 years of age (Berger, et al. 1977; Bunch and Raiford 1931; Jerger, et al. 1993; Post 1964; Royster, et al. 1980; Royster and Thomas 1979). The differences noted between male and female auditory sensitivity include the following:

- Hearing threshold level curves for women exhibit almost no age effects (AEs), such as increases in the threshold level due to aging, before age 30, which is not true for men.
- In general, women have larger AEs in the lower frequencies with advancing age, whereas men have larger AEs in the higher frequencies (Royster and Thomas 1979).

Table 11-3   Mean Hearing Threshold Levels at 4,000 Hz for White and Black Women and Men in the United States Not Exposed to Industrial Noise as a Function of Age

	Age (in years)				
	20–29	30–39	40–49	50–59	60–69
White men (Royster and Thomas 1979)	10.8	19.3	27.7	37.4	37.7
White women (Royster and Thomas 1979)	4.5	8.7	12.4	17.4	30.5
Black men (Royster, et al. 1980)	4.0	8.3	14.6	17.6	31.9
Black women (Royster, et al. 1980)	3.8	8.4	8.6	12.7	13.2

- The same pattern of gender differences holds true for both black and white populations. Studies also indicate better auditory sensitivity for black men across all frequencies compared to white men. Black women have better auditory sensitivity than white women (Royster, et al. 1980; Royster and Royster 1982) (Table 11-3).

Audiologic norms, therefore, actually may vary as a function of gender and race. Data still need to be collected from other racial groups.

Linguistic Factors

Use of English-language speech test materials with individuals who do not speak English with native or near-native proficiency is inappropriate. Spanish-language materials are available, along with materials in a few other languages. Audiologists should not use these materials unless they are qualified to provide services in the dialect and language of the client or unless they hire a dialect and language-appropriate interpreter. Alteration in the pronunciation of the dialect of the client could alter test results. Further, audiologists must remember to look at the norming of any non-English tests used and determine the country of origin, language, and dialect of the speaker, if using recorded materials.

When hiring an interpreter, audiologists should seek an individual who meets the following qualifications: (1) high degree of oral and written proficiency in both the first and second languages, (2) ability to convey meaning from one language to the other, (3) sensitivity to the speaker's style, (4) ability to adjust to linguistic variations within different communities (dialects exist), (5) knowledge about the cultures of the people who speak the languages, (6) familiarity with the specific terminology used in audiology, (7) understanding of the function and the role of the interpreter on the team, and (8) flexibility (Roseberry-McKibbin 1995). Family members or those not trained in aspects of the assessment should not be used as interpreters.

For audiologists who speak only English, a promising area of research is examining the use of multimedia in speech testing. McCullough and colleagues (1994) described a prototype Spanish picture-identification task using a multimedia approach that incorporates a simple language-to-place transformation on a computer monitor. The audiologist selects the target word and presentation level from a menu on a control monitor. The patient then responds to the stimulus by pointing to the picture in the quadrant that represents the target word on another monitor.

Cultural Factors

Among the cultural factors to consider in assessment is touching. This may become a factor in immittance, auditory brain stem response, or electronystagmography testing, as well as in general interactions. Cultures view touching or physical displays differently. In cultures that view physical displays favorably, physical displays usually signal friendship; there are no sexual connotations. Examples of "don't touch," "touch," and "middle ground" cultures are indicated below (Axtell 1991).

Don't touch	Middle ground (i.e., touching is appropriate in some situations but not in others)	Touch
Japan	France	Middle Eastern countries
United States	China	Latin countries
Canada	Ireland	Italy
England	India	Greece
Scandinavia		Spain
Other Northern		Portugal
European countries		Some Asian countries
Australia		Russia
Estonia		
Korea		

Differences in touching may also exist between women and men, and between adults versus adults and children.

There is one absolutely universal gesture that is rarely, if ever, misunderstood and that scientists believe actually releases chemicals called endorphins into the body thus creating a feeling of mild euphoria—the smile (Axtell 1991). Use it freely and often to communicate.

Cross-Racial Variables in Hearing Disorders

Otitis Media

Differences have been found in the incidence rates of otitis media among racial groups (National Center for Health Statistics 1986). American Indians, Alaskan Eskimos, and Aborigines have the highest rates, and blacks have the lowest rates among racial groups. Hispanic and white incidence rates fall between the two. Asian and Pacific islander rates match American Indian rates, possibly because of a common gene pool. These differences in rates of otitis media may be caused in part by differences in the structure and function of the eustachian tube among racial groups. Evidence exists in support of this hypothesis (Beery, et al. 1980; Doyle 1977). Anatomic differences in length, width, and angle of the eustachian tube have been reported by Doyle in Alaskan Eskimo, American Indian, white, and black adult populations. In addition, differences in eustachian tube function have been found between a group of White Mountain Apache Indians and a group of whites, both with a history of otitis media (Beery, et al. 1980).

Intraracial differences also exist. Not all American Indian tribes have the same incidence rates of otitis media nor do all peoples of African descent (e.g., Nigerians, black South Africans, and black Americans). Individual variability must be taken into account in examining incidence or prevalence rates of otitis media, as well as familial or genetic factors, climate, and exposure to antibiotics.

Otosclerosis

Otosclerosis is a genetic disease found primarily among whites worldwide. The disease is transmitted in an autosomal dominant manner with variable expression and is thought to be more common in women than men (Bess and Humes 1990). It has been estimated that the disease is 2.5 times more common in women than men and may be exacerbated during pregnancy (Bess and Humes 1990). Histologic or nonclinical otosclerosis (otosclerosis observed in temporal bones) has a prevalence of 8–12% in whites (Schuknecht 1974) and approximately 0.9% in blacks (Guild 1944). The prevalence of clinical otosclerosis (otosclerosis manifested by a hearing loss) is probably less than histologic otosclerosis. According to Causse and Causse (1985), Sakai and Miyake (1977) have estimated the prevalence rate of clinical otosclerosis is 0.3% in Japan.

Sickle-Cell Disease and Hearing Loss

Sickle-Cell Disease: Definition and Incidence

Sickle-cell disease (SCD) is recognized as a world health problem predominantly affecting people of African descent in the United States, Africa, and the Caribbean. To a lesser extent, it affects Latins and selected populations generally adjacent to the Mediterranean Sea and Indian Ocean.

SCD is a genetically inherited abnormality of the hemoglobin molecule, which is responsible for carrying oxygen in red blood cells. More than 500,000 black Americans have SCD. One in 375 Americans of African ancestry is born with SCD (HbSS). One in 12 carries the sickle cell gene (HbAS). Approximately one in 835 black Americans is born with an HbS and an HbC gene, referred to as sickle cell–hemoglobin C disease; it is milder than SCD. Approximately one in 1,667 black Americans is born with an HbS gene, and beta thalassemia gene, referred to as sickle cell–beta thalassemia disease. This disease is variable, ranging from being indistinguishable from ordinary SCD to being almost symptom-free, depending on the nature of the thalassemia mutation (Bloom 1995).

One of the clinical manifestations of the disease is that sickle-shaped cells tend to occlude smaller veins and capillaries, possibly including those supplying blood to the cochlea. In addition, central nervous system (CNS), which includes the auditory pathways, manifestations are frequent in SCD. It is postulated that CNS involvement could be due to small-vessel obstruction, although angiographic studies have revealed people with SCD who have partial or complete occlusion of such major intracranial vessels as the internal carotid, middle, and anterior cerebral arteries. The exact incidence of CNS involvement is unknown; however, a review of the literature reveals incidence figures of 4–40% (Sarniak, et al. 1979).

SCD has periods when it is more active, referred to as crises. These episodes often occur with colds and other infections and are more frequent in early childhood. At such times, the individual becomes listless and complains of pain, usually in the back, extremities, or abdomen. Crisis episodes can necessitate hospitalization. Treatment generally involves the provision of pain medication and, occasionally, blood transfusions. The disease tends to become milder as individuals grow into adulthood. Crises are usually less frequent and often less severe after adolescence (Scott and Kessler 1977).

Auditory Involvement in Sickle-Cell Disease

Considering the vaso-occlusive nature of SCD, the potential for auditory involvement is not unexpected. There are reports of individuals under extreme physiologic stress due to SCD who suffer severe to profound sensorineural hearing losses, with partial or complete recovery of their hearing in some cases. These reactions are similar to what happens during a vasospasm of the internal auditory artery. Studies with larger samples of patients with SCD have shown prevalence rates of sensorineural hearing loss associated with SCD of 4–22% (Scott 1986).

The aim of a study conducted at Howard University by D. Scott (Crawford, et al. 1995) was to longitudinally assess auditory function in a group of pediatric patients (ages 5 months to 16 years) with SCD. Twenty-four subjects received comprehensive audiologic evaluations (pure tone and speech audiometry and immittance measurements), whereas eight subjects received electrophysiologic testing. Six children exhibited a mild bilateral conductive hearing impairment, one exhibited a slight high-frequency sensorineural hearing impairment, and one exhibited both a mild conductive impairment in the low frequencies and a slight sensorineural impairment in the high frequencies. Some children also exhibited abnormalities on acoustic reflexes and acoustic reflex decay, and auditory brain stem response waveforms and latencies. Tables 11-4 and 11-5 compare the results of the Howard University study to previous studies involving children and adults as subjects.

There is evidence of peripheral and central auditory dysfunction in children with SCD. Permanent peripheral dysfunction is most likely to manifest itself as a high-frequency sensorineural hearing impairment. Central auditory dysfunction is not uncommon, but shows no consistent pattern. There appear to be differences in the prevalence of sensorineural hearing impairment in children versus adults with SCD (with a greater prevalence in adults) but not in the presence and variability of central auditory dysfunction. If damage due to SCD occurs mainly in the cochlea and is associated with crisis episodes, greater hearing impairment over time would be expected, resulting in higher prevalence rates of hearing loss in adults.

Future study of the impact of SCD should include more longitudinal studies, the use of otoacoustic emissions to examine cochlear function, and the use of magnetic resonance imaging to examine central auditory anatomy.

Human Immunodeficiency Virus, Acquired Immunodeficiency Syndrome, and Hearing Loss

Human Immunodeficiency Virus and Acquired Immunodeficiency Syndrome: Definition and Incidence

The human immunodeficiency virus (HIV) causes acquired immunodeficiency syndrome (AIDS). HIV is an RNA retrovirus that infects white blood cells, the brain, the bowel, the skin, and other tissues. The most severe manifestation of HIV infection is AIDS (Simonds and Rogers

Table 11-4   Crawford, et al.'s and Gould, et al.'s Study of the Prevalence of Hearing Impairment in Adults with Sickle-Cell Disease

Hemoglobin Type	Number	Number with Sensorineural Hearing Loss	Percent of Hearing Loss by Hemoglobin Type (%)
Sickle cell-disease (HbSS)	50	18	36
Sickle cell–C disease (HbSC)	13	9	69
Sickle cell–beta thalassemia (HbS$_{b+}$–thal)	8	4	50
Sickle cell–beta thalassemia (HbS$_{bO}$–thal)	4	0	0
Total	75	31	41

Note: Sensory auditory system abnormalities were found, but there was no consistent pattern of abnormality.

Sources: Adapted from H.J. Gould, M.R. Crawford, W.R. Smith, et al. (1991). Hearing disorders in sickle cell disease: Cochlear and retrocochlear findings. *Ear and Hearing, 12,* 352; and M.R. Crawford, H.J. Gould, W.R. Smith, et al. (1991). Prevalence of hearing loss in adults with sickle cell disease. *Ear and Hearing, 12, 349.*

Table 11-5   Audiological Studies of Children with Sickle-Cell Disease

Researcher(s)	Number	Age	Number and Percentage of Sensorineural Loss	Number and Percentage of Conductive Loss
Friedman, et al. (1980)[a]	43	73	5 (12%)	0 (0%)
Forman-Franco, et al. (1982)[b]	54	Mean = 12 years	2 (3.7%)	4 (7.4%)
Scott (1995)[c]	24	5 months to 16 years	2 (8%)	7 (29%)

[a]All of the children had sickle-cell disease. Three of the five subjects with sensorineural hearing loss had history of cerebrovascular accidents of varying severity.

[b]All of the children had sickle-cell disease. Thirteen of 28 children tested showed evidence of mild central auditory dysfunction.

[c]Seventeen children had sickle-cell disease, four children had sickle cell–C disease, two children had sickle cell–beta thalassemia, and one had sickle cell–D disease.

1992). The AIDS-infected individual's immune system is significantly compromised. Since 1981, when the first report on AIDS was published by the Centers for Disease Control (1990), the number of people who have died from AIDS-related conditions is 295,473, with another 181,426 people living with AIDS. More recently, the Centers for Disease Control estimates that 1 million Americans are infected with HIV (Centers for Disease Control and Prevention 1995).

Six thousand infants are born to HIV-positive women each year, with 25–35% becoming HIV-positive themselves (Ellerbrock, et al. 1991). HIV infects children from all cultural groups, socioeconomic levels, family structures, and regions of the country. The majority of children with HIV infection are born to mothers who were intravenous drug users or to mothers who were sexual partners of intravenous drug users. A disproportionate number of these women and their children are blacks, Hispanics, and members of lower socioeconomic groups. In 1989, 57% of the children with reported perinatally acquired AIDS were black, 33% were Hispanic, and 12% were white (Simonds and Rogers 1992). Fifty percent of these children were male, and 42% were diagnosed before 1 year of age (Simonds and Rogers 1992). The percent of cumulative pediatric AIDS cases reported through June 1991 by ethnicity included 52.7% blacks, 21.3% whites, 25.1% Hispanics, 0.5% Asians and Pacific islanders, and 0.2% American Indians (Fleming, et al. 1992). Most women (73%) and children (78%) with AIDS are black or Hispanic (Centers for Disease Control 1990). It is projected that racial and ethnic minorities will account for an increasing proportion of cases among women and children in the coming years (Centers for Disease Control 1990).

Auditory Function in Human Immunodeficiency
Virus and Acquired Immunodeficiency Syndrome

A large portion of patients with HIV present with head and neck symptoms. The most common otologic and audiologic manifestations of HIV and AIDS include Kaposi's sarcoma of the ear, otitis caused by *Pneumocystis carinii*, eustachian tube obstruction caused by nasopharyngeal mass, serous otitis media, abnormal auditory response in the brain stem, sensorineural hearing loss, and facial palsy (Lalwani and Sooy 1992).

Hearing impairment associated with HIV and AIDS is generally viewed as a secondary disorder arising from at least three primary etiologies: (1) effects of immunosuppression caused by HIV and direct infection of the hearing mechanism by HIV itself; (2) other opportunistic infections that attack the hearing mechanism; and (3) damage to the hearing mechanism due to toxic side effects of medications prescribed to treat the HIV or any associated opportunistic infections (Madriz and Herrera 1995; Lalwani and

Sooy 1992). The hearing impairment can be manifested as a conductive, sensorineural, or central auditory disorder. In addition, a high prevalence of tinnitus has been reported in people with HIV and AIDS (Lalwani and Sooy 1992). Estimates of the prevalence of hearing loss in this population vary widely. Lalwani and Sooy (1992) estimated that sensorineural hearing loss in HIV-positive and AIDS patients ranged from 20.9% to 49%. The National Institute on Deafness and Other Communication Disorders (NIDCD), on the other hand, estimated that "75% of adult AIDS patients and 50% of ARC [AIDS-related complex] patients show clinical auditory system abnormalities" (National Institute on Deafness and Other Communication Disorders 1989).

At a university-affiliated program, a special multiprofessional team was established to serve children with HIV infections and their families (Diamond and Cohen 1989). Fifty percent of the children seen had conductive hearing loss, and 5% had severe to profound sensorineural hearing impairment.

Reasons for the variability in hearing impairment prevalence rates could include (1) nonrandom subject samples (subjects evaluated present with otologic and audiologic symptoms), (2) nondifferentiation of AIDS patients from HIV-positive patients, (3) differing definitions of hearing impairment, and (4) fluctuating and transient hearing loss in many people with HIV or AIDS (Friedman 1996). More research is needed, including a well-planned epidemiologic study.

Noise-Induced Hearing Loss

Differences in rates of hearing loss based on sex and race have been found in industrial noise-exposed populations. The differences are similar to the differences found in nonindustrial noise-exposed populations, as discussed in "Assessment." Black women tend to show the least effects of noise on auditory thresholds, followed by white women and black men, then white men (Jerger, et al. 1986). Black women therefore show the least standard threshold shift on annual tests, and white men show the most (Royster and Royster 1982). Audiologists must be aware of these differences in judging the effectiveness of hearing conservation programs.

It has been postulated that inner ear melanin (a biological polymer responsible for pigmentation) may serve to protect the ear from excessive noise (Barrenäs and Lindgren 1990). In addition to having more melanin content in the skin and eyes, individuals with darker skin have more melanin in the inner ear (La Ferriere, et al. 1974). Some studies (Hood, et al. 1976; Tota and Bocci 1967) have found brown-eyed individuals to have less temporary threshold shift (TTS) than blue-eyed individuals when exposed to noise; Karlovich (1975) did not. Barrenäs and Lindgren (1990) conducted an experiment using 44 white male Swedish subjects with three different skin types and found the least pigmented subjects showed the greatest TTS and the most pigmented subjects showed the least TTS.

Presbycusis

Decline in hearing acuity with advancing age is a fact of life, but the speed of decline seems to be affected by both sex and race. Women tend to hear better than men, and blacks tend to hear better than whites. More research is needed. As a start, population audiologic studies are needed for all racial groups. It will be difficult, if not impossible, to separate the various factors contributing to changes in auditory sensitivity over time. These factors include physiologic aging, diet, stress, noise exposure, disease processes, and racial and genetic factors (Scott 1993).

Intervention for Hearing Disorders

An individual's culture is not a diagnostic category. Cultural heritage does not wholly explain how an individual thinks and acts, but it can help audiologists anticipate and understand how and why individuals and families make certain decisions. Audiologists must keep in mind an individual's and family's view of disability. Three almost universal issues have been identified concerning the social implications of chronic illness and disability (Groce and Zola 1993):

1. The culturally perceived cause of a chronic illness or disability is significant in all cultures. The reason why an illness or disability is believed to have occurred in an individual plays a significant role in attitudes toward that individual. In some cases, the illness or disability is viewed as a form of punishment, a family curse, evidence of a past transgression, or an indication of an imbalance within the body. If a disability is viewed as unacceptable by a culture, the individual or family may feel pressured not to seek services even though they know they exist. In addition, the concept of early intervention is not known in many countries.

2. The expectations for survival (usually conceptualized as actual physical survival) for the individual with an illness or disability affect both the immediate care the individual receives and the amount of effort expended in planning for future care and education. The accepted body of folk knowledge plays a role in families' understanding of survivability.

3. The social role(s) deemed appropriate for children or adults with disability help determine the amount of resources a family and community invest in an individual. This includes education, training, and social life. As an example, a sex bias in favor of males is found in many cultures. Fewer resources and attention may be given to girls and young women with chronic illness or disability in traditional families.

Part of the audiologic intervention process usually involves the selection and use of hearing aids and assistive listening devices. The following are examples of cultural influences that audiologists should keep in mind during this process:

- The color of hearing aids and ear molds is important. Hearing aids and ear molds will be more acceptable to people of color if the aids and ear molds more closely match their skin color.
- Elders in a community may need to give permission before intervention services can begin and a hearing aid is accepted.
- The Deaf community does not view the use of cochlear implants on young deaf children as appropriate. The Deaf community does not believe a Deaf child's hearing needs to be "fixed."

Other forms of aural rehabilitation also must be culturally appropriate. The definition of family needs to include single parents, gay and lesbian parents, and large extended families. A choice of language for (re)habilitation needs to be made by the family. Too often in the past, English has been the language of intervention, with little or no consideration given to the home language or signing system.

Hearing disability among racial and ethnic minority groups has received little attention. Hanyak (1992) conducted a study to determine the utility of a modified Hearing Handicap Inventory for the Elderly—Screening Version (HHIE-S) for the assessment of hearing handicap and the incidence of self-reported hearing handicap in Hispanic adults. The Spanish version of the HHIE-S was shown to be a useful screening tool with Hispanic adults. In his conclusions, Hanyak recommended that the HHIE-S Spanish version be administered by bilingual interpreters rather than through self-administration due to the limited reading levels of Hispanic elderly.

The Future

A 1992 NIDCD working group examined the issue of research and research training of minorities. The report made many recommendations regarding multicultural research needs. Among the recommendations were that the NIDCD should provide support for research into (1) racial differences and influence of differing linguistic structures in normal auditory function, (2) epidemiologic studies of auditory disorders across all racial and cultural groups, (3) hearing deficits as a function of aging across all racial and cultural groups, (4) the effects of noise exposure, (5) disorders that affect general circulation, (6) otitis media, (7) SCD, and (8) the underuse of hearing health care services by blacks and other racial and ethnic minority groups (National Institute on Deafness and Other Communication Disorders 1992). These studies have yet to be completed.

Access to hearing services in racially and ethnically diverse communities is an important issue. In a survey of hearing health care needs among racial and ethnic minorities, Jones and Richardson-Jones (1987) found that only 9% of 230 respondents knew that they should seek an audiologist for hearing health care, and none knew where they could find an audiologist in their communities. They also found that 73% of the respondents rated hearing health care as a low priority. In 1986, Jones had found that African American populations use hearing aids at a rate that is only one-fifth that of the majority population in the United States (Jones 1986). Jones and Richardson-Jones (1987) stated that there are a number of reasons for the underuse of hearing health care services, including the need for more effective hearing health education in racial and ethnic minority communities, the costs of hearing services, and the nonpromotion of hearing services by hearing aid manufacturers in racial and ethnic minority communities. Jones (1988) also emphasized the need for more audiologists from racially and culturally diverse backgrounds to serve racial and ethnic minority communities.

Jones and Richardson (1995) discussed the need, in this case, to market to African American communities, which many audiologists do not do. Audiologists could initially target other community health care services that are already being used, such as family physician offices, drugstores, neighborhood health clinics, and health ministries of community churches. Providing hearing screenings, hearing aid service and sales, and hearing health care counseling at community day care centers also would be a good starting point.

Conclusion

Cultural competence generally is defined as consisting of three areas—knowledge, affect, and skills. A person who is culturally competent possesses a willingness and capability to draw on community-based values and customs and to work with others in developing focused interventions, communications, and other supports. Cultural incompetence, which is manifested as having no knowledge of cultural issues, apathy in caring about cultural issues, and no skills, can be destructive. Audiologists may not physically harm another person by being culturally incompetent, but those denied culturally appropriate hearing services may not return to such an audiologist or any hearing health care provider. Those individuals may then never receive the hearing services that could improve their quality of life. When detection of a life-threatening auditory disease, such as cancer or tumor on the auditory pathway, could have been detected early by an audiologic examination, those individuals who do not receive culturally competent audiologic services could face the shortening of their life.

Acknowledgments

I wish to acknowledge the assistance of Jerry Friedman in gathering the information on adults with HIV/AIDS and on the relationship between HIV/AIDS and hearing impairment.

References

American Speech-Language-Hearing Association, Research Division. (1994). *Survey of income and program participation estimates for United States, 1991–92. Number of people who have difficulty or are unable to hear normal conversation and whose speech is understood only with difficulty or not at all, by race and Hispanic origin.* Rockville, MD: American Speech-Language-Hearing Association.

Anderson, P.P., & Fenichel, E.S. (1989). *Serving culturally diverse families of infants and toddlers with disabilities.* Washington, DC: National Center for Clinical Infant Programs.

Axtell, R.E. (1991). *Gestures: The do's and taboos of body language around the world.* New York: Wiley.

Barrenäs, M.L, & Lindgren, F. (1990). The influence of inner ear melanin on susceptibility to TTS in humans. *Scandinavian Audiology, 19,* 97–102.

Beery, Q.C., Doyle, W.J., Cantekin, E.I., et al. (1980). Eustachian tube function in an American Indian population. *Annals of Otology, Rhinology, and Laryngology, 89(Suppl 68),* 28–33.

Berger, E.H., Royster, L.H., & Thomas, W.G. (1977). Hearing levels of nonindustrial noise exposed subjects. *Journal of Occupational Medicine, 19,* 664–670.

Bess, F.H., & Humes, L.E. (1990). *Audiology: The fundamentals.* Baltimore: Williams & Wilkins.

Bloom, M. (1995). *Understanding sickle cell disease.* Jackson, MS: University Press of Mississippi.

Bunch, C.C., & Raiford, T.S. (1931). Race and sex variations in auditory acuity. *Archives of Otolaryngology, 13,* 423–434.

Causse, J.R., & Causse, J.B. (1985). The genetics of the otospongiotic-otosclerotic disease. In V. Colletti, & S.D.G. Stevens (Eds.), *Disorders with defective hearing* (pp. 128–314). New York: Karger.

Centers for Disease Control. (1990). Estimates of HIV prevalence and projected AIDS cases: Summary of a workshop, October 31–November 1, 1989. *Morbidity and Mortality Weekly Report, 39,* 110–119.

Centers for Disease Control and Prevention. (1995). *HIV/AIDS surveillance report, 1995.* Atlanta: Centers for Disease Control and Prevention.

Crawford, M.R., Gould, H.J., Smith, W.R., et al. (1991). Prevalence of hearing loss in adults with sickle cell disease. *Ear and Hearing, 12,* 349–351.

Crawford, M.R., Burch-Sims, G.P., Scott, D.M., et al. (1995, April). *Audiologic considerations in sickle cell disease.* Paper presented at the annual convention of the American Academy of Audiology, Dallas.

Diamond, G.W., & Cohen, H.J. (1989). *Guidelines on developmental services for children and adults with HIV infection.* Silver Springs, MD: American Association of University Affiliated Programs.

Doyle, W.J. (1977). *A functiono-anatomic description of eustachian tube vector relations in four ethnic populations—an osteologic study.* Ph.D. dissertation, University of Pittsburgh.

Ellerbrock, T., Bush, T., Chamberland, M., & Oxtoby, M. (1991). Epidemiology of women with AIDS in the U.S., 1981–1990. *Journal of the National Medical Association, 265,* 2971.

Fleming, P., Gwinn, M., & Oxtoby, M. (1992). Epidemiology of HIV infection. In R. Yogev, & E. Connor (Eds.), *Management of HIV infection in infants and children.* St. Louis: Mosby–Year Book.

Forman-Franco, B., Karayalcin, G., Mandel, D.D., & Abramson, A.L. (1982). The evaluation of auditory function in homozygous sickle cell disease. *Otolaryngology-Head and Neck Surgery, 89,* 850–856.

Friedman, J. (1996). *Prevalence of hearing problems for people with HIV/AIDS.* Unpublished report.

Friedman, E.M., Luban, N.L.C., Herer, G.R., & Williams, I. (1980). Sickle cell anemia and hearing. *Annals of Otology, Rhinology, and Laryngology, 89,* 342–349.

Gould, H.J., Crawford, M.R., Smith W.R., et al. (1991). Hearing disorders in sickle cell disease: Cochlear and retrocochlear findings. *Ear and Hearing, 12,* 352–354.

Groce, N.E., & Zola, I.K. (1993). Multiculturalism, chronic illness, and disability. *Pediatrics, 91(Suppl)*, 1048–1055.

Guild, S. (1944). Histologic otosclerosis. *Annals of Otology, 53*, 246–266.

Hanyak, R.E. (1992, November). *Perdida de audicion en los adultos Hispanos (Hearing handicap in Hispanic adults)*. Paper presented at the annual convention of the American Speech-Language Hearing Association, San Antonio, TX.

Hood, J.D., Poole, J.P., & Freedman, L. (1976). The influence of eye color upon temporary threshold shift. *Audiology, 15*, 449–464.

Jerger, J., Jerger, S., Pepe, D., & Miller, R. (1986). Race difference in susceptibility to noise-induced hearing loss. *American Journal of Otology, 7*, 425–429.

Jerger, J., Chmiel, R., Stach, B., & Spretnjak, M. (1993). Gender affects audiometric shape in presbycusis. *Journal of the American Academy of Audiology, 4*, 42–49.

Jones, R.C. (1986). *Does the hearing aid industry discriminate against minorities?* Unpublished report.

Jones, R.C. (1988). Minority audiologists: A critical need to establish a professional/community identity. *ASHA, 30(8)*, 35–37.

Jones, R.C., & Richardson-Jones, J.T. (1987). Strategies for marketing hearing healthcare services to minority populations. *Hear Journal, 40(1)*, 13–16.

Jones, R.C., & Richardson, J.T. (1995). A study of the availability of hearing healthcare services in African-American communities. *ECHO, Fall*, 29–32.

Karlovich, R.S. (1975). Comments on the relation between auditory fatigue and iris pigmentation. *Audiology, 14*, 238–243.

La Ferriere, K.A., Kaufman-Arenberg, I., Hawkins, J.E., & Johnson, L.G. (1974). Melanocytes of the vestibular labyrinth and their relationship to microvasculature. *Annals of Otology, Rhinology, and Laryngology, 83*, 685–694.

Lalwani, A., & Sooy, D. (1992). Manifestaciones otológicas y neuro-otológicas del SIDA. *Clínicas Otorrinolaringologicas de Norte América, 6*, 1239–1254.

Madriz, J.J., & Herrera, G. (1995). Human immunodeficiency virus and acquired immune deficiency syndrome: AIDS-related hearing disorders. *Journal of the American Academy of Audiology, 6*, 358–364.

McCullough, J.A., Wilson, R.H., Birck, J.D., & Anderson, L.G. (1994). A multimedia approach for estimating speech recognition of multilingual clients. *American Journal of Audiology, 3*, 19–22.

National Center for Health Statistics. (1986). *Current estimates from the National Health Interview Survey, United States 1984. (Vital and*

Health Statistics. Series 10, No. 156. DHHS Pub. No. [PHS] 86-1584. Public Health Service). Washington, DC: U.S. Government Printing Office.

National Institute on Deafness and Other Communication Disorders. (1989). *A Report of the Task Force on the National Strategic Research Plan.* Bethesda, MD: National Institutes of Health.

National Institute on Deafness and Other Communication Disorders. (1992). *Report from the Working Group: Research and research training needs of minority persons and minority health issues.* Bethesda, MD: National Institutes of Health.

Orque, M., Block, B., & Monrroy, L. (1983). *Ethnic nursing care: A multicultural approach.* St. Louis: Mosby.

Post, R.H. (1964). Hearing acuity variation among Negroes and whites. *Eugenics Quarterly, 11,* 65–81.

Roberts, R.N. (1990). *Workbook for developing culturally competent programs for children with special needs.* Washington, DC: Georgetown University Child Development Center.

Roseberry-McKibbin, C. (1995). *Multicultural students with special language needs: Practical strategies for assessment and intervention.* Oceanside, CA: Academic Communication Associates.

Royster, L.H., & Thomas, W.G. (1979). Age effect hearing levels for a white nonindustrial noise-exposed population (NINEP) and their use in evaluating industrial hearing conservation programs. *American Industrial Hygiene Association Journal, 40,* 504–511.

Royster, L.H., & Royster, J.D. (1982). Methods of evaluating hearing conservation program audiometric databases. In P.W. Alberti (Ed.), *Personal hearing protection in industry* (p. 571). New York: Raven.

Royster, L.H., Driscoll, D.P., Thomas, W.G, & Royster, J.D. (1980). Age effect hearing levels for a black nonindustrial noise-exposed population (NINEP). *American Industrial Hygiene Association Journal, 41,* 113–119.

Sakai, M., & Miyake, H. (1977). Primary otosclerosis in the stapes of a Japanese. *Japan Auris Nasus Laryngology, 4,* 97–105.

Sarniak, S., Soorya, D., Kim, J., et al. (1979). Periodic transfusions for sickle cell anemia and CNS infarction. *American Journal of the Diseased Child, 133,* 1254–1257.

Schuknecht, H.F. (1974). *Pathology of the ear.* Cambridge, MA: Harvard University Press.

Scott, D. (1986). Sickle-cell anemia and hearing loss. In F.H. Bess, B.S. Clark, & H.R. Mitchell (Eds.), *Concerns for minority groups in communication disorders* (p. 69). Rockville, MD: American Speech-Language-Hearing Association (ASHA Reports 16).

Scott, D.M. (1993). Aging and hearing loss: Race and gender differences in African Americans and Euro-Americans. *Howard Journal of Communications, 4,* 369–379.

Scott, R.B., & Kessler, A.D. (1977). *A child with sickle cell anemia in your class.* Washington, DC: Howard University Center for Sickle Cell Disease.

Simonds, R., & Rogers, M. (1992). Epidemiology of HIV infection in children and other populations. In A.C. Crocker, H.J. Cohen, & T.A. Kastner (Eds.), *HIV infection and developmental disabilities: A resource for service providers* (pp. 3–14). Baltimore: Brookes.

Tota, Y., & Bocci, G. (1967). The importance of the colour of the iris on the evaluation of resistance to auditory fatigue. *Rev Oto-Neuro-Ophthalmology, 42,* 183–192.

U.S. Bureau of the Census. (1990). *Statistical abstract of the United States: 1990 (110th ed.).* Washington, DC: U.S. Bureau of the Census.

U.S. Bureau of the Census. (1992). *Population projections for states by age, sex, race, and Hispanic origin: 1992 to 2050, current population reports* (pp. 25–1092). Washington, DC: U.S. Bureau of the Census.

U.S. Bureau of the Census. (1993). *Language spoken at home and ability to speak English for United States, regions, and states: 1990, CPH-L-133.* Washington, DC: U.S. Bureau of the Census.

U.S. Bureau of the Census. (1995). *Statistical abstract of the United States (115th ed.).* Washington, DC: U.S. Bureau of the Census.

12

Multicultural Aspects of Deafness

Njeri Nuru-Holm
and Dolores E. Battle

Deafness transcends decibels and embraces Deaf people, their communities, and their culture. It is important to recognize that within the Deaf community at large, cultural diversity traditionally has meant Deaf culture and Hearing culture, not ethnic diversity. Deafness has taken precedence over ethnicity in the Deaf community. As a result, minorities have been virtually invisible in the study of Deaf people in America. The history and current situation of Deaf people from ethnic, linguistic, and racial minority backgrounds is more than a colorized version of the history of the Deaf in America. The body of information needed to understand the behaviors and problems of non–English-speaking and ethnic minority Deaf in the United States is still in its early stages of development.

Throughout this chapter, *Deaf* is capitalized to signify inclusion of the cultural aspects of deafness; *deaf* is used to connote hearing loss. *Hearing* is used to signify audiocentricity (hearing-centered world view); *hearing* refers to hearing status.

Demographics

The Deaf population is decreasing. As shown in Figure 12-1, the number of hearing-impaired students younger than age 21 years decreased from 88,732 in 1978–1979 to 59,071 in 1988–1989 (Gallaudet University, unpublished data, 1980–1990). Data from the 1989–1990 Annual Survey of Hearing-Impaired Children and Youth (Gallaudet University, unpublished data, 1980–1990) indicated that 46,000 hearing-impaired children in the United States were receiving special education services in 1989–1990. A 10-year comparison of these data also indicates a decrease in the overall number of Deaf children (Table 12-1 and Figure 12-1).

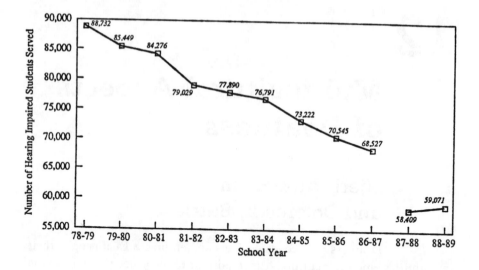

Figure 12-1 Number of hearing-impaired students younger than age 21 years as reported to be served by special education programs during the 1978–1979 to 1988–1989 school years. Note that before the 1987–1988 school year, the figures represented children 0–21 years of age served under Public Law 89-313 and children 3–21 years of age served under Public Law 94-142. (Data from the Office of Special Education and Rehabilitative Services. *Annual Reports to Congress on Implementation of the Education of All Handicapped Children Act.*)

Although the total number of Deaf and hard-of-hearing children is decreasing, the representation of minority children among the Deaf is increasing. Deafness among minority groups increased by 14.1%, from 22.5% in 1980 to 36.6% in 1990 (Gallaudet University, unpublished data, 1980, 1985, 1990; Harris and Moran 1986). Comparative data on hearing-impaired children younger than age 6 years show more minority hearing-impaired children in 1984 compared with 1977 and a decrease in the number of the white deaf children in the population (Cohen, et al. 1990).

Deafness in the white population decreased 14.1% between 1980 and 1990. Deafness in the African American population decreased by only 2.2% during the same period. In contrast, there was an increase in deafness among Hispanics, Asians and Pacific islanders, and American Indians, with the increase among Hispanics being the most significant. Deafness among the Hispanics showed a 4.9% increase between 1980 and 1990 (Gallaudet University 1980-1990). The largest number of Deaf Hispanics have been found among the Hispanic population in California, Texas, and New York (Schildroth and Hotto 1993), as would be expected considering the demographic

Table 12-1 Annual Survey of Hearing-Impaired Children and Youth
(by Ethnicity): 1980–1990

Ethnicity	1979–1980		1989–1990		Percentage Change
	Number	*Percentage*	*Number*	*Percentage*	
White	36,621	77.5	29,178	63.4	–14.1
Black	9,098	19.2	7,817	17.0	–2.2
Hispanic*	[4,985]	[9.1]	6,257	14.0	+4.9
Asian Pacific	547	1.2	1,542	3.0	+2.8
American Indian	221	0.5	328	0.7	+0.2
Other	784	1.7	923	2.0	+0.3
Total population	47,271		46,045		

*Represents 1980–1981 data. Hispanics were not designated as a separate ethnic group in the 1979–1980 survey. Hispanic representation was included among the black, white, and other groupings.
Source: Data from the Gallaudet University Center for Assessment and Demographic Studies. Annual surveys of hearing-impaired children and youth, 1979–1990.

distribution of Hispanics in the United States (U.S. Bureau of the Census 1996). As shown in Figure 12-2, the Deaf Asian and Pacific island population more than doubled from 1.2% in 1980 to 3.0% in 1990. This could be related to the large number of immigrants from refugee camps in southeast Asia, where hearing impairment was not prevented.

Demographic patterns of the Deaf are consistent with population patterns across the United States. In his testimony before the Commission on the Education of the Deaf, Cohen (1987) described strong ethnic minority representation across the United States. Along the Middle Atlantic and Southeast coast and across the southern states to Texas and California, Hispanics and African Americans represent 49% of Deaf students. He also indicated that ethnic diversity is strong among the Deaf population in the inner cities in large metropolitan areas, where ethnic, cultural, and linguistic minorities are predominant in the 25 largest urban school systems.

In 1979–1980, white Deaf constituted a large majority in all regions (67–85%). Deaf from ethnic minorities constituted the majority in only one continental state (Missouri) and in Washington, DC. According to data from the Gallaudet University Center for Assessment and Demographic Studies, because

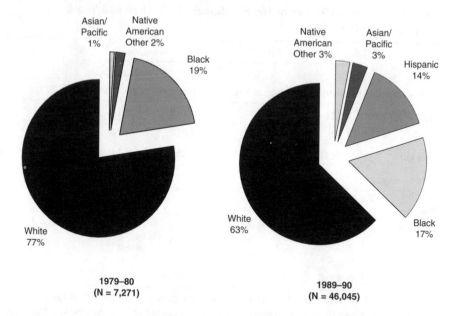

Figure 12-2 Annual survey of hearing-impaired children and youth (by ethnicity): 1980–1990. (Data from the Gallaudet University Center for Assessment and Demographic Studies. Annual survey of hearing-impaired children and youth.)

of the decrease in deafness among the white population between 1980 and 1990, as well as smaller decreases and increases among the minority populations, in 1989 minority Deaf constituted the majority of the Deaf population in five continental states (California, Missouri, New Mexico, New York, and Texas) and in Washington, DC (Cohen, et al. 1990).

During the 1980s, the proportion of white Deaf children has decreased by 28% in the West and by more than 10% in 15 states in the Northeast (Cohen, et al. 1990). Deafness among the white population decreased by from 20% to 46% in some other states (Cohen, et al. 1990). The percentage of white Deaf has decreased by 13% in Washington, DC, and by 2% in four states, all in the South (Cohen, et al. 1990). Approximately two-thirds (63%) of the white Deaf population live in the Midwest and South (Gallaudet University, unpublished data, 1980, 1985, 1990).

More than half (55%) of the African American Deaf population now lives in the South, where African Americans are a large proportion (approximately one-third or more) of the total population. The African American Deaf population in Washington, DC, decreased by 26% between 1980 and 1990 but by only 1–6% in 20 other states (Cohen, et al. 1990).

The smallest representation (9%) of African American Deaf population is in the West. In contrast, nearly half (48%) of the Asian Deaf population and 40% of Deaf Hispanics live in the West. The other half (52%) of the Asian Deaf population is equally distributed between the South (27%) and the Northeast (25%). Almost half of the Deaf American Indian population lives in the West and the other half lives in the Midwest and South (Cohen, et al. 1990).

Etiology

In 1970, maternal rubella, mumps, and measles ranked as the major causes of hearing impairment. By 1980, mumps and measles had nearly disappeared, but rubella still occurred (Figure 12-3). The incidence of rubella decreased by 7% from 1980 to 1985, and it is now the second primary cause of deafness among the school-aged population (Schildroth 1986).

Schildroth and Hotto (1993) analyzed the results of the 1989–1990 National Survey of Hearing-Impaired Children and Youth (Gallaudet University, unpublished data, 1990). They concluded that with rubella nearly eliminated (less than 5%) as a major cause of deafness and the rubella bulge population having almost left school, heredity and meningitis are the primary causes of deafness (Figure 12-4). They speculated that hereditary causes were previously underreported due to the large numbers of students included as "undetermined" causes or for whom no data were available. Within the "other" category, Schildroth and Hotto (1993) noted the persistence of cytomegalovirus (a herpes virus known to cause a complex of physical problems among newborns, including hearing loss) as a cause of deafness.

Data from the 1979–1980 and 1989–1990 Annual Survey of Hearing-Impaired Children and Youth were reanalyzed by the author for ethnicity information (Figures 12-3 and 12-4). Major etiology varied by ethnicity. Although meningitis and heredity were primary causes of hearing loss across all populations (5–16%), the incidence of meningitis disproportionately increased among African Americans and American Indians. Heredity disproportionately affected the white, Hispanic, and American Indian populations. The incidence of meningitis had increased for whites and American Indians, as well (Nuru 1993).

Heredity was the primary cause of deafness among whites (15.8%), Hispanics (13.2%), and Asian- and Pacific island–Americans (6.6%). However, even as a primary cause among Asians, heredity affected a lower percentage of the Asian population than it did as a secondary cause among Native Americans and African Americans. Deafness due to heredity was half as prevalent in African Americans (7.9%) as whites (15.8%) (Nuru 1993).

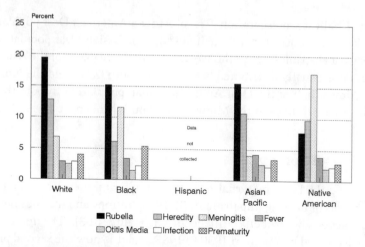

Figure 12-3 Causes of hearing loss in children and youth by ethnicity: 1979–1980. (Data from the Gallaudet University Center for Assessment and Demographic Studies. Annual survey of hearing-impaired children and youth.)

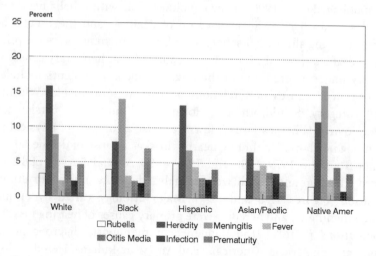

Figure 12-4 Causes of hearing loss in children and youth by ethnicity: 1989–1990. (Data from the Gallaudet University Center for Assessment and Demographic Studies. Annual survey of hearing-impaired children and youth.)

Meningitis was the primary cause of deafness among American Indians (16.2%) and African Americans (14%) and approached the incidence rate of deafness caused by rubella more than a decade ago. This disproportionate incidence is nearly double that for the white (8.8%) and Hispanic (6.8%) populations, for whom it is the secondary cause. It is four times more prevalent for African Americans and Hispanics than for Asians or Pacific Americans (4%) (Nuru 1993). Meningitis, however, is a preventable disease and should be addressed with the same level of vigor as rubella was. It is a primary issue related to prevention, early identification, and health care delivery to minority populations.

Across ethnic groups, the incidence of other etiologies (including rubella) is less than 5%, with the exception of prematurity in the African American population. Prematurity has increased across all groups but is highest among the black population (7%) (National Center for Health Statistics 1994). The increase in the number of minority children who are Deaf probably reflects the increase of prematurity, which is a cause of deafness in African Americans (Brown 1986). It is the third highest cause of deafness in African American and white children and the second highest for Asians and Pacific Americans. Rubella is highest among Hispanics. Otitis media has also increased slightly across all groups but is lowest for blacks (2%) (Nuru 1993). Otitis media is highest among the American Indian population and has long been reported by the Indian Health Service as a major nonmortal disease and health care problem among American Indians. The continued high incidence of meningitis in the American Indian population is speculated to be influenced by otitis media (Hammond and Meiners 1993).

Hearing loss is present at birth for approximately 75% of the population (Padden and Humphries 1988). Approximately 11–30% of Deaf school children inherit their deafness; however, less than 10% are born to Deaf parents (Padden and Humphries 1988). Accordingly, most deaf people were not a part of the Deaf community at birth. There is a higher incidence of adventitious hearing loss among African Americans and American Indians (Christensen and Delgado 1993). This may be associated with the higher incidence of meningitis among these populations. In the American Indian population, it also may be the result, to some degree, of otitis media and untreated infection. It is noteworthy that, with the exception of high fever and otitis media, the incidence of adventitious hearing loss was lowest among the Asians and Pacific islanders (Cheng 1993). The reasons for this lower incidence need to be investigated. It is possible, for example, that other causes do not emerge due to deaths among infants and children before they reach school age. It is important to be aware that in 1979–1980 data were not collected for Hispanics (Gallaudet University, unpublished data, 1980).

Incidence data may reflect improved diagnostics or outreach and service delivery to previously underserved ethnic populations. It is also believed that increased awareness of genetically linked hearing loss has resulted in better categorization of causes in the "other" category that previously were attributed to heredity.

Education for the Deaf

Current data show that across all ethnic groups Deaf students continue to be educated primarily in special education classes and secondarily in residential schools. In a study by Andrews and Johnson (1993), more than half of the white and Asian and Pacific American Deaf students reported integration with hearing students, whereas more than half of their African American, Hispanic, and American Indian counterparts did not. More than half of all Deaf students are educated in programs that combine the use of sign and speech (MacNeil 1990). More than half of Deaf African Americans (70%) and Hispanics (66%) are enrolled in special education programs that use a combination of sign and speech, whereas only 42% of Deaf whites are enrolled in such programs (MacNeil 1990). A sign-language interpreter is used by 93% of the students enrolled in combined sign and speech programs (Gallaudet University, unpublished data, 1980).

Understanding Differences

In the Deaf community, Deaf culture, as opposed to Hearing culture, is emphasized so much that the ethnic aspect traditionally has been ignored. Even "educators of deaf children and youth have had a tendency to accept the erroneous proposition that deafness in some ways precludes ethnic and racial minority group membership and status" (Cohen, et al. 1990).

Culturally diverse Deaf people experience the same cultural behaviors and problems as others of their culture do. At the same time, they also experience the behaviors and problems related to deafness as do other Deaf people. For the Deaf minority child, hearing loss introduces another layer of complexity to be negotiated. This layer includes the multicultural aspects of linguistic and cultural code switching that need to be successfully negotiated to facilitate communication, mobility, development, and achievement (Gomperz 1971, 1982). The increase in Deaf minorities signals an increase in the number of children for whom it is probable that the sign language used at school, oral language used at school, or both are different from the language used in the home. The challenge to the Deaf child is to come to terms with the culture of the home and the culture of school and peers and to effectively negotiate both.

Environment, body awareness, and social attitude are influenced by cultural differences. The use of space and time varies widely among different ethnic groups, and it is important to clarify and define the importance of these elements for social interaction and business (e.g., concepts of time and being on time) (Vernon and Mindel 1971; Otterbein 1977; Koo 1982; Condon and Jousef 1985). Eye contact, stance, touch, and gestures, all of which are also important elements in Deaf culture, reflect differences in rules regarding the body and body awareness between Deaf culture and ethnic cultures. These elements may be in or out of phase. Social attitudes also vary according to gender, status, and age (e.g., male dominance, birth order, revered age, and extended family).

Social acceptance of hearing loss and other hearing disabilities varies across cultures and can differ from the Western model. Educators need to be sensitive to and nonjudgmental of culturally determined reactions. Such reactions can be perceived as defensiveness, denial, avoidance, or rationalization; "shopping" for someone who will say what they want to hear activism (if it concerns people fluent in English and familiar with the education and the social services systems); increased religious activity and the belief that the Deaf child is given by God as a cross to bear; or embarrassment (often reflected in missed appointments due to not wanting to be seen in the special facility). Although such reactions can be disruptive and inconvenient to intervention, they also can be a source of family strength.

The American Indian Deaf

Although cultural and behavioral differences have been identified that affect education and health care services (e.g., eye contact, aggressiveness, and silence), research specific to the American Indian Deaf has not been available. Counter's audiologic research (1986) on Amerindians in the nontechnologic noise-free rain forest in Surinam (South America) resulted in identification of conductive and sensory-neural hearing impairment, primarily sequelae to otitis media, aging, and what is speculated to be ototoxicity from ingestion of large quantities of the manioc cassava, which has high concentrations of cyanide. Deafness, however, was not reported (Counter 1986).

The powers of medicine men continue to be a part of American Indian culture. A child with a handicap may be accepted by parents and into society as the will of the gods. Navajo Deaf are valued as sheepherders. In contrast, the use of a device, such as a hearing-aid, may not be easily accepted. Because the family is a strong and close-knit unit in American Indian culture, parents do not send their children away for prolonged periods of time. Accordingly, not many American Indian children attend schools for the Deaf (Stewart 1985).

The Asian Deaf

The Asian family in America symbolizes the multicultural complexity of the environment a Deaf Asian child faces with the verbal and nonverbal differences of two languages and two cultures. For example, Japanese children are taught to show respect through silence and a bowed head, with little or no direct eye contact. (Direct eye contact represents defiance and disrespect to an adult.) On the other hand, in American culture, children are taught to look directly at a person and to express themselves verbally. The Asian hearing-impaired child, who must depend heavily on the visual channel to facilitate communication therefore has opposite expectations of communication from those prevalent in most schools and also misses the incidental learning and communication that occurs based on rules of a different culture. To avoid confusion, therefore, the child needs guidance in learning the different rules of communication in school. It is important that the reasons for different communicative and behavioral expectations in different settings are pointed out to the child in a constructive manner (Yacobacci-Tam 1987).

The African American Deaf

Immersed in both African American and Deaf cultures, the African American Deaf are affected educationally, vocationally, and socially by both the issues facing the Deaf population and those facing the African American population. In a hearing- and color-conscious society, African American Deaf are a minority within a minority and continue to be disadvantaged and powerless along with other nonwhite minorities in America, even more than their nondeaf counterparts (Vernon and Makowsky 1970; Lombardo 1976; Anderson 1972). Although conditions have improved to some degree in recent years, African American Deaf people still labor under a legacy of generations of discrimination and a lack of awareness of the extent of deafness in the African American population, even among educators of the Deaf (Moores and Oden 1977).

Fischgrund and colleagues (1987) believe that to facilitate the effectiveness of educational, vocational, and parent intervention programs, one must first understand the African American Deaf population. Crucial to that understanding is an understanding of the social and economic realities of life in most African American communities. The African American population in America represents Caribbean cultures, African cultures, and African American experiences. Most Africans and Caribbeans come from countries and islands where they are the majority and hold political and economic power. This background influences their response to the U.S. white power structure and their perspective as African Americans and minorities.

The African American Deaf population historically has been a neglected and multidisadvantaged group characterized by poverty, social isolation, lack of communication skills, unemployment or underemployment, and undereducation (Lombardo 1976; Anderson and Bowe 1972; Bowe 1971; Smith 1972; Whiting 1975). The problems and needs of the African American Deaf population were rarely talked about in open meetings before the 1972 Fourth Biennial Conference of Professional Rehabilitation Workers with the Adult Deaf. At this meeting, a panel of four African American Deaf professionals in education and rehabilitation identified four major problems: (1) the high unemployment rates of African American Deaf compared with white Deaf; (2) the limited number of African American Deaf going beyond the eighth grade; (3) the lack of awareness among African American Deaf and their parents of available facilities and services, education, scholarships, and training programs; and (4) the paucity of African American Deaf professionals, resulting in a lack of role models for African American Deaf children (Hairston and Smith 1983). The number of African American Deaf completing secondary school has increased since that time; however, the other problems persist.

Education of African American Deaf Children

Before the Education of Handicapped Children Act of 1975, education and service systems had largely been unsuccessful in reaching and serving the African American Deaf population (Furfey and Harte 1968; Hairston and Bachman 1967). For the African American Deaf community, this resulted in a general lack of success, poor communication skills, and a mistrust of government (i.e., the white power structure), which resulted in a call for the use of paraprofessionals from within the African American community to bridge this distrust (Bowe 1972). In examining the school records of African American Deaf adolescents in Baltimore, Furfey and Harte (1968) found the African American Deaf students who had average IQs were identified as educationally deprived. Many African American Deaf children started school late, some as late as 8–9 years of age. Ries and colleagues (1975) reported under-representation of African American hearing-impaired children (younger than 6 years old) in preschool programs compared with those in programs for children ages 6 years and older. Reasons for this under-representation included (1) late identification of hearing loss attributed to lack of awareness among African American parents of available services, (2) frustration in trying to identify services, (3) historical inadequacy of services for children 6 years of age and younger, (4) a higher rate of acquired deafness in African American children, and (5) a disproportionately high identification of African American deaf children as mentally retarded.

The Individuals with Disabilities Education Act of 1990 had a significant impact on the availability of educational services for all Deaf children, including African American Deaf. The Education of the Handicapped Amendments of 1976 created early identification and intervention programs for infants and toddlers 0–2 years of age. The legislation made early identification of deafness and early education and intervention available to Deaf children at no cost to the parents.

African American Deaf children, as with African American hearing children, are disproportionately identified as mentally retarded (e.g., 13–17% of the deaf population is misdiagnosed as mentally retarded, but 22–24% of the African American Deaf population is misdiagnosed as mentally retarded.) (Gallaudet University, unpublished data, 1990; Babbidge 1965; Bowe 1974). Misdiagnosis of mental retardation can result from (1) misunderstanding due to lack of cultural awareness, knowledge, and sensitivity to the African American child in educational and clinical settings; (2) misinterpretation of delayed development of communication skills as functional retardation; (3) higher incidence of prematurity as an etiology, which increases susceptibility to brain damage and mental retardation (Moores and Oden 1977; Babbidge 1965; Vernon 1968); and (4) ambiguous and subjective interpretations rooted in the same practices found in regular and special education (Babbidge 1965; Bowe 1974; Hamayan and Damico 1991; Mattes and Omark 1991; Battle and Grantham 1997). It is noteworthy that, although identification procedures have improved and incidence decreased, mental retardation and hearing disabilities continue to be identified disproportionately as additional disorders among minority Deaf when compared with white Deaf.

The Individuals with Disabilities Education Act of 1990 also had a significant impact on the types of educational programs available to Deaf children. African American Deaf children are now able to attend educational programs in their neighborhood rather than be moved to residential schools where they are often immersed in white culture. Being able to attend the public school with their cultural peers has reduced the isolation felt by many Deaf children and increases their ability to function in the community (O'Connell 1997; O'Connell and Huffman 1997). Many members of the Deaf community have been less than enthusiastic about the move to increased community schooling. There has been a movement toward Deaf pride, similar to movements within other groups (Solomon 1994). This movement has not affected the African American Deaf because they continue to exist as a minority within a minority and are without voice in the political arena of the Deaf.

African American Sign Language

Before 1970, African American and white Deaf children in the South were educated in segregated schools. Although African American children knew the white variety of American Sign Language (ASL), a distinct variety called Black- or African American ASL developed. Its relationship to ASL is analogous to the relationship between Standard American English (SAE) and African American English (Woodward 1976; Maxwell and Smith-Todd 1986).

The linguistic features of African American ASL were perceived by others as poorly developed communication skills, which served as a communication barrier and a reason for rejection at Deaf social and cultural activities (Anderson and Bowe 1972). African American Deaf children who attended schools for white Deaf were especially mindful of the white variety of ASL. For this reason, African American Deaf children were sometimes chided by their peers as "signing white" when using SAE, similar to the manner in which their hearing counterparts were chided as "talking white."

Linguistic switching by African American signers has been observed within their own milieu similar to code switching by speakers of African American English (e.g., when in the company of family or friends or in clubs) (Smith 1972; Whiting 1975; Woodward 1982). Regional differences were noted analogous to spoken regional dialects. The historical roots for these differences were the societal attitudes and educational policy in the South, especially in Georgia, North and South Carolina, Florida, Alabama, and Virginia. Compared with standard signs, these African American Deaf regional or local signs were generally "more colorful and demonstrative with non-verbal expressions and body language, or shortcut versions of standard signs" (Hairston and Smith 1983). In his book *How You Gonna Get to Heaven if You Can't Talk with Jesus!* Woodward (1982) attempts to depathologize deafness through a sociolinguistic analysis of dialectal differences of African American sign language. Lucas and Valli (1989) examined the sociolinguistic factors related to the dynamics of contact signing between deaf and hearing African American and white dyads and described the morphologic, syntactic, and lexical structures of the contact signing and the nature of code switching.

African American Family and Community

Parents of Deaf African American children have the same reaction as other parents when they learn of a child's deafness or hearing loss. Many of these parents, however, are additionally challenged by stressors such as poverty, immigration, and other inequalities historically experienced by African Americans, American Indians, and Hispanics.

In seeking the factors that contribute to the low educational achievement of African American Deaf students, some researchers typically have looked to the family and the local community. Insensitive to differences and values related to family structure, they have identified factors about the African American family as negative variables. Examples of such factors are (1) the single-parent family (which may be a strong positive unit compared to a dysfunctional two-parent unit); (2) living with grandparents or in a foster home (neither of which is inherently negative); (3) median family size of 5.3, which may include the extended family; and (4) minimally educated parents (Grier and Cobbs 1968; Lerman and Cortez 1987).

African Americans and whites in the adult Deaf community are relatively unintegrated. Whether this is the result or the manifestation of indirect or overt discrimination, the majority of African American Deaf do not freely associate socially or on an equal basis with white Deaf people. It is not unusual, however, for African American Deaf to enjoy social support from one another (Hairston and Smith 1983). When they do attend social events where whites are also present, they often stay together. As a result, their experiences are often not reflected in the information related to the Deaf community.

Many African American Deaf are therefore disadvantaged due to limited contact with professionals. They are also limited in association with their hearing counterparts in the African American hearing community.

The Hispanic Deaf

The needs of Deaf children from linguistic minority groups were largely unrecognized in deaf education until population demographics began to change rapidly in the past two decades. The Gallaudet Center for Assessment and Demographic Studies data indicate significant growth in the number of Hispanic hearing-impaired students (Schildroth and Hotto 1993). Of 54,774 hearing-impaired children and youth in the 1981–1982 Annual National Survey of Hearing-Impaired Children and Youth, 5,185, or 9.5%, were Hispanic. This percentage grew to 11.1% in the 1984–1985 survey and to 14% in 1989–1990. African Americans and Hispanics alone represent nearly one-third (31%) of hearing-impaired youth in the United States (Schildroth and Hotto, 1993). Sixty-eight percent of Hispanic Deaf children were from California, Texas, and New York (Schildroth and Hotto 1993), as is expected, since these states also have the highest number of Hispanic residents (U.S. Bureau of the Census 1996). Lerman and Cortez (1987) revealed that Hispanics make up 26% of Deaf youth in Texas, 28% of Deaf youth in regional day school programs in Texas, and 16% of the students at the Texas School for Deaf Hispanics. In addition, Lerman and Fischgrund (1980) reported that 40% of the hearing-impaired students in New York City were Hispanic.

Lerman and Cortez (1980) reported that 30% of Hispanic Deaf children become deaf after birth, as compared with 22% of the white Deaf population. This is primarily due to heredity (13%) and secondarily to meningitis (7%). Hispanic Deaf children primarily attend day school and nonintegrated local schools.

Education

As a group, Deaf Hispanic children have low academic achievement. A disproportionate number of Deaf Hispanic children in schools for the Deaf are placed in groups for the low-achieving or learning-disabled students (Gallaudet University, unpublished data, 1980, 1985; McCahill 1974; Christensen 1985). Studies report that Hispanic Deaf children score significantly lower on tests of language development, computation, and social-emotional status compared with non-Hispanic children (De Garcia 1993). Delgado (1984) reported on a survey of hearing-impaired children from non-English language homes conducted by Gallaudet University in 1979–1980. The 62% response rate represented 41,489 hearing-impaired children, of which 12,237, or 29%, had additional handicaps. Three thousand (7%) of the children were from non–English-speaking homes where Spanish was the predominant first language. Fifteen hundred (51%) of the non–English-speaking group reportedly had additional handicaps, such as mental retardation and learning disabilities. The low achievement of the Hispanic Deaf is related to the difficulty doing an unbiased assessment with a child who cannot use hearing to process linguistic cues. All the problems identified for the speech-language nonbiased assessment of bilingual children are multiplied for the speech-language and other assessments of the Hispanic Deaf child (Mattes and Omark 1991).

Bilingualism and Trilingualism

Parent-child interaction and communication are important in the development of communicative competence (Corsaro 1981). However, Christensen (1985) found that less than 1% of Hispanic families with deaf children were fluent in the sign language the children were learning and using at school. In Texas, 75% of Hispanic Deaf students come from Spanish-speaking homes (Christensen 1985). Trybus and colleagues (1978) found that Spanish was used in 19% of the homes of Hispanic Deaf in the United States. When the language of the family is different from the language of academic instruction, the problems inherent to acquisition of conceptual sign language are compounded. Similar to the conflict that arises when children from Spanish-speaking homes are immersed in English-only education programs, conflict arises when a Deaf Hispanic child receives Spanish linguistic cues at home and English linguistic cues at school with a structured sign system. This conflict manifests as low achievement scores in the development of communication skills of the Hispanic Deaf (Cortez 1975; Delgado 1984) and as problems in communication at home reported by mothers (Schlesinger and Meadow 1972).

The Hispanic Deaf child in a Spanish-speaking home has particular problems learning to communicate. Their problems are similar to those of other children in Spanish-speaking homes, with the added dimension of the inability to use hearing to develop a linguistic system in either English or Spanish. ASL, based on SAE, is difficult for the Hispanic child whose home language is based on Hispanic language concepts. The Deaf child from a Spanish-speaking family must not only learn to communicate in Spanish at home but also must learn to communicate in ASL at school. This requires the development of English-based language (Paul 1996; Stuckless 1991). The child must be trilingual, a task difficult even for those in the hearing world. Unlike the culturally diverse hearing individual who is bilingual, the Deaf individual is faced with complex cognitive "differences in receptive and expressive modes of sign [versus] spoken language [that are] greater than the phonologic and linguistic differences [of] disparate spoken languages" (Kopp 1984). Teachers have raised serious questions and concerns regarding the challenges posed by Deaf children from non–English-speaking homes (Jensema 1975; Blackwell and Fischgrund 1984). If the natural sign language theory is extended to children of Spanish-speaking families, it follows that instruction and speech-language intervention should be conducted in the sign language that is natural to any given culture (e.g., Spanish sign language for children from Spanish-speaking homes). However, the lack of bilingual or Spanish-speaking educators of the deaf or educational audiologists and the nearly total absence of trilingual professionals make the challenge of providing appropriate clinical or educational services particularly difficult.

Conceptual sign language (CSL) can serve as an alternative visual gestural mode of communication that can bridge the disparate linguistic and phonologic boundaries of oral English and Spanish and lead to effective communication among parents, Deaf children, and teachers. CSL can be acquired more easily than a second language of different or arbitrary structure for several reasons: (1) Some of the syntactic structures in Spanish and ASL are similar (e.g., noun-adjective construction: "house white") (Leutke 1976), (2) the lexical items in ASL are iconic in nature, (3) lexical functioning is separate from syntactic processes in ASL (McCahill 1974), and (4) kinesthetic involvement facilitates second-language learning (Christensen 1985). The following is an example of the contrasts between English, Spanish, ASL, and CSL:

English	Spanish	ASL	CSL
white house	*casa blanca*	[house] + [white]	[white] + [house]

Because the icon (or sign) is understood as a concept, and syntax is not a bound process, the meaning is clear regardless of word order in both ASL and CSL.

Speech-Language Development and Intervention for the Hispanic Deaf

Speech-language pathologists and teachers of the Deaf often ask the following questions when making decisions about the education and clinical intervention for the Hispanic Deaf child from a Spanish-speaking hearing family:

1. What are the reasonable expectations for Deaf children who have "no language"?
2. Because Deaf children have so much difficulty in the acquisition of one language, would the acquisition of two languages not be inordinately difficult?
3. If learning two languages is out of the question (and given that this is an English-speaking society), shouldn't our efforts to teach the children English include discouraging the use of Spanish?
4. If the goal is to teach the children to communicate in an English-speaking society, shouldn't we ask the parents to speak English at home, especially to their Deaf children? We do not want the use of Spanish in the home to confuse Deaf children and hinder their understanding of English.
5. With the language development curriculum, shouldn't we begin by working on the English or ASL vocabulary for things already familiar to the child (e.g., food, clothing, body parts, furniture, and rooms in the house)?
6. Shouldn't the educational program for Deaf children contain only a minimum of basic skills until they are old enough to be in a vocational training program that includes a life-skills component?

These questions reflect a racial and ethnic bias; a monocultural perspective and experience; and dubious assumptions based on lack of understanding of the process of language acquisition, the nature of bilingualism, and the role of culture in education and learning. They are the same questions that speech-language pathologists ask when considering intervention for a hearing child from a non–English-speaking family. What is needed is an understanding of the concepts that underlie the teaching of English as a second language and the development of language in bilingual children. Instruction should take place via total communication in the language spoken at home and the sign language able to be used by the parents. The Deaf child should be fully immersed in the culture of the Deaf and the ethnic community of the individual. Only then can minority Deaf people hope to obtain their rightful place in the American mainstream.

Conclusion

The Americans with Disabilities Act of 1990 mandated a societal accessibility for the Deaf population that is unprecedented. Along with the Telecommunications Decoder Act and the Civil Rights Act of 1964 (Section 504), the Individuals with Disabilities Education Act of 1990 provided the groundwork for greater accessibility and equal opportunities for the hearing impaired. It is now incumbent upon educators, health care professionals, and the public, individually and collectively, to move inspirational mottoes, symbolism, and political rhetoric into the reality of human resources and systems. To do this in the challenging and diverse multicultural society that is ours, we must personally address that which cannot be legislated—the ethical foundations that undergird and guide our own human behavior.

References

Anderson, G.B. (1972). Vocational rehabilitation services and the black deaf. *Journal of Rehabilitation of the Deaf, 6,* 126–128.

Anderson, G.B., & Bowe, F.G. (1972). Racism within the deaf community. *American Annals of the Deaf, 117,* 617–619.

Andrews, J.F., & Jordan, D.L. (1993). Minority and minority deaf professionals: How many and where are they? *American Annals of the Deaf, 138(5),* 388–396.

Babbidge, H.D. (1965). *Education of the deaf: A report to the Secretary of Health, Education, and Welfare by his advisory committee on the education of the deaf.* Washington, DC: U.S. Department of Health, Education, and Welfare.

Battle, D.E., & Grantham, R. (1997). Serving culturally and lingustically diverse students. In P. O'Connell (Ed.), *Speech language hearing programs in schools: A guide for students and practitioners* (pp. 305–344). Gaithersburg, MD: Aspen.

Blackwell, P.M., & Fischgrund, J.E. (1984). Issues in the development of culturally responsive programs for deaf students from non–English-speaking homes. In G.L. Delgado (Ed.), *The Hispanic deaf: Issues and challenges in bilingual special education.* Washington, DC: Gallaudet University Press.

Bowe, F.G. (1971). Nonwhite deaf personnel: Educational, psychological, and occupational considerations. *American Annals of the Deaf, 188,* 357–361.

Bowe, F.G. (1972). Role of the paraprofessional in inner city services to deaf persons. *Journal of Rehabilitation of the Deaf, 6,* 120–122.

Bowe, F.G. (1974). Deafness and mental retardation. In J. Schein (Ed.), *Education and rehabilitation of deaf persons with other disabilities* (pp. 26–58). New York: University Deafness Research and Training Center.

Brown, S. (1986). Etiology trends, characteristics and distribution. In A.N. Schildroth, & M.A. Karchmer (Eds.), *Deaf children in America* (pp. 15–27). San Diego: College Hill.

Cheng, L. (1993). Deafness: An Asian-Pacific Island perspective. In K.M. Christensen, & G.L. Delgado, (Eds.), *Multicultural issues in deafness* (pp. 113–126). White Plains, NY: Longman.

Christensen, K.M. (1985). Conceptual sign language as a bridge between English and Spanish. *American Annals of the Deaf, 130,* 244–249.

Christensen, K.M., & Delgado, G.L. (1993). *Multicultural issues in deafness.* White Plains, NY: Longman.

Cohen, O. (1987, May). *Current and future needs of minority learning-impaired children and youth.* Testimony presented at the Commission on the Education of the Deaf. Washington, DC.

Cohen, O.P., Fischgrund, J.E., & Redding, R. (1990). Deaf children from ethnic, linguistic and racial minority backgrounds: An overview. *American Annals of the Deaf, 153,* 67–73.

Condon, J.C., & Jousef, F.S. (1985). *An introduction to intercultural communication.* New York: Macmillan.

Corsaro, W. (1981). The development of social cognition in preschool children: Implications for language learning. *Topics in Language Disorders, 2,* 77–95.

Cortez, E. (1975). *Meeting the needs of Hispanic deaf children.* New York, NY: Lexington School for the Deaf: Lexington Reports.

Counter, S.A. (1986). Audiological screening of American Indians of the Suriname rainforest. *Scandinavian Audiology, 15,* 57–64.

De Garcia, B.G. (1993). Assessing the needs of Hispanic deaf children. In K.M. Christensen & G.L. Delgado (Eds.), *Multicultural issues in deafness* (pp. 69–88). White Plains, NY: Longman.

Delgado, G.L. (1984). Hearing-impaired children from non-native language homes. In G.L. Delgado (Ed.), *The Hispanic deaf: Issues and challenges in trilingual special education* (pp. 45–72). Washington, DC: Gallaudet University Press.

Fischgrund, J.E., Cohen, O.P., & Clarkson, R.L. (1987). Hearing-impaired children in black and Hispanic families. *Volta Review, 89,* 59–67.

Furfey, P., & Harte, T. (1968). *Interaction of deaf and hearing in Baltimore City, MD.* Washington, DC: Catholic University of America Press.

Gallaudet University Center for Assessment and Demographic Studies. (1980–1990). The annual survey of hearing impaired children and youth: 1980 to 1990 school years (unpublished reports). Washington, DC: Gallaudet University.

Gomperz, J.J. (1971). *Language in social groups.* Stanford, CA: Stanford University Press.

Gomperz, J.J. (1982). *Discourse strategies.* London: Methuen.

Grier, W.H., & Cobbs, P.M. (1968). *Black rage.* New York: Basic Books.

Hairston, E., & Bachman, J. (1967). *A study of a segment of the Negro deaf population in the Los Angeles area.* Los Angeles: Leadership Training Program in the Area of the Deaf.

Hairston, E., & Smith, L. (1983). *Black and deaf in America: Are we that different?* Silver Springs, MD: TJ Publishers.

Hammond, S.A., & Meiners, L.H. (1993). American Indian deaf children and youth. In K.E. Christensen, & G.L. Delgado (Eds.), *Multicultural issues in deafness* (pp. 143–166). White Plains, NY: Longman.

Hamayan, E.V., & Damico, J. (1991). *Limiting bias in the assessment of bilingual students.* Austin, TX: PRO-ED.

Harris, P.R., & Moran, R.T. (1986). *Managing cultural differences (2nd ed.).* Houston, TX: Gulf Publishing.

Jensema, C. (1975). *The relationship between academic achievement and the demographic characteristics of hearing impaired children and youth.* Washington, DC: Gallaudet University Office of Demographic Studies.

Koo, L.C. (1982). *Nourishment of life: Health in Chinese society.* Hong Kong: Commercial Press.

Kopp, H.G. (1984). Bilingual Problems of the Hispanic Deaf. In G.L. Delgado (Ed.), *The Hispanic Deaf: Issues and challenges in bilingual special education* (pp. 73–96). Washington, DC: Gallaudet University Press.

Lerman, A., & Cortez, E. (1980). *Discovering and meeting the needs of hearing impaired children. Report CREED VII Project.* New York: Lexington School for the Deaf.

Lerman, A., & Cortez, E. (1987). *Discovering and meeting the needs of Hispanic hearing impaired children. Report CREED VII Project.* New York: Lexington School for the Deaf.

Lerman, A., & Fischgrund, J. (1980, April). *Improving services of Hispanic hearing-impaired students and their families.* Paper presented at the Ninth Annual Meeting of National Association of Bilingual Education, Anaheim, CA.

Leutke, B. (1976). Questionnaire results from Mexican-American parents of hearing impaired children in the United States. *American Annals of the Deaf, 121,* 565–568.

Lombardo, A.S. (1976). An examination of the difficulties encountered by the black deaf. *Deaf Americans, 7,* 23–26.

Lucas, C., & Valli, C. (1989). Language contact in the American deaf community. In C. Lucas (Ed.), *The sociolinguistics of the deaf community* (pp. 103–119). San Diego: Academic Press.

MacNeil, B. (1990). Educational needs for multicultural hearing-impaired students in the public school system. *American Annals of the Deaf, 135,* 75–82.

Mattes, L.J., & Omark, D.R. (1991). *Speech and language assessment for the bilingual handicapped.* Oceanside, CA: Academic Communication Associates.

Maxwell, M., & Smith-Todd, S. (1986). Black sign language and school integration in Texas. *Language in Society, 15,* 81–94.

McCahill, P.A. (1974). A case of disinterest: The deaf in Puerto Rico. *American Annals of the Deaf, 116,* 413–414.

Moores, D., & Oden, H. (1977). Educational needs of black deaf children. *American Annals of the Deaf, 122,* 313–318.

National Center for Health Statistics. (1994). *Healthy United States: 1993.* Hyattsville, MD: Public Health Service.

Nuru, N. (1993). Multicultural aspects of deafness. In D. Battle (Ed.), *Communication disorders in multicultural populations* (pp. 287–305). Butterworth–Heineman: Boston.

O'Connell, P. (1997). History of school services: Speech-language and hearing. In P. O'Connell (Ed.), *Speech, language, hearing programs in schools: A guide for students and practitioners* (pp. 3–13). Gaithersburg, MD: Aspen.

O'Connell, P., & Huffman, N. (1997). Speech-language pathology and audiology in the educational setting: Professional qualifications, roles, and services. In P. O'Connell (Ed.), *Speech, language, hearing programs in schools: A guide for students and practitioners* (pp. 66–103). Gaithersburg, MD: Aspen.

Otterbein, K.F. (1977). *Comparative cultural analysis.* San Francisco: Holt, Rinehart, and Winston.

Padden, C., & Humphries T. (1988). *Deaf in America.* Cambridge, MA: Harvard University Press.

Paul, P.V. (1996). First and second-language English literacy. *The Volta Review, 98(2),* 5–16.

Ries, P., Bateman, D., & Schildroth, A. (1975). *Characteristics of impaired students in the United States.* Washington, DC: Gallaudet University Office of Demographic Studies.

Schildroth, A.N. (1986). Hearing impaired children under age 6: 1977 and 1984. *American Annals of the Deaf, 111,* 85–90.

Schildroth, A.N., & Hotto, S.A. (1991). Annual survey of hearing impaired children and youth: 1989–90 school year. *American Annals of the Deaf, 136,* 155–163.

Schlesinger, H, & Meadow, K. (1972). *Sound and sign.* Berkeley, CA: University of California Press.

Smith, L.D. (1972). Work-study programs and black deaf people. *Journal of Rehabilitation of the Deaf, 6,* 116–119.

Solomon, J.A. (August 28, 1994). Defiantly deaf. *New York Times Magazine, 98,* 38–45.

Stewart, J.L. (1985). Provision of health care to underserved populations. *Volta Review, 77,* 64–71.

Struckless, E.R. (1991). Reflection on bilingual bicultural education for deaf children: Some concerns about current advocacy and trends. *American Annals of the Deaf, 136,* 270–272.

Trybus, R., Rawlings, B., & Johnson, R. (1978). *State survey of hearing-impaired children and youth. A new approach to statewide planning, monitoring, and evaluation of special education programming.* Washington, DC: Gallaudet University Office of Demographic Studies.

U.S. Bureau of the Census. (1996). *Statistical abstract of the United States: 1996 (116th ed.).* Washington, DC: U.S. Bureau of the Census.

Vernon, M. (1968). *Multiply handicapped deaf children: Medical, educational and psychological considerations.* Washington, DC: Council for Exceptional Children.

Vernon, M., & Mindel, E. (1971). *They grow in silence.* Silver Springs, MD: National Association for the Deaf.

Whiting, H.A. (1975). *Services to the black deaf adult.* Ph.D. dissertation, University of Wisconsin.

Woodward, J. (1976). Black southern signing. *Language in Society, 5,* 211–218.

Woodward, J. (1982). *How you gonna get to Heaven if you can't talk with Jesus?* Silver Springs, MD: TJ Publishers.

Yacobacci-Tam, P. (1987). Interacting with the culturally different family. *Volta Review, 89,* 46–58.

Additional Resources

Christensen, C., & Delgado, G.L. (1993). *Multicultural issues in deafness.* White Plains, NY: Longman.

Lucas, C. (1989). *The sociolinguistics of the deaf community.* San Diego: Academic.

13

Assessment Issues with Multicultural Populations

Toya Wyatt

When working with multicultural populations, it is important to provide services that are both culturally sensitive and appropriate. To accomplish this goal, speech-language pathologists and audiologists must understand how cross-cultural differences in communication styles; views toward health, illness, and disability; the nature and prevalence of communication disorders; and language differences affect the diagnostic evaluation process. This applies to every aspect of the assessment process, including obtaining the case history, test administration, interpretation, diagnosis, and report writing. The purpose of this chapter is to discuss how some of the cross-cultural variables addressed in this book affect each of these components of the speech-language hearing assessment process.

The Case History and Factors to be Considered in the Case History Interview

The assessment process usually begins with obtaining information about the client's background and history of the problem. This is often accomplished through the taking of an oral case history or the completion of a written case history supplemented by an oral history. The oral case history is a significant communication event affected by all parameters of interpersonal communication. When the communication event takes place between two people, clinician and client, who are from different cultural or language backgrounds, the cultural and linguistic variables discussed in previous chapters become significant. These variables can have an impact on the client's willingness to participate in the assessment process, on the eventual diagnosis of the problem, or on both.

There are a number of factors that must be taken into consideration when preparing for and obtaining case history information from clients from culturally and linguistically diverse backgrounds. These include but are not limited to culturally based differences in (1) beliefs concerning the most appropriate topics; (2) the interpretation of questions and requests for information; (3) norms for greeting and addressing individuals; (4) norms for initiating, sustaining, and terminating conversations; (5) nonverbal communication behaviors; (6) turn-taking; (7) communication style; (8) the familiarity and acceptability of proposed clinical procedures and recommendations; (9) views of health, handicap, illness, disorder, and disability; and (10) the prevalence and incidence of communicative disorders. Other factors, such as a client's degree of familiarity with English and the clinical service delivery process, must also be taken into consideration.

Client's Familiarity with the Clinical Process

A client's degree of familiarity and experience with the clinical process should also be taken into account when working with clients from culturally diverse populations. In many cases, culturally diverse clients have had less exposure to clinical procedures used in speech pathology and other health-related fields than mainstream clients. Clinicians should therefore take more time to explain the purpose of the diagnostic evaluation process and documents that need to be signed, such as the informed consent form. They should also explain what takes place during the assessment and what information clients should expect to accomplish at the conclusion of the session. Clinicians should realize that terms such as *confidentiality* and *informed consent* may be less familiar to clients from nonmainstream backgrounds. This makes the assessment process less intimidating to clients who are less familiar with the traditional Western model of health care delivery.

In addition, when communicating with clients who have limited English proficiency, clinicians should be certain that the clients understand information requested on forms. All written documents requiring the client's signature should be presented in the client's native language. If documents written in English are to be translated, it is important to give the translator sufficient time to prepare the translation so that the client can understand the content and intent of the forms (Kayser 1995; Roseberry-McKibbin 1995). Roseberry-McKibbin (1995) stated that one of the most common complaints of interpreters is not being given enough time to prepare for diagnostic evaluations and translating paperwork. The translation of paperwork is especially important when documents, case history interview questions, or both, which are to be translated, contain terms that are fairly technical in nature or not typically found in the native language of the client.

In addition to the language barrier, there are other barriers that may be encountered by clinicians when asking clients or family members to give their written consent for certain procedures. Clients from some religions may, for example, feel uncomfortable about giving permission for themselves or family members (e.g., children) to be videotaped, because to capture an individual's visual image in photographs or videotapes may be equated with control (e.g., control over one's soul). Clinicians may also find that some clients object to videotaping because of cultural mistrust and fear of lack of confidentiality. As Terrell and Terrell (1996) indicated, cultural mistrust can cause clients to refuse to participate in assessment because of concern about the use of the information. These concerns are rooted in a historical past, where information obtained was used to substantiate claims about linguistic and intellectual inferiority. The use of information may also be of concern when informed consent is requested to provide an agency with the opportunity to use clinical records for research purposes. Clinicians may find that they must answer a number of questions about how the information will be used, as well as assure clients that the information will be used in a manner that protects their privacy.

Verbal Communication

Topics and Questions

The establishment of rapport can be affected by the type of topics addressed, questions asked, and the manner in which each question is asked. Frequently asked case history questions, such as birth history, place of residence, and the nature of the client's communication difficulties, can be perceived by some clients as being too personal, intrusive, inappropriate, or irrelevant. In some Native American communities, for example, the mere mention or discussion of an individual's disability can be viewed as potentially putting that person at risk for greater difficulties (Harris 1993). For some clients, fairly neutral questions such as "Where do you live?" can be viewed with suspicion. For example, clients who have a high level of cultural mistrust, as defined by Terrell and Terrell (1996), may misinterpret this type of question as an indirect attempt to obtain private information, such as the client's socioeconomic or immigration status (i.e., illegal or legal). Either of these can have a negative impact on the amount of information that clients are willing to disclose. It may be helpful, therefore, to ask someone from the same cultural background as the client or someone who is knowledgeable about the client's cultural community to review case history questions before the interview to determine their cultural appropriateness.

During the interview, clinicians should explain the purpose and use of questions that may be sensitive or intrusive. For example, the clinician might introduce a question such as "Where do you live," which might be viewed with suspicion by some clients, with, " Mrs. Jones, I realize that the next question may be a little personal, but it is important so that I know where to send our final report." Other introduction statements such as "Some of the questions I will need to ask you are necessary for me to understand the problem" help the client understand the intent of the questions and minimize concerns they may have about responding. It can also help build trust at an early stage in the assessment process.

Greetings and Social Address

Social norms for greetings and social address are a key issue that must be considered when conducting the case history interview. For example, in some communities where formality and status play a significant role in interpersonal communication, clinicians need to pay more attention to how initial introductions with a client are made. According to Matsuda (1989), in Asian cultures it is important to know the social status of another when interacting in social situations so that the appropriate form of address is used. One must know, for example, "whether the person to be addressed is of higher, equal or lower status before speaking" (Matsuda 1989). Knowing another's status helps to determine how one is to be addressed and how communication is to proceed.

Matsuda (1989) suggests that, as a result, clinicians need to be "status conscious" when working with individuals from Asian or Asian American backgrounds. Clinicians should establish their role, as well as that of the family or parent, during initial introductions. For example, when working with a team of professionals in a clinical setting, one member of the team should introduce all other members of the team by name, title, and professional role (clinical responsibilities) before beginning the assessment or team meeting. Whenever possible, formal introductions should be made by a third party familiar to or respected by the client. Third-party introductions are likely to be viewed more positively than personal introductions. Third-party introductions also serve as an important mechanism for establishing a clinician's initial credibility. The introductions are best carried out by the individual who has had the most contact with the family before the evaluation or by the person with the highest status in the agency or on the team.

Clinicians should also give some consideration to the terms of address used with clients and family members. In recent years, American society has begun the practice of addressing individuals by their first name during professional interactions. In many minority communities, however, addressing strangers by their first name, even after the first meeting, is more likely to be viewed as socially inappropriate and in some cases disrespectful, particularly when the individual being addressed is older and has had much more life experience than the addresser. Many African Americans consider this practice to be presumptuous and a form of disrespect. Clinicians should greet and address clients and family members using titles (e.g., "Mr." or "Mrs.") and last names, until and unless a client indicates that it is acceptable to do otherwise. When working with Spanish-speaking clients, it is also important for clinicians to use the more proper form of *you* (*usted* versus *tu*) when addressing parents, adults, or older patients (Langdon 1992a).

Initiating, Sustaining, and Terminating Conversation

Once the interview begins, clinicians should use their knowledge about cross-cultural differences in communication to facilitate the case history interviewer process. This includes being aware of cross-cultural differences in how one initiates, maintains, and terminates conversation. For example, in Hispanic communities, conversations, even those that are professional in nature, always begin on a personal note with discussion of family and other nonclinical matters. It is considered rude and an invasion of privacy to initiate conversation with business talk (Langdon 1992a). Clinicians should also be aware that in some Native American communities, social rules dictate that one remains silent at the beginning of initial social encounters (Saville-Troike 1986). To deal with this issue, clinicians may want to plan two meetings instead of one for conducting diagnostic evaluations. The first meeting should be used to establish rapport, and the second should be used to elicit important case-history and assessment information.

Turn Taking

Cross-cultural differences in turn taking must also be taken into consideration when working with individuals from differing cultural and linguistic backgrounds. In some cultures, the length of time expected between conversational turns either exceeds or is considerably less than that typically seen in mainstream Euro-centered discourse. For example, it is common to see longer periods of silence and greater pausing between conversational turns in Native American and Asian discourse, where silence is highly valued (Harris 1993; Mattes and Omark 1991; Matsuda 1989; Roseberry-McKibbin 1995). Listeners are expected to reflect on what has been said before responding. Clinicians who experience these prolonged periods of silence between their questions and the interviewee's response may misinterpret such pauses as a sign of noncomprehension or a refusal to answer. Some clinicians might respond to this situation by repeating or reformulating questions before interviewees have had an opportunity to respond. Clinicians who patiently wait for the interviewee's response, however, generally find that the client understood the question and that the client was simply responding in the manner that he or she considered to be socially and culturally appropriate. Silence on the part of the client may also indicate that a certain question was inappropriate.

Clinicians also need to be aware that in cultures in which turns occur more rapidly, it is common for several individuals to be speaking at the same time and for one speaker to overlap another (Schieffelin and Eisenberg 1984; van Kleeck 1994). Kochman (1981) states that in the African American speech community, it is allowable for a speaker to interrupt another, once the former has made at least one good point. This can create problems for clinicians who are used to a more Euro-centered style of turn taking in which listeners generally wait for the speaker to yield the floor. Clinicians who are more familiar with Euro-centered discourse patterns may misinterpret interruptions from an African American client using an overlapping turn-taking style as rude and possibly hostile.

Clinicians should also be aware that cultural communities differ with respect to other communication style differences, such as the use of directiveness. When interacting with clients from certain cultural backgrounds, clinicians who have a Euro-centered communication style may be viewed as being too direct and probing in their questions. This can occur with clients who have a more Asian-centered style of communication. According to Matsuda (1989), an indirect communication style is more highly valued in the Asian community than in American mainstream communities. As a result, American communicators who are direct in their communication are often viewed by Asian speakers as making embarrassing critical remarks and asking prying questions. This type of conversational-style mismatch can create difficulties during the case history interview process and destroy the harmony of the communication process.

Group harmony is highly valued in many Asian communities. It is so important that some Asian communicators refrain from saying "no" or indicating any disagreement with statements or suggestions made by others. They may even say "yes" or "okay" when they are not in agreement, so as not to appear rude (Matsuda 1989). Consequently, it can be beneficial for clinicians to use a more indirect manner of asking questions of their Asian clients, particularly when these questions deal with sensitive topics and information. The use of indirect and open-ended questions can preserve group harmony during the interview process. Clinicians may also find it helpful to use the key discourse strategies used within the cultural community of their client (e.g., more pausing between turns and allowing more time for reflection) to improve the information sharing or disclosure process.

Bilingual Language Issues

When preparing to evaluate bilingual clients, there are additional considerations that must be taken into account when planning the case history interview. The language that the interview should be conducted in is of primary importance. Naturally, the interview should be conducted in the native language of the client. If a clinician with native or near-native use of the client's language is not available, a trained interpreter should be used.

During the information-gathering process, it is also important to ask about the client's language history and development for both languages spoken. Determining this information applies regardless of whether the suspected communication disorder is the result of developmental or acquired factors. Furthermore, a comprehensive review of the client's abilities in all languages spoken should be conducted, regardless of whether the client presents a fluency, voice, articulation, expressive language, receptive language, or aphasia disorder. Examples of information to be obtained include (1) the age at which the client was exposed to each language, (2) conditions under which each language was acquired, (3) the course of development in each language, (4) the perceived level of proficiency in both languages, (5) current language-use patterns (i.e., when, where, with whom, and how often), (6) the nature of communicative difficulties in each language, (7) current level of proficiency in both languages (speaking, understanding, reading, writing), and (8) client and family attitudes toward the language of intervention or instruction.

In the case of acquired disorders such as aphasia, it is also important to ask questions about language use and communicative skills before onset of the disorder. Determining the client's degree of educational training in each language is also important when printed (written language) materials are being considered for use during the evaluation process. Clinicians should be aware that the overall literacy level of clients from some cultural communities is lower than that in other communities. For example, Reyes (1995) stated that elderly Hispanics are six to seven times more likely to be functionally illiterate (to have less than 5 years of schooling) than elderly whites. In addition, only 10% of Hispanics 25 years of age or older have completed 4 or more years of college, as compared with 21% of non-Hispanics. It is also possible that schooling was in the first language, making reading in a second language more difficult. For other clients, reading proficiency in the second language may be greater than speaking proficiency because literacy skills were first developed in the second language instead of the first language. These factors suggest that clinicians must determine a client's levels of literate, as well as oral, language proficiency before selecting or administering diagnostic procedures or conducting the case history interview. Readers are directed to the parent, teacher, and client questionnaires presented in Cheng (1991) Kayser (1995), Langdon (1992b), Mattes and Omark (1991), and Roseberry-McKibbin (1995) for examples of questions that should be included in a bilingual case history interview.

Nonverbal Communication

Eye Gaze

During communicative interactions, there are also differences in how listeners signal to the speaker that they are attending to what is being said. When communicating with a Euro-centered style of communication, sustained eye gaze is used to signal attentiveness. Diverted eye gaze is often interpreted as a sign of disinterest, disrespect, or both. In many cultures, diverted eye gaze is viewed as a sign of respect, and direct eye gaze is viewed as rude or an attempt to challenge the speaker. As a result, sustained eye gaze occurs less often during communicative interactions with African American, Asian, Native American, Pacific islander, and Hispanic listeners (Conklin and Lourie 1983; Roseberry-McKibbin 1995; Terrell and Terrell 1993). When working with clients from these cultures, clinicians must be careful of misinterpreting differing eye-gaze patterns as a sign of disinterest, nonattentiveness, or as an "attitude problem."

Head Nodding

Other culturally based nonverbal differences that can be misinterpreted include head nodding. In the Asian community, head nodding is often used as a sign of respect or attention rather than of agreement (Matsuda 1989). Misinterpretation of this nonverbal signal by clinicians can lead to misunderstanding between the clinician and family regarding a family's acceptance or understanding of the matters discussed as well as the client's intention to follow through on recommendations.

Client's View of Health, Illness, and Disorder

Another factor that clinicians should consider during the interview process is the differing views that clients may have about health, illness, and disorder. According to Maestas and Erickson (1992), perceived causes of disability in the Mexican-American community vary substantially from those perceived by parents in non–Mexican-American communities. In their study of 27 Mexican-American immigrant mothers, Maestas and Erickson asked mothers of children receiving special education services to identify common causes of disability. Some of those reasons cited by more than 50% of the respondents interviewed were (1) mother had a big fright (*sustos*), (2) punishment for bad behavior, (3) mother is too old, (4) mother has had too many children, or (5) someone cast a spell. In addition, 15% or more respondents attributed disability to the following possibilities: (1) an earthquake, (2) an eclipse, (3) mother is too young, or (4) *mal ojo* (evil eye).

Clinicians need to expect similar types of responses from some of their clients during the case history process. Clinicians should never respond to these beliefs in a manner that suggests, even indirectly, that the client's ways of viewing disorder are inappropriate. This can have a negative effect on the establishment of rapport and the information disclosure process.

Clinicians may also encounter clients who come from a cultural community in which disorders are concealed. In such cases, clinicians may find that clients are reluctant to respond to any questions that focus on the origins, nature, or course of a disorder. In minority communities in which adults have become wary of how society has traditionally labeled their children, clinicians may also find that commonly used terms such as "language disorder," "language handicap," or "language impairment" are viewed as offensive or that these terms are likely to be more readily associated with mental retardation or illness (Roseberry-McKibbin 1995). Terms such as "problem" may also be equated with more serious conditions and be rejected by clients. Clinicians are encouraged to be more neutral in their use of terminology. This can include using a phrase such as "communication difficulties" rather than "communication disorder." Clinicians must also take more time to explain these terms and their clinical and educational implications.

Nature and Prevalence of Communication Disorders

Another important cross-cultural difference that must be considered during the interview is the difference that exists in the nature and prevalence of certain communicative disorders. There are a number of communication disorders that have a higher incidence in some cultures and racial and ethnic groups than others. For example, several studies have documented the higher incidence of hearing-related disorders, such as otitis media, in Pacific islander and Native American populations (Buchanan, et al. 1993; Pang-Ching, et al. 1995). There are also certain medical conditions, such as sickle cell anemia, that occur more frequently in certain racial groups and put individuals in those groups at a slightly higher risk for sensorineural and central auditory nervous system disorders (Buchanan, et al. 1993; Scott 1986). Clinicians need to be remain cognizant of these differences when planning what information to obtain during the interview. Specifically, when working with clinical populations likely to be at greater risk for these conditions, clinicians must include questions that probe issues that are related to these concerns.

Test Administration

Test Bias

In addition to thinking about the type of questions to be used during the case-history interview, clinicians must give a great deal of thought to the type of assessment procedures to be used. One of the first issues that must be addressed by any clinician before engaging in the assessment process is the possibility of test bias. According to Taylor and Payne (1983), Vaughn-Cooke (1986), and Chamberlain and Medeiros-Landurand (1991), there are a number of factors that can have a negative impact on the collection or interpretation of test information and lead to a possible misdiagnosis of communicative impairment. These include but are not limited to (1) situational bias, (2) format bias, (3) value bias, and (4) linguistic bias.

Situational Bias

Situational bias can occur whenever there is a mismatch in the communicative styles of the client and clinician. Differences in the interpretation of sustained eye gaze, for example, can lead to the misdiagnosis of a pragmatic disorder in clients who normally divert eye gaze during listening as a sign of respect. It is not uncommon to find diagnostic reports that cite lack of sustained eye gaze as evidence of pragmatic deficit in African American clients. Many communication assessment protocols used to identify pragmatic disorders list sustained eye gaze as an important aspect of communicative competence. These protocols, however, have been based primarily on research findings obtained from individuals from white, middle-class mainstream communication backgrounds. Often, researchers are not sensitive to the differing use of eye contact in communication among other cultures.

Situational bias can also occur when there is a mismatch in the communicative expectations of the clinician and client regarding the conversational roles of children. For example, Heath (1982), Langdon (1992a), Kayser (1993), Schieffelin and Eisenberg (1984), van Kleeck (1994) and Anderson and Battle (1993) have noted that in some minority communities, children learn early that they are not to initiate conversation with adults and that they are to speak only when spoken to. Children are also taught to respond to the questions of adults minimally. As a result, it is common for minority children to say little during the testing process with adult examiners or to initiate conversation much less often than their nonminority peers. These children may also be less elaborate in their descriptions of action pictures, not because of limited language abilities but because of their socialization. This is in contrast to middle class nonminority children who are encouraged to initiate conversation with adults and encouraged to be verbal in their responses to questions.

Format Bias

Format bias occurs when clinicians use testing procedures, picture stimuli, topics, or vocabulary that are unfamiliar to the client. Heath's (1982, 1983, 1986) research on African American and Mexican-American communities revealed that children in both of these communities are less likely than their Euro-American peers to engage in label quests and to answer known-information questions. This includes responding to requests to identify pictured objects in the view of both the examiner and client (e.g., "Show me the ball") or answering questions about stories that have just been read or a picture that has just been seen. Such requests were rarely made by adults in the children's communities. In addition, in Mexican-American families, children use label quests only in a limited number of contexts (i.e., labeling distant objects, body parts, and family member names). Labeling differences have also been noted during book reading. Anderson-Yockel and Haynes (1994) found, for example, that African American mothers were less likely than white mothers to ask their children *wh-* and yes-and-no questions during book-reading tasks. Because of these differences, it is possible that some minority clients may respond more slowly to requests to label pictures and objects.

In some communities, known-information questions are also rarely used. Furthermore, when assessing clients of cultures in which discussions about the obvious rarely take place, clinicians may find their clients responding to questions with responses that focus more on events and topics outside of the immediate situational context. In other words, responses tend to focus more on new, rather than shared or old, information (information that is not already known to the listener). Clinicians should avoid labeling such responses as tangential or irrelevant to the topic.

Clinicians should be careful about using topics or vocabulary items that are unfamiliar to clients from a certain cultural background. For example, it may be inappropriate for clinicians to ask clients who live in desert areas to label pictures of items such as ocean or seashells. They should also avoid asking clients to define vocabulary terms or discuss topics not typically found in their home communities. Inability to label such concepts could be a function of limited exposure rather than limited vocabulary or cognitive abilities. Similarly, clinicians should recognize that clients who have newly arrived from other countries or who have not assimilated well into the mainstream culture may have had less exposure to objects, events, and items that are typically associated with American culture. Cheng (1991) provides some examples of American concepts that are likely to be unfamiliar to children coming from Asian countries. Examples include household objects commonly found in American kitchens and homes (e.g., certain cooking utensils [blenders] or furniture items), vehicles that are not common in a child's home community (e.g., fire engines), American sports, musical instruments (e.g., banjo, harmonica), clothing, historical events, people (e.g., Abraham Lincoln), buildings (e.g., Empire State Building), and holidays (e.g., Halloween, Christmas). Many items contained within standardized speech and language tests are culture bound.

Dialect differences that occur in the vocabulary or pronunciation of sounds in the English and other non-English languages can result in bias. Merino (1992) and Goldstein (1995) both present examples of speech sound and vocabulary differences that can occur in the various dialects of Spanish. For example, it is not uncommon for Puerto Rican Spanish speakers to produce *puerta* as "*puelta*" or to produce final /s/ as /h/ in a word such as *gatos*. In addition, either *naranja* or *china* can be used to refer to an orange, dependent on one's native Spanish dialect. Geographically based language differences can exist even within the same dialect of Spanish. This would explain some of the differences between the various Southwestern varieties of Spanish (e.g., the Mexican-American Spanish spoken in New Mexico versus that spoken in Southern California and Texas).

Value Bias

Value bias in testing results when test items reflect the traditional views, attitudes, opinions, social norms, or values of one group versus another. Value bias is frequently seen in tests that attempt to assess a client's comprehension abilities through the use of logical or problem-solving questions. Such questions typically begin with the phrases "What should you do if...?" or "What should you do when...?" For example, if a child who is raised in a more rural community is asked "What should you do when you run out of milk?," he or she may respond "You should go to the barn and milk one of the cows." This may be viewed as an inappropriate response by the clinician if he or she is not aware that the client lives on a farm. This type of bias can also occur on items that ask a client to identify the right or correct way of doing something. For example, when the question "Why should you brush your teeth?" from the Preschool Language Scale-3 (PLS-3) (Zimmerman, et al. 1992) is administered to African American and Hispanic children residing in urban southern California communities, this author has found that it is not uncommon for many of the children to say, "'Cause my momma tell me to." It is possible that many of those children are less likely to hear an explanation like that provided in the scoring manual of the PLS-3 (e.g., "If you don't, you'll get cavities") than their mainstream American peers because of the social rule within their communities that prohibits children from questioning adults about doing things that they are told to do. Such responses should not be considered incorrect. This type of response, however, would be considered wrong by the standard scoring conventions of the PLS-3.

Linguistic Bias

Linguistic bias occurs when tests used are based on a language system different from that used by the client. At present, all of the English-language tests used by speech-language pathologists are based on Standard American English (SAE). Therefore, the client who uses African American English (AAE) or any other dialect is likely to be misdiagnosed as presenting a language disorder even when they are using the normal rules of their dialect. This is because many of the grammatical features of nonstandard English dialects, such as the occasional absence of the copula and frequent absence or devoicing of final consonant sounds, are similar to the features exhibited by SAE speakers with communicative disorders. Linguistic bias also occurs when clinicians use SAE tests to assess the language skills of non-English or limited English proficient speakers. In most cases, the administration of an English test to a nonnative English speaker provides more information about their level of English proficiency than about the presence or absence of a communicative disorder.

This issue is equally important when discussing certain audiologic assessment procedures, such as speech reception and discrimination testing. There are some studies that suggest that monolingual non-native English speakers can be at a significant disadvantage when speech discrimination testing is conducted in English using English word stimuli (Danhauer, et al. 1984). In a study comparing the performance of monolingual English, monolingual Spanish, and bilingual Spanish-English speakers on a 25-item nonsense syllable test originally designed for English-speaking populations, Danhauer and colleagues (1984) found that monolingual Spanish subjects performed considerably poorer than the other two groups. Part of the problem with using non-native language stimuli is that stimuli used in most English-based speech reception tests consist of spondee words (two-syllable words with equal stress applied to each syllable). According to Mattes and Omark (1991), however, the use of such stimuli would be considered inappropriate for individuals who speak languages other than English, due to linguistically based differences in word-stress patterns. For example, with native Spanish speakers, trochaic stress patterns (words with stressed first syllables and unstressed second syllables) would be more appropriate to use because they are more common in Spanish.

In general, test bias occurs whenever clinicians attempt to use tests that have been normed on populations that differ in cultural, social, or language background from the individuals taking the tests. In most cases, tests in the field of speech-language pathology have been normed on individuals from white, middle-class, SAE-speaking backgrounds. These include translated versions of tests such as the Boehm Test of Basic Concepts (Boehm 1971), Expressive One-Word Picture Vocabulary Test-Revised (Gardner 1990), PLS-3 (Zimmerman, et al. 1992), Receptive One-Word Picture Vocabulary Test (Gardner 1985), and the Screening Test for Auditory Comprehension of Language (Carrow 1974), all of which have Spanish translations normed on English-speaking populations.

In recent years, several test developers have attempted to correct this situation by ensuring that the ethnic make-up of the normative sample reflects that of the general U.S. population. Even this fails to adequately address the situation, however, because the bulk of the normative sample continues to be composed of children from white middle-class SAE-speaking backgrounds. In addition, test developers rarely provide information about the language status of minority individuals participating in the sample (e.g., as speakers of SAE or AAE or as Spanish dominant, English dominant, or bilingual Spanish-English).

In addition, there are few efforts taken to ensure that the test performance of minority children in the normative sample does not differ from that of other children included in the sample. It is possible for an African American client to receive the same average test score as African American individuals included in the standardization sample. However, this fact is likely to be obscured by the fact that the scores of African Americans participating in the standardization sample are averaged in with those of individuals from other cultural backgrounds. Furthermore, it is possible that many African American individuals in the normative sample are from middle-class SAE-speaking backgrounds. This could be problematic when attempting to use the test with African American clients from lower socioeconomic non-SAE–speaking backgrounds.

Another common weakness of standardized speech and language tests for children is that the majority of these tests are based on theories of monolingual versus bilingual language development. This is significant when one considers that bilingual individuals may have labels for some concepts in one language but have labels for other concepts in another language. It is very common for bilingual children exposed to English for the first time after entering school to know the labels for school-related concepts in English but to know the labels for home-related concepts (e.g., food items) in their native language (Langdon and Merino 1992). There are really no tests, however, that make accommodations for this type of language use and possible response pattern.

Reducing the Effects of Test Bias

Several different solutions have been proposed for addressing the issue of test bias, including (1) using tests that are normed on or developed for minority clients, (2) using translated versions of existing tests, (3) establishing local norms for a test based on the population with which it is being used, (4) removing potentially culturally biased items, and (5) using alternative scoring procedures (Vaughn-Cooke 1986). The following are three limitations to many of these solutions:

1. Unavailability of culturally and linguistically appropriate norms. Few tests have been developed for and normed on culturally and linguistically different populations. Furthermore, the majority of those tests developed for culturally and linguistically different populations have been developed for Spanish-speaking (primarily Mexican-American Spanish-speaking) populations. To date, there are no published standardized assessment tools that have been developed exclusively for children who speak AAE or one of the many Native American or Asian languages.

2. Limitations of using translated tests. A large number of translated tests continue to be normed on English-speaking populations. For example, in a survey of the Spanish speech and language tools used by Southern California speech-language pathologists, Albertson, et al. (1993) found that more than one-third of the tests used to assess the language abilities of Spanish-speaking children from Mexican-American backgrounds were normed on English-speaking populations.

3. Limitation of establishing local norms. The establishment of local norms often results in test scores that are lower than those of nonminority populations. Vaughn-Cooke (1986) criticized this approach because it perpetuates a deficit view of the minority individual's communicative abilities. One should also be aware that the use of local norms does not minimize the cultural bias of test items. The use of alternative scoring procedures, the removal of potentially biased test items, or both, are more effective; however, use of these strategies affects the internal reliability and validity of a standardized measure, making the reporting of normative test scores inappropriate.

Alternative Assessment Procedures

In response to test bias concerns, a number of scholars have advocated the use of other alternative strategies, such as parent-teacher interviews, language samples, observational data, and criterion-referenced and dynamic assessment measures.

Parent or Family Report

The value of a parent report is that most parents who have children with true communication impairments know that their child's communication skills are not in line with those of children from similar backgrounds. The same can be said of spouses of adult clients who are able to recognize that their loved one's communicative abilities are different from what they were before the stroke. It is always useful, therefore, for clinicians to ask family members to describe how a client's development differs from that of other individuals of the same age in the same family or community. In many cases, minority children with true communication disorders, like their nonminority peers, are generally slower in their speech and language development when compared to their siblings. They are also more likely to use nonverbal rather than verbal means of communication, are often difficult for family members to understand (in the case of articulation disorders), and are beginning to exhibit signs of frustration (e.g., crying, throwing tantrums, withdrawing) as a result of their communication difficulties. There is likely to be some evidence or history of disorder in the family.

Teacher Report

Teacher reports can also serve as an effective means for identifying those children with communication disorders, when the teacher has had a great deal of experience working with children from the same ethnic, cultural, or language background as the client in question. In a study of speech sound errors made by African American preschoolers with communication disorders, Bleile and Wallach (1992), for example, were able to note significant differences in the type of speech sound errors made by children labeled by classroom teachers as having "trouble talking" versus those who had "no trouble talking." Statistical confirmation of these differences provided strong validation for teachers' clinical intuitions.

Observation of Peers

Observation of peer interactions is another useful tool suggested by researchers such as Mattes and Omark (1991). According to Mattes and Omark (1991), clinicians can use key observational criteria such as the following when attempting to identify children with true communicative impairments: (1) rarely initiates verbal interactions with peers, (2) generally uses gestures rather than speech to communicate, and (3) produces utterances that appear to have little or no effect on the actions of peers. In addition, clinicians should also look for evidence that peers (1) rarely initiate verbal interactions with the client and (2) use facial expressions, actions, or both that indicate that they have difficulty understanding the child's communication. This strategy can also be used with adult clients involved in communicative interactions with other adults from similar cultural and language backgrounds.

Language Sampling

The primary value of using language sampling is that it enables clinicians to avoid many of the pitfalls associated with the use of standardized tests, primarily because language sample data can be collected in a variety of different authentic communication situations and because the data can be interpreted in light of existing normative information on the language development of children from culturally and linguistically different backgrounds. Language sampling in a variety of different contexts with a variety of different individuals also provides the opportunity for clinicians to examine language-use patterns and the code-switching behavior of individuals who are bilingual or bidialectal. Knowing these language use patterns gives clinicians a more comprehensive view of a client's communicative repertoire. It can also provide clinicians with an informal measure of a client's language dominance.

Modified Standardized Testing

If a clinician must use standardized assessment measures for any reason, the following steps should be taken to reduce bias: (1) examine the test manual and stimuli for evidence of potential test bias and (2) modify the test administration process.

Identifying potential test bias can be accomplished by administering a given test to parents, normally developing peers, or other individuals from the same cultural and language background as the client and identifying those items where alternative responses (responses other than those listed as acceptable) are given. Terrell and colleagues (1992) provided an excellent example of how this approach can be used with clients who speak an unfamiliar or uncommon language or dialect of English.

Interpreters, translators, and professionals who have had experience with individuals from a client's cultural and language community can also help to identify those test items that are most likely to be difficult for normally developing individuals from that community. In a sense, these individuals can serve as cultural informants in helping clinicians to identify those test items that present some form of cultural or linguistic bias.

Test modifications that can also be used to minimize test bias include the following: (1) eliminating potentially culturally biased items; (2) rewording test instructions; (3) allowing extra time for responses; (4) increasing the number of practice items; (5) recording all responses, particularly when a client changes an answer, explains, comments, or uses nonverbal gestures to respond; (6) using alternative scoring procedures; and (7) continuing to test beyond the ceiling or recommended stopping points.

Eliminating potentially culturally and linguistically biased test items can also help reduce the effect of cultural and linguistic differences in test administration. Items that have potential bias can be identified and eliminated by a clinician familiar with cultural and linguistic differences between the language of the client and the linguistic and cultural basis of the test. If items are eliminated, obviously the traditional scoring norms and procedures cannot be used. As an alternative, the client could be given credit for items known to be culturally or linguistically biased.

Rewording test instructions can help to reduce the effects of format bias by providing clients with prompts that represent those more likely to be used in eliciting the desired response. In some communities, for example, it may be more effective to use a prompt such as to "Put your finger on the _____" instead of "Show me the _____." In most cases, the change in wording should not affect the primary goal of the task being administered. If the primary goal of a test item is to determine how many concepts a client is able to identify through pointing, it makes little difference whether "Show me" or "Put your finger on" is used.

Changing a stimulus from a less familiar sentence completion format (e.g., "An elephant is big, a lady bug is _____.") to a more familiar question format (e.g., "If an elephant is big, what is a lady bug?") can also reduce the effect of format bias. By using a different elicitation prompt that is perhaps more familiar, the clinician may obtain more valid test data. Increasing the number of practice items can also help reduce format bias by providing clients with more experience with testing formats (e.g., naming pictures within the view of the examiner) that involve procedures rarely used in the client's home community.

Allowing a client extra time to respond is another appropriate modification, if a test is being administered in a language other than the client's native language. It is reasonable to expect that a client needs more processing time when being tested in the less-dominant language. In such cases, language processing delays should not be viewed as evidence of receptive language delays.

Continuing to test beyond the ceiling is another technique that can be used for identifying the possible existence of cultural bias. On tests that represent valid measures of a client's abilities, clients should not be able to correctly answer most of the test items beyond the ceiling. However, clients correctly answer several items beyond the ceiling when lack of exposure, rather than linguistic or cognitive deficits, serves as the reason for test errors.

Asking clients to explain responses that do not appear to be correct according to the test manual or to what a clinician has determined to be culturally or linguistically correct can also be useful in identifying potential test bias. A few years ago, one of this author's student clinicians used this approach when working with an African American aphasic client. The clinician, who was attempting to work on the classification of food terms, observed that her client repeatedly failed to identify a sandwich as a food item. When the clinician asked the client why she was not including sandwich on her list of foods, the client responded, "Honey, a sandwich ain't food. Food is things like greens, chicken, potato salad. Now that's real food." Just this explanation, alone, was sufficient to demonstrate the inherent cultural bias of the classification task as well as the client's ability to categorize related vocabulary items.

Recording all of a client's responses instead of using a simple plus and minus scoring system can help increase the information available from test analysis. Writing down a client's entire response enables a clinician to check the accuracy of responses later with someone who is able to determine what is culturally and linguistically appropriate. This also enables a clinician to provide a more descriptive, qualitative versus quantitative description of a client's performance strengths and weaknesses. The latter often provides a more accurate view of client performance when test scores are considered to be invalid.

Using a criterion-referenced framework for reporting standardized test results as a means for reducing test bias can serve as an alternative strategy for evaluating test performance. For example, if a clinician is interested in evaluating a child's comprehension of commands, the Oral Directions subtest of the Clinical Evaluation of Language Fundamentals–Revised could be administered using procedures outlined in the test manual. However, test results could be reported in terms of percentage of items passed, instead of using the suggested standard and percentile-rank scores. The scoring grid that appears at the bottom of the subtest scoring page can also be used to analyze a client's performance in terms of the percentage of one- versus two- and three-step commands correctly answered. It also enables the clinician to determine how well the client performs on commands involving serial orientation versus left-right orientation terms. This type of information can then be used to identify relative language strengths and weaknesses by comparing performance across a number of different tasks. This intrapersonal versus interpersonal approach avoids the problem of comparing a client's performance to that of other individuals from differing cultural and language backgrounds. It also provides information relevant to the establishment of appropriate intervention goals. The downside of this approach is that it forces clinicians to rely on their own knowledge of culturally based differences in language development and use to determine when an apparent language weakness is the result of true communicative impairment rather than language exposure.

Using a dynamic assessment approach to assessment can minimize the inherent bias of using static scores for identifying disorder. This involves the use of a test-teach-retest paradigm for determining an individual's learning potential. One key underlying assumption of the dynamic assessment approach, when used with culturally different clients with suspected communication disorders, is that those individuals who test poorly as a result of culturally based communication and learning style differences demonstrate significant improvement on the same test after a brief mediated learning experience. This is in comparison to individuals whose poor performance is the result of true communication deficits.

In a study that investigated African American and Puerto Rican preschoolers' performances on the Expressive One-Word Picture Vocabulary Test (EOWPVT), Peña and colleagues (1992) were able to demonstrate the effects of using dynamic assessment as a means for distinguishing between difference and disorder. Part of their subject pool consisted of children identified as having possible language disorders on the basis of classroom language observations, teacher interview, and parent report. All other children were determined to be free from communicative impairment. At the beginning of the study, the EOWPVT was administered to all children participating in the study. Pretest results revealed that more than 80% of the children scored at least one standard deviation below the mean. There were no significant differences in the performances of normal versus possibly language-disordered subjects. The authors of this study hypothesized that part of the poor testing performance could be attributed to the children's less frequent use of object labels and more frequent use of descriptions when responding to picture stimuli.

All subjects were then involved in a mediated learning experience, in which they were seen for two 20-minute small-group classroom intervention sessions. The purpose of these sessions were to increase children's use of labels versus category and functional descriptions when responding to EOWPVT stimuli. After the two 20-minute sessions, the EOWPVT was readministered. Post-test results revealed a significant improvement in normal subjects' test performance in comparison to their possibly language-disordered peers. In addition, differences in the post-test scores of the two groups were found to be statistically significant (Peña, et al. 1992). These results provided support for the use of a test-teach-retest approach that (1) examines clinical gains made after mediated learning experiences as a method for ruling out cultural experience as a factor in test performance and (2) helps distinguish between language difference and true language disorder. This same assessment approach can be immensely helpful during the diagnostic evaluation process for accomplishing the same with either child or adult clients.

Testing in the Client's Native Language

When working with clients who are more proficient (dominant) in a language other than English, it is always important to conduct part of the speech and language evaluation process in the client's most dominant language. If the client is monolingual in a language other than English, testing should be done exclusively in that language. Clinicians who work in the public schools are legally bound to follow these procedures. The Individuals with Disabilities Education Act of 1990 requires that assessment procedures be administered in a child's native language or mode of communication used in addressing the child at home. In addition, the American Speech-Language-Hearing Association (ASHA) (1985) takes the position that "assessment and intervention of speech and language disorders of limited English proficient speakers should be conducted in the client's primary language."

To determine the primary language of assessment, clinicians must first determine a bilingual client's most dominant language. In some school districts, this determination is made through the use of language-dominance testing. The testing is usually conducted by professionals other than the speech-language pathologist. Many of the tests that are traditionally used for achieving this goal, however, have been criticized for focusing on only one aspect of language use and development (generally vocabulary). According to Mattes and Omark (1991) and Hamayan and Damico (1991), this creates a problem with test validity because it is possible for a bilingual individual to be dominant in one language in one domain (e.g., vocabulary) or modality (e.g., reading), but dominant in another language in other domains (e.g., articulation or grammar) or modalities (speaking or listening).

In addition to using traditional language-dominance testing procedures, clinicians should use information from the case history interview to help establish a client's language profile. Clinicians can obtain some idea about a client's language dominance by determining, for example, (1) the age at which the client (if a child) said his or her first words in each language, as well as the age at which he or she began to form two-word sentences in both languages, (2) the current length of sentences in both languages, and (3) the most frequently used language. The frequency with which each language is used and the situational contexts in which each language is used are also important to determine when working with adult clients.

Any preliminary determinations of language proficiency from the case history interview should be validated by observations of language-use patterns during naturalistic language or conversational sampling procedures. Observations of a client's ability to respond to questions and to express himself or herself in English (e.g., with an English-speaking clinician) can be compared with his or her ability to accomplish these same communicative goals in conversational exchanges with non-English speakers (e.g., family members, peers, bilingual paraprofessional). Clinicians should also pay attention to cues such as the number of times the client needs to have questions repeated in one language versus the other, the length of sentences produced in both languages, evidence of more word-finding difficulties in one language versus the other, evidence of more code switching or mixing when speaking in one language versus the other, and so forth. All of these observations should provide the clinician with an intuitive sense of the client's strongest language.

Once it has been determined that a client is more dominant in a language other than English, it is clear that at least some aspects of the assessment process must be conducted in that language. If clinicians do not possess the necessary competencies to conduct assessment in the client's native language, they must find some other alternative strategy for accomplishing this goal. In most cases, this involves employing the services of a bilingual professional or paraprofessional who can serve as an interpreter or translator (American Speech-Language-Hearing Association 1985). The lack of personnel resources for conducting a bilingual assessment is not sufficient reason for conducting the evaluation of the limited English proficient client in English. In some cases, the individual serving as the bilingual paraprofessional may be a family member or friend of the client. Use of a family member or friend of the client as an interpreter is not encouraged, however, because such individuals are not typically trained in the assessment process. In addition, they may not give an accurate interpretation of the clinician's requests nor of the client's responses, preferring to alter the question or response to present the family in a more favorable light.

According to Roseberry-McKibbin (1995), Kayser (1995), and Mattes and Omark (1991), there are a number of skills and abilities that an interpreter must possess if he or she is to be used effectively. First, interpreters must be sufficiently trained to carry out the roles and responsibilities they have been given. They must possess good oral and written skills in English and be proficient in the use of the language in which assessment is being completed. They must have a solid understanding of professional ethics and they must be able to relate culturally to the individual(s) they are assisting. Interpreters and translators should also meet the minimum educational standards and clinical competencies outlined by the ASHA for support personnel (American Speech-Language-Hearing Association Task Force on Support Personnel 1995). He or she must also undergo some degree of training. In a recent survey of Southern California public school speech-language pathologists regarding the use of paraprofessionals with low-incidence language populations (children speaking languages other than English and Spanish), McCann and colleagues (1996), found that the issue of training was an area of concern expressed by more than 40% of survey respondents. More than 40% of respondents also expressed concerns about the validity and reliability of information obtained during the assessment process with the assistance of paraprofessionals.

As part of their training, interpreters should receive information on topics such as (1) the characteristics of normal and disordered speech, language, voice, and fluency disorders; (2) the first and second language acquisition process; (3) guidelines for distinguishing between disorder and difference; (4) professional terminology in the field of speech-language pathology; (5) procedures for administering and scoring diagnostic procedures; (6) structural differences between English and other languages; and (7) professional ethics in the field of speech-language pathology. A number of other training topics are recommended by Langdon (1992b), Mattes and Omark (1991), and Matsuda and O'Connor (1993). A basic outline of the training curriculum modules recommended by Langdon (1992b) and Matsuda and O'Connor (1993) can be found in Kayser (1995).

According to Langdon (1996) and Kayser (1995), interpreters should meet with the diagnostic clinician, the team, or both on at least three separate occasions during the diagnostic process. The purpose of the first meeting (briefing) is to provide the interpreter with background information about the client to be tested, including the presenting problem, an overview of the diagnostic evaluation session goals, and an introduction to the tests and materials to be used during the assessment process. The purpose of the second meeting is to conduct the diagnostic evaluation (interaction), and the purpose of the third meeting (debriefing) is to discuss results and observations from the testing session.

Although interpreters are invaluable during the assessment process, there are a number of potential problems that can occur when using an interpreter (Kayser 1995; Roseberry-McKibbin 1995; Cheng 1991). Examples include (1) the natural desire on the part of some interpreters to protect the client by hiding or minimizing the extent of the client's communicative problems or failing to share information from the case history interview that is perceived as being potentially damaging and (2) errors in translation, including omitting, adding, or substituting words, phrases, or sentences. In many cases, translation errors occur when (1) the interpreters believe that a certain word, phrase, or sentence is not important to relay; (2) certain concepts are difficult to translate; (3) translators have difficulty retaining the original message or keeping up with the pace of the speaker; (4) there is a desire to editorialize or be more elaborate; or (5) they are confused about a certain term (Kayser 1995; Cheng 1991). These potential problems can be avoided by providing interpreters with adequate training and sufficient time to prepare for a diagnostic evaluation. Clinicians can also help by making adjustments such as speaking in shorter units and avoiding professional jargon (Roseberry-McKibbin 1995).

Once the need to conduct an assessment in two or more languages is determined, clinicians must determine which parts of the assessment process should be conducted in one language versus the other. It is beneficial to administer all tests in both languages to determine relative language strengths and weaknesses in both languages. The goal of this procedure is to identify weaknesses that cut across both languages (e.g., word-retrieval difficulties, reduced sentence length, articulation errors that cannot be explained on the basis of first-language influences or normal development). This procedure is extremely time consuming, however, and requires a great deal of effort on the part of the translator. Some suggestions for modifying this process while still obtaining information crucial to diagnosis include (1) collecting language or conversational sample data in both languages, (2) conducting assessment in both languages in those areas considered to be most affected by the disorder, and (3) re-administering any subtests or test items failed in English in the native language of the client. The value of language sampling is that clinicians can quickly determine, usually in less than 30 minutes, a client's relative proficiency in several different communication

areas, including semantics, syntax, pragmatics, phon
guage, fluency, voice, and receptive language. The v̇
third approaches are that they enable the clinician tc
apparent weakness in one language (e.g., matching p'
lish) is also a weakness in the other language.

Interpretation and Diagnosis

Diagnosing Language Impairment in Nonstandard English Dialect Speakers

Perhaps the most important aspect of the evaluation process is the interpretation and analysis of diagnostic findings. It is at this stage of the evaluation process when clinicians must identify any test results that appear to be the result of cultural or linguistic differences or bias. This section provides some suggestions for how clinicians can accomplish this and effectively differentiate normal speech and language differences from disorder.

When working with clients who speak a dialect of English other than SAE, proposed solutions include focusing on nondialect specific aspects of speech and language development and use (California Speech-Language-Hearing Association Task Force on the Assessment of the African American Child 1994; Cole 1983; Stockman 1996). When attempting to ascertain whether speech sound differences are the result of phonologic delay, clinicians should "determine first if AAE speakers are delayed on phonological features that do not differ from SAE" (Stockman 1996). Examples of features that can be examined include the following speech sounds in initial word position: /m/, /n/, /p/, /k/, /g/, /h/, /j/, /t/, /f/, /b/, /s/, /f/, /w/, /l/, and /r/.

When Stockman and Settle (1991) compared the initial speech sound productions of normally developing African American and white children, they found that this minimal core of sounds was produced by 80–100% of the children in both groups by the age of 3 years. The examination of initial consonants in the speech of AAE speakers is further supported by the findings of Bleile and Wallach (1992), who found that one of the most significant differences between the speech sound productions of children who had trouble talking compared to children who had no trouble talking was the frequency of speech sound errors in initial and medial word positions. There was little difference between the groups in the production of final sounds. The latter can be explained by the fact that there are several rules in AAE that allow for the absence or devoicing of final consonant sounds. These findings suggest that, as in the case of SAE speakers, clinicians should be concerned about AAE speakers who omit initial speech sounds.

ther examples of non–dialect-specific structures that can be examined ing the differential diagnosis stages include complex syntactic construc-ions such as infinitive clauses (e.g., "He don't need *to stand up*" and "The bus driver told the kids *to stop*"), noun phrase complements (e.g., "I told you *there's a Whopper*"), relative clauses (e.g., "That's the noise *that I like*"), and gerunds and participles (e.g., "It get *rainy*"). According to Craig and Washington (1994) and Washington (1996), these structures provide larger syntactic unit analyses that are less likely to be affected by the morphosyntactic differences between AAE and SAE. Similarly, clinicians can focus on grammatical forms such as *a* and *the*, which are obligated in both AAE and SAE speech. Focusing on adjective and noun word ordering can also be helpful. This is because the word order rules for adjectives and nouns are the same in both AAE and SAE. In both dialects, adjectives must always precede the nouns they modify. Clinicians should suspect disorder in a child who is only exposed to AAE and SAE and says phrases such as "car orange," "kittens three," or "teeth baby."

Clinicians can also focus on those aspects of language that appear to be more universal, such as semantics and pragmatics, particularly when working with AAE child speakers younger than age 3 years. This is because the morphosyntactic development of AAE child speakers differs little from that of other English-speaking children (including SAE child speakers) before the age of 3 years. Dialect differences become more of an issue with children between the ages of 3 and 5 years, when there is a marked increase in the use of nonstandard English features (Cole 1980; Stockman 1986). Although AAE speakers and African Americans who use a more Afro-centered discourse style sometimes express meanings or use language in ways that differ somewhat from SAE and Euro-centered communicators, there are also some important similarities between these four groups of speakers during the earliest stages of development. For example, researchers have found that African American children go through the same stages of semantic and pragmatic development as other children (Stockman and Vaughn-Cooke 1982; Bridgeforth 1987). Specifically, these researchers found that African American children acquire the same semantic and pragmatic categories at the same stages of development and in the same sequence as other children. The only difference is the linguistic code (e.g., AAE or SAE) used to code these meanings and functions.

These research findings have important implications for clinicians involved with the assessment of children younger than age 3 years. Given these findings, clinicians should feel comfortable using existing semantic and pragmatic language development information to identify younger African American children with communicative impairments. Clinicians should attempt to identify those children who use a restricted range of semantic meanings or language functions when compared to other age peers. The latter conclusion must be based, of course, on reliably obtained language sample data.

One final suggestion is to focus on grammatical contexts that require or obligate the presence of a given dialectal form when attempting to analyze the more variable aspects of dialect feature use. According to the earlier sociolinguistic studies, there are a number of features in AAE, such as the copula verb *is*, that can be variably absent in contexts in which they are normally required in SAE (Labov, et al. 1968; Labov 1969; Wolfram 1969). For example, in AAE, there are a number of grammatical environments in which the copula can be expressed (e.g., "She *is* sick") or absent ("She sick"). There are also contexts, however, in which the copula must appear. These contexts include (1) past-tense contexts (e.g., "They *were* sick" or "They *was* sick"), (2) final clause position (e.g., "Yes, he *is*"), (3) first-person singular contexts (e.g., "I *am* sick"), and (4) in emphatic utterances ("Yes he *is* sick").

The research of Wyatt (1991, 1996) revealed similar patterns of copula production in AAE child speech. In addition, Stockman and colleagues (1982) found that young AAE speakers employed the same variable rules for producing final nasals as adult AAE speakers. The implications of these research findings are that clinicians should be able to identify language impairment in AAE-speaking populations in the same way that language impairment is often identified in SAE, by examining feature use within obligatory grammatical contexts. The only difference is that the identification of obligatory contexts requires some knowledge of the dialect-specific variable rules associated with AAE grammar.

When attempting to differentiate between disorder and dialect difference in African American client populations, the range of linguistic variability that exists in the African American population must be considered. For example, although the term *AAE* might seem to imply that there is a single variety of English common to all African American speech, not every African American speaks AAE, even within working-class African American communities where AAE is presumed to be most widely spoken (Wyatt 1995). Clinicians must take this factor into account before attempting to analyze and categorize the language productions of African American speakers. Specifically, it is important to first determine whether an individual is an AAE speaker before identifying an apparent language difference as dialect based. If one determines an African American client to be a native SAE speaker, one cannot attribute certain language productions, such as absence of the copula, to dialect differences. The determination of the latter can only be reliably achieved by examining language-use patterns in a variety of different communicative settings with a variety of different communicative partners (Wyatt 1995; Wyatt and Seymour 1990).

Diagnosing Language Impairment in Bilingual Speakers

Just as clinicians must have some prior understanding of dialect features and rules to distinguish between disorder and difference in nonstandard English-speaking populations, they must also be familiar with the grammatical and phonologic structure of languages other than English when working with non-native English speakers. Knowledge of these language differences enables a clinician to determine whether any differing productions of English sounds or grammatical structures can be attributed to normal first-language influences, normal dialect differences, universal second-language errors, or (in the case of children) developmental influences. Clinicians must rule out each of these factors when attempting to determine whether apparent English "errors" are the result of normal language differences or true disorder.

When attempting to rule out normal first-language influences, clinicians should try to identify those speech sounds or grammatical omissions and substitutions that can be explained by the absence of that linguistic feature in a client's native language. It is common, for example, for many non-native English–speaking clients to substitute some other sound for the *th* sound in English, because this sound does not exist in many non-English languages, including Spanish, several Asian languages, Polynesian languages, and the majority of Arabic dialects (Cheng 1993; Langdon and Merino 1992; Kayser 1995; Roseberry-McKibbin 1995; Adler 1993; Ruhlen 1975). The lack of inflectional markers in Chinese and many other Asian languages help to explain why native Asian speakers are likely to omit final past tense *-ed*, plural *-s*, and possessive *-s* markers (Cheng 1993). In some cases, omission of substitution of a speech sound can be attributed to the fact that it never occurs in a certain word position in a client's native language. For example, even though /b/, /p/, /g/, /m/, /t/, /k/, /tʃ/, and /f/ are sounds that exist in both Spanish and English, it would be normal for Spanish speakers to omit these sounds in the final position of English words, because they never occur in word final positions in Spanish (Langdon and Merino 1992).

In addition to ruling out "errors" that appear to be the result of first-language influences, the grammatical and phonologic differences that can occur among different dialects of the same language must be considered. Clinicians must be familiar with the dialect-specific rules of their client's native tongue before identifying a speech sound or grammatical difference as a true communicative error. The latter is key when examining speech and language productions made in the first, as well as second, language.

Diagnosing Articulation/Phonologic Disorders in Bilingual Speakers

When working with child clients, clinicians have the formidable task of attempting to determine whether some speech sound or grammatical differences are the result of normal developmental processes. For example, it is common in all speech communities for children to produce errors that differ from those generally produced by adults. This is because their language systems are developing. As a result, whenever such information is available, clinicians should attempt to examine first and second language errors in accordance with existing normative data on child populations. At present, Spanish is the only language other than English on which there is extensive developmental data. Much of this data can be found in Merino (1992), Goldstein (1995), Anderson (1995), and Gutierrez-Clellen (1995). In the absence of developmental data, clinicians are encouraged to take time to observe the typical speech and language patterns of children who are from the same language background as their clients, but who appear to be normal in their speech and language development. It is also important for clinicians to recognize that many of the English errors made by children acquiring English as a second language are similar to those made by children acquiring English as a first language who have had the same degree (number of years) of language exposure. It is not unreasonable, therefore, for nonnative English child speakers with less than 3 years of English-language exposure to omit grammatical forms, such as the copula, that are generally omitted by monolingual English speakers younger than 3 years of age.

There are also a number of English grammatical forms that have been found to be universally difficult for individuals acquiring English as a first language. For example, according to the research of Dulay and Burt (1974) and Dulay, et al. (1982) all second-language learners have difficulty with certain English grammatical forms, such as copula and auxiliary *be*, irregular past tense verbs, possessive *-s*, and the third person singular *-s* regardless of their native language background. Dulay and colleagues (1982) also proposed that these various structures are acquired in a predictable order by second-language speakers, regardless of second-language background.

Identifying the Impact of First Language on Second Language

The first step in any evaluation of second-language productions, therefore, is to identify those speech sound or language "errors" that appear to be the result of first language, universal, developmental, and dialect influences. It is important to recognize, however, that it is not always possible to attribute the source of these productions exclusively to one factor. In many cases, differing productions can be the result of more than one factor. For example, in their analysis of the grammatical productions made by the native Chinese speaker acquiring English as a second language, Gee and Wyatt (1994) believed that the substitution of *him* for *he* could be equally attributed to either first-language influences (misuse of English pronouns is common among native Chinese speakers according to Roseberry-McKibbin 1995), normal development (pronoun case errors are common in the early language development of all children acquiring English, including monolingual English speakers), or universal second-language learning errors (see Dulay and Burt 1974 and Dulay, et al. 1982).

Interlanguage

After ruling out each of these possible influences, clinicians may be left with a number of remaining features that cannot be explained. Clinicians should not automatically assume that remaining differences are an indication of possible disorder. It is common for second-language learners to go through a transitory stage of second-language acquisition in which attempts to produce target sounds and grammatical structures result in idiosyncratic approximations that cannot be clearly attributed to first-language or second-language structure. This transitory language system is often referred to as *interlanguage*. As the second-language learner gains more experience with the second language, these productions may change in nature, eventually becoming more similar to the target language structure. However, these productions can also become fossilized (become a permanent part of the speaker's communicative repertoire). The type of interlanguage errors that are made by individual speakers, even those from the same language background, are usually unique.

Even when faced with the possibility that some errors can be attributed to normal interlanguage phenomenon, it is also important to determine the relative frequency of these errors (Gee and Wyatt 1994). Although it is reasonable to expect errors that cannot be attributed to developmental, dialect, or first-language influences, clinicians should be concerned when the majority of speech sound and grammatical errors cannot be explained on the basis of either of these criteria. A final diagnosis of impairment, however, must be based on indications of difficulty from other sources of data, including the case history interview and testing completed in the first language of a client.

Code Switching

An analysis of bilingual code-switching patterns may also have potential value for identifying individuals with underlying communication disorders. For example, when working with the bilingual aphasic client, it can be useful to consider case history information about a client's code mixing or code switching patterns before and after the stroke. Although code mixing and switching represent natural and normal patterns of language use in bilingual clients, a substantial increase in code-mixed utterances after a stroke could serve as evidence of true disorder-based expressive language difficulties. Reyes (1995) stated that "although certainly not all lexical switches are indicative of lexical unavailability, switches of single words may be a red flag to clinicians that perhaps the patient is experiencing word-retrieval difficulties." An increased frequency of code-switching could also have clinical implications. According to Cheng and Butler (1989), as cited in Langdon (1992b), it is possible for an overabundance of code-switching to signal possible lack of competence in either language. It is for this reason that Reyes (1995) emphasizes the importance of inquiring about a patient's pre-morbid code-switching abilities and patterns and making comparisons to post-insult code-switching.

Additional Diagnostic Considerations

When working with clients who exhibit voice, neurologically based, and fluency disorders, one key signal of true communicative impairment is the existence of similar problems when communicating in both languages. For example, individuals who appear to demonstrate evidence of speech apraxia, dysarthria, or both in one language as a result of neurologically based impairments should exhibit evidence of the same type of problem in any other languages spoken. In addition, individuals with true fluency difficulties are likely to exhibit similar patterns of dysfluency in each language, even though the similarities may not at first be readily apparent. For example, in a study of a bilingual Spanish-English speaker's dysfluency patterns, Bernstein-Ratner and Benitez (1985) found the subject to be more dysfluent on sentence initial constituents in Spanish than English. However, a more in-depth analysis of the speakers' dysfluencies revealed that he also tended to stutter more on verbs than nouns in both languages. This explained the higher frequency of dysfluent sentence initial constituents in Spanish than English. This pattern of dysfluency was directly related to the fact that a greater number of sentences in Spanish begin with verbs. Spanish allows for the optional deletion of subject-noun phrases. In essence, the loci of stuttering instances were the same in both languages. On first inspection, however, this similarity was masked by grammatical differences between English and Spanish.

Before making a definite diagnosis of disorder, clinicians must also consider the possible cross-cultural variations that can occur in fluency and voice productions. DeJarnette and Holland (1993) and Salas-Provance (1996) cited a number of studies that suggest that the average fundamental frequency of black men and women is lower than that generally reported for their white counterparts. This has significant implications for the diagnosis of vocal-pitch disorders in black clients. The findings also suggest that clinicians need to be wary of using existing fundamental voice norms derived from research conducted primarily on nonminority speakers with individuals from other cultural backgrounds.

Cross-cultural differences in the use of prosody and fluency have also been noted during narrative assessment tasks (Gutierrez-Clellen and Quinn 1993; Hyter and Westby 1996). These parameters, as well as other aspects of narrative ability (e.g., topic, content, structure, and organization), must therefore be evaluated in light of culturally based criteria. In addition, when working with individuals who are acquiring English as a second language, it is important to recognize that the presence of fillers, interjections, whole-word repetitions, unfilled pauses, and other typical dysfluencies in the second language are a normal consequence of second-language learning.

Least-Biased Report Writing

The diagnostic evaluation process is not complete without a final written report of evaluation findings. It is equally important during the report-writing process that clinicians attempt to present final evaluation results in a manner that is culturally sensitive and accurate. This includes using nondeficit terminology for describing normal language differences. Speech sound or language productions that appear to be the result of normal first-language influences versus disorder should be clearly distinguished from true errors by using phrases such as "speech sound/grammatical differences" or "nonstandard productions."

To provide the most comprehensive picture of a client's communicative abilities, all diagnostic reports on bilingual clients should also provide sufficient information on the client's language background, language-use patterns, and level of language proficiency in both languages as determined from the case history interview and observations of language use during formal observation, language sampling, and testing procedures. A balanced description of test performance in both should be provided and communicative strengths, as well as weaknesses, should be delineated for both languages (see Appendix 13A).

In cases in which the clinician has decided to modify standardized testing or scoring procedures, it is important for the clinician to discuss the type of testing or scoring modifications made (see Appendix 13B). This enables other professionals to replicate testing in a manner that allows for later evaluation of client progress. Discussion of test modifications can also help other professionals recognize why they do not obtain the same findings, if a test is given in a more standardized fashion at a later time. To avoid the issue of test scoring bias altogether, clinicians should provide more qualitative rather than quantitative descriptions of client performance. Another alternative is to use a criterion-referenced reporting format in which percentages rather than standardized test scores are used to identify areas of communicative strengths and weaknesses (see Appendix 13C).

Scoring bias can also be minimized by reporting scores in terms of age ranges, percentile ranks, or both, using the widest confidence intervals possible (e.g., 90% rather than 68%). This reporting ensures that only clients with the most significant communication differences are identified, thereby reducing the likelihood of misdiagnosis (see Appendix 13D). In cases in which clinicians have used normal standardized testing procedures, scores, or both that are potentially biased, a cautionary statement about the reliability or validity of test results should be included. Examples of reports of potential test bias can be found in Appendix 13E.

Finally, when discussing speech sound and language "errors," clinicians should ensure that those productions related to normal first language, developmental, or dialect influences be clearly differentiated from those resulting from probable language disorder, using interpretive statements such as those provided in Appendix 13F. Distinguishing error patterns that are the result of true disorder are also important in establishing appropriate therapy goals and targets (see Appendix 13C).

Conclusion

This chapter provides a framework for structuring the diagnostic evaluation process with clients from culturally and linguistically diverse populations. Clinicians must recognize that there are a number of cultural and linguistic factors that can potentially impact the nature, accuracy, and extent of information obtained during the case history interview and assessment process. Part of being culturally sensitive, competent, and responsible is acknowledging that there are differences that must be considered when working with clients from linguistically and culturally different backgrounds, as well as making those adjustments necessary to minimize cultural and linguistic test bias. This applies regardless of the presenting communicative problem(s) of the client (e.g., voice, fluency, neurologically based speech and language disorders, hearing disorders, developmentally delayed speech and language skills).

A number of strategies are presented in this chapter for structuring the diagnostic evaluation process so that potential cultural and linguistic bias is minimized. Such strategies include (1) consulting individuals who have had experience working with cultural and language communities that represent the background of clients before and after the diagnostic evaluation process; (2) carefully considering the type of questions and tests to be used as well as the manner in which questions are asked and tests are administered; (3) reviewing tests for evidence of potential situational, linguistic, value, and format test bias; (4) using interpreters, translators, and other bilingual paraprofessionals to assist with the test administration and analysis process; (5) modifying standardized tests or using alternative assessment procedures such as parent report, teacher interview, observation, and naturalistic language sampling; (6) conducting speech and language testing in the native language of the client when the client speaks a primary language other than English; (7) making a differential diagnosis that clearly distinguishes difference and disorder; and (8) presenting test findings in a least-biased manner.

References

Adler, S. (1993). *Multicultural communication skills in the classroom.* Boston: Allyn & Bacon.

Albertson, L.L., Alvarado, D.Y., & Wyatt, T.A. (1993, November). *An evaluation of Spanish speech and language assessment tools.* Presented at the annual meeting of the American Speech-Language-Hearing Association, Anaheim, CA.

American Speech-Language-Hearing Association. (1985). Clinical management of communicatively handicapped minority language populations. *ASHA, 27,* 29–32.

American Speech-Language-Hearing Association Task Force on Support Personnel. (1995). Position statement for training, credentialing, use and supervision of support personnel in speech-language pathology. *ASHA, 37(Suppl 14),* 21.

Anderson, R.T. (1995). Spanish morphological and syntactic development. In H. Kayser (Ed.), *Bilingual speech-language pathology* (pp. 41–74). San Diego: Singular.

Anderson, N.B., & Battle, D.E. (1993). Cultural diversity in the development of language. In D.E. Battle (Ed.), *Communication disorders in multicultural populations* (pp. 158–186). Boston: Butterworth–Heinemann.

Anderson-Yockel, J., & Haynes, W.O. (1994). Joint book-reading strategies in working-class African-American and white mother-toddler dyads. *Journal of Speech and Hearing Research, 37,* 583.

Bernstein-Ratner, N., & Benitez, H. (1985). Linguistic analysis of a bilingual stutterer. *Journal of Fluency Disorders, 10*, 211–219.

Bleile, K.M., & Wallach, H. (1992). A sociolinguistic investigation of the speech of African American preschoolers. *American Journal of Speech-Language Pathology, 1(2)*, 54–62.

Boehm, A.E. (1971). *Boehm test of basic concepts.* New York: The Psychological Corporation.

Bridgeforth, C. (1987). *The identification and use of language functions in the speech of 3- and 4 1/2 year-old black children from working class families.* Ph.D. dissertation, Georgetown University.

Buchanan, L.H., Moore, E.J., & Counter, S.A. (1993). Hearing disorders and auditory assessment. In D.E. Battle (Ed.), *Communication disorders in multicultural populations* (pp. 256–286). Boston: Butterworth–Heinemann.

California Speech-Language-Hearing Association Task Force on the Assessment of the African-American Child (1994). CSHA position paper: Assessment of the African-American child. *CSHA, 21(3)*, 1–17.

Carrow, E. (1974). *Screening test for auditory comprehension of language.* Austin, TX: Learning Concepts.

Chamberlain, P., & Medeiros-Landurand, P. (1991). Practical considerations for the assessment of LEP students with special needs. In E.V. Damico, & J.S. Damico (Eds.), *Limiting bias in the assessment of bilingual students* (pp. 111). Austin, TX: PRO-ED.

Cheng, L.L. (1991). *Assessing Asian language performance (2nd ed.).* Oceanside, CA: Academic Communication Associates.

Cheng, L.L. (1993). Asian-American cultures. In D.E. Battle (Ed.), *Communication disorders in multicultural populations* (pp. 38–77). Boston: Butterworth–Heinemann.

Cheng, L.L, & Butler, K. (1989). Code switching: A natural phenomenon versus language deficiency. *World English, 8*, 293–309.

Cole, L. (1980). A developmental analysis of social dialect features in the spontaneous language of preschool black children. *Dissertation Abstracts International, 41(6)*, 2132B.

Cole, L. (1983). Implications of the position of social dialects. *ASHA, 25*, 25–27.

Conklin, N.F., & Lourie, M.A. (1983). *A host of tongues: Language communities in the United States.* New York: The Free Press.

Craig, H.K., & Washington, J.A. (1994). The complex syntax skills of poor, urban, African-American preschoolers at school entry. *Language, Speech, and Hearing Services in Schools, 25(3)*, 181–190.

Danhauer, J.L., Crawford, S., & Edgerton, B.J. (1984). English, Spanish, and bilingual speakers' performance on a nonsense syllable test (NST) of speech sound discrimination. *Journal of Speech and Hearing Disorders, 49,* 164–168.

DeJarnette, G., & Holland, R.W. (1993). Voice disorders. In D.E. Battle (Ed.), *Communication disorders in multicultural populations* (pp. 212–238). Boston: Butterworth–Heinemann.

Dulay, H.C., & Burt, M.K. (1974). Natural consequences in child second language acquisition. *Language Learning, 24,* 37–53.

Dulay, H.C., Burt, M.K., & Krashen, S. (1982). Language two. New York: Oxford University.

Gardner, M.F. (1985). *Receptive one-word picture vocabulary test.* Novato, CA: Academic Therapy Publications.

Gardner, M.F. (1990). *Expressive one-word picture vocabulary test [revised].* Novato, CA: Academic Therapy Publications.

Gee, B., & Wyatt, T. (1994, November). *The acquisition of English by a preschool-aged native Chinese speaker.* Paper presented at the annual meeting of the American Speech-Language-Hearing Association, New Orleans.

Goldstein, B.A. (1995). Spanish phonological development. In H. Kayser (Ed.), *Bilingual speech-language pathology* (pp. 17–40). San Diego: Singular.

Gutierrez-Clellen, V.F. (1995). Narrative development and disorders in Spanish-speaking children: Implications for the bilingual interventionist. In H. Kayser (Ed.), *Bilingual speech-language pathology* (pp. 97–128). San Diego: Singular.

Gutierrez-Clellen, V.F, & Quinn, R. (1993). Assessing narratives of children from diverse cultural/linguistic groups. *Language, Speech, and Hearing Services in Schools, 24(1),* 2–9.

Hamayan, E.V., & Damico, J.S. (1991). Developing and using a second language. In E.V. Hamayan, & J.S. Damico (Eds.), *Limiting bias in the assessment of bilingual students.* Austin, TX: PRO-ED.

Harris, G.A. (1993). American Indian cultures: A lesson in diversity. In D.E. Battle (Ed.), *Communication disorders in multicultural populations* (pp. 78–113). Boston: Butterworth–Heinemann.

Heath, S.B. (1982). Questioning at home and school: A comparative study. In G. Spindler (Ed.), *Doing the ethnography of schooling: Educational anthropology in action* (pp. 102). New York: Holt, Rinehart, and Winston.

Heath, S.B. (1983). *Ways with words: Language, life, and work in communities and classrooms.* London: Cambridge University Press.

Heath, S.B. (1986). In Bilingual Education Office, California State Department of Education (Ed.), *Beyond language: Social and cultural factors in schooling language minority students* (pp. 143–186). Los Angeles:

Evaluation, Dissemination, and Assessment Center, California State University.

Hyter, Y.D., & Westby, C.E. (1996). Using oral narratives to assess communicative competence. In A.G. Kamhi, K.E. Pollock, & J.L. Harris (Eds.), *Communication development and disorders in African-American children* (pp. 247–284). Baltimore: Brookes.

Kayser, H. (1993). Hispanic cultures. In D.E. Battle (Ed.), *Communication disorders in multicultural populations* (pp. 114–257). Boston: Butterworth–Heinemann.

Kayser, H. (1995). Interpreters. In H. Kayser (Ed.), *Bilingual speech-language pathology* (pp. 207–222). San Diego: Singular.

Kochman, T. (1981). *Black and white styles in conflict*. Chicago: University of Chicago Press.

Labov, W., Cohen, P., Robins, C., & Lewis J. (1968). *A study of nonstandard English of Negro and Puerto Rican speakers in New York City*. Washington, DC: U.S. Office of Education (Final report, Cooperative Research Project No. 3288).

Labov, W. (1969). Contraction, deletion, and inherent variability of the English copula. *Language, 45,* 715–762.

Langdon, H.W. (1992a). Language communication and sociocultural patterns in Hispanic families. In H.W. Langdon, & L.L. Cheng (Ed.), *Hispanic children and adults with communication disorders: Assessment and intervention* (pp. 99–131). Gaithersburg, MD: Aspen.

Langdon, H.W. (1992b). Speech and language assessment of LEP/bilingual Hispanic students. In H.W. Langdon, & L.L. Cheng (Ed.), *Hispanic children and adults with communication disorders: Assessment and intervention* (pp. 201–271). Gaithersburg, MD: Aspen.

Langdon, H.W. (1996). Teaming with interpreters/translators. In H.W. Langdon, & T.I. Saenz (Eds.), *Language assessment and intervention with multicultural students: A guide for speech-language-hearing professionals* (pp. 89). Oceanside, CA: Academic Communication Associates.

Langdon, H.W., & Merino, B.J. (1992). Acquisition and development of a second language in the Spanish speaker. In H.W. Langdon, & L.L. Cheng (Eds.), *Hispanic children and adults with communication disorders: Assessment and intervention* (pp. 132–167). Gaithersburg, MD: Aspen.

Maestas, A.G., & Erickson, J.G. (1992). Mexican immigrant mothers' beliefs about disabilities. *American Journal of Speech-Language Pathology, 1,* 5–10.

Matsuda, M. (1989). Working with Asian parents: Some communication strategies. *Topics in Language Disorders, 9,* 45–53.

Matsuda, M., & O'Connor, L.C. (1993, March). *Creating an effective partnership: Training bilingual communication aides.* Presented at the annual meeting of the California Speech, Language, and Hearing Association, Palm Springs, CA.

Mattes, L., & Omark, D. (1991). *Speech and language assessment for the bilingual handicapped (2nd ed.).* Oceanside, CA: Academic Communication Associates.

McCann, M.K., Napoli, M.C., & Wyatt, T.A. (1996, March). *Use of bilingual paraprofessionals with low-incidence language populations: A survey.* Presented at the annual meeting of the California Speech-Language-Hearing Association, Monterey, CA.

Merino, B.J. (1992). Acquisition of syntactic and phonological features in Spanish. In H.W. Langdon, & L.L. Cheng (Eds.), *Hispanic children and adults with communication disorders: Assessment and intervention* (pp. 57–98). Gaithersburg, MD: Aspen.

Pang-Ching, G., Robb, M., Heath, R., & Takumi, M. (1995). Middle ear disorders and hearing loss in native Hawaiian preschoolers. *Language, Speech, and Hearing Services in Schools, 26(1),* 33–38.

Peña, E., Quinn, R., & Iglesias, A. (1992). The application of dynamic methods to language assessment: A nonbiased procedure. *The Journal of Special Education, 26(3),* 269–280.

Reyes, B.A. (1995). Considerations in the assessment and treatment of neurogenic communication disorders in bilingual adults. In H. Kayser (Ed.), *Bilingual speech-language pathology* (pp. 153–182). San Diego: Singular.

Roseberry-McKibbin, C. (1995). *Multicultural students with special language needs: Practical strategies for assessment and intervention.* Oceanside, CA: Academic Communication Associates.

Ruhlen, M. (1975). *A guide to the languages of the world.* Stanford, CA: Stanford University Language Universals Project.

Salas-Provance, M.B. (1996). Orofacial, physiological, and acoustical characteristics: Implications for the speech of African-American children. In A.G. Kamhi, K.E. Pollock, & J.L. Harris (Eds.), *Communication development and disorders in African-American children* (pp. 155–188). Baltimore: Brookes.

Saville-Troike, M. (1986). Anthropological considerations in the study of communication. In O.L. Taylor (Ed.), *Nature of communication disorders in culturally and linguistically diverse populations* (pp. 47–72). San Diego: College Hill.

Schieffelin, B.B., & Eisenberg, A.R. (1984). Cultural variations in children's conversations. In R. Schiefelbusch, & J. Pickar (Eds.), *The acquisition of communicative competence* (pp. 377–420). Baltimore: University Park Press.

Scott, D. (1986). Sickle cell anemia and hearing loss. In F. Bess, B. Clark, & H. Mitchell (Eds.), *ASHA Reports No. 16: Concerns for minority groups in communication disorders* (pp. 52–57). Rockville, MD: American Speech-Language-Hearing Association.

Stockman, I. (1986). Language acquisition in culturally diverse populations: The black child as a case study. In O.L. Taylor (Ed.), *Nature of communication disorders in culturally and linguistically diverse populations* (pp. 117–155). San Diego: College Hill.

Stockman, I. (1996). Phonological development and disorders in African-American children. In A.G. Kamhi, K.E. Pollock, & J.L. Harris (Eds.), *Communication development and disorders in African-American children* (pp. 117–154). Baltimore: Brookes.

Stockman, I., & Vaughn-Cooke, F. (1982). Semantic categories in the language of working-class black children. *Proceedings of the Second International Child Language Conference, 1,* 312–327.

Stockman. I., & Settle, S. (1991, November). *Initial consonants in young black children's conversational speech.* Poster presented at the annual meeting of the American Speech-Language-Hearing Association, Atlanta.

Stockman, I., Vaughn-Cooke, F., & Wolfram, W. (1982). *A developmental study of black English—Phase I [final report].* Washington, DC: Center for Applied Linguistics. (ERIC Document Reproduction Service No. ED 245 555).

Taylor, O.L., & Payne, K. (1983). Culturally valid testing: A proactive approach. *Topics in Language Disorders, 3,* 8–20.

Terrell, S.L., & Terrell, F. (1993). African-American cultures. In D.E. Battle (Ed.), *Communication disorders in multicultural populations* (pp. 3–37). Boston: Butterworth–Heinemann.

Terrell, S.L., & Terrell, F. (1996). The importance of psychological and socio-cultural factors for providing clinical services to African American children. In A.G. Kamhi, K.E. Pollock, & J.L. Harris (Eds.), *Communication development and disorders in African-American children* (pp. 55). Baltimore: Brookes.

Terrell, S.L., Arensberg, K., & Rosa, M. (1992). Parent-child comparative analysis: A criterion-referenced method for the nondiscriminatory assessment of a child who spoke a relatively uncommon dialect of English. *Language, Speech, and Hearing Services in Schools, 23(1),* 34–42.

van Kleeck, A. (1994). Potential cultural bias in training parents as conversational partners with their children who have delays in language development. *American Journal of Speech-Language Pathology, 3,* 67–78.

Vaughn-Cooke, F.B. (1986). The challenge of assessing the language of non-mainstream speakers. In O.L. Taylor (Ed.), *Treatment of communication disorders in culturally and linguistically diverse populations* (pp. 23–48). San Diego: College Hill.

Washington, J.A. (1996). Issues in assessing the language abilities of African-American children. In A.G. Kamhi, K.E. Pollock, & J.L. Harris (Eds.), *Communication development and disorders in African-American children* (pp. 35–54). Baltimore: Brookes.

Wolfram, W. (1969). *A sociolinguistic description of Detroit Negro speech.* Washington, DC: Center for Applied Linguistics.

Wyatt, T.A. (1991). Linguistic constraints on copula production in black English child speech. *Dissertation Abstracts International, 52,* 781B.

Wyatt, T.A. (1995). Language development in African-American English child speech. *Linguistics and Education, 7(1),* 7–22.

Wyatt, T.A. (1996). Acquisition of the African-American English copula. In A.G. Kamhi, K.E. Pollock, & J.L. Harris (Eds.), *Communication development and disorders in African-American children* (pp. 95–116). Baltimore: Brookes.

Wyatt, T.A., & Seymour, H.N. (1990). The implications of code-switching in Black English speakers. *Equity & Excellence [Special issue: Language and discrimination], 24(4),* 17–18.

Zimmerman, I.L., Steiner, V.G., & Pond, R.E. (1992). *Preschool language scale–3.* San Antonio, TX: The Psychological Corporation.

Appendix

13A: Analysis of Communication Abilities in Both Languages Based on Case History Interview and Testing Results

Sample Report 1: Bilingual Arabic- and English-Speaking Child with Suspected Articulation and Language Delay (Chronologic Age = 4 Years, 10 Months)

G's parents, Mr. and Mrs. S, first became concerned with G's speech when he was 2 years old. According to both parents, G progressed through the normal stages of cooing and babbling. He said his first word in Arabic at approximately 9 months and his first word in English at approximately 12 months. Although G produced his first words at a normal age, he did not start putting two words together in English or Arabic until he was 4 years old.

G has been exposed to both Arabic and English since birth, but Arabic is the primary language spoken at home. Both parents reported that G often mixes the two languages but that most of his switching occurs when speaking Arabic. They also reported that G speaks mostly Arabic with family members but that he speaks only English at school and with his friends. At present, they consider G's level of proficiency to be "about the same" in both languages, although his sentences are slightly longer in English.

When asked to describe G's communication difficulties in English, Mr. and Mrs. S reported that G has difficulty producing the /l/ and /v/ sounds and that he substitutes /w/ for /r/. He also has problems with English plural and past-tense endings and negatives.

In addition, G has difficulty using pronouns correctly in both English and Arabic, and he often leaves words out of his sentences in both languages.

Sample Report 2: Bilingual Arabic- and English-Speaking Adult with Aphasia

An analysis of MQ's communicative abilities in English, as revealed through informal administration of subtests from the Minnesota Test for Differential Diagnosis of Aphasia and the Western Aphasia Battery, revealed strengths in recognizing common spoken words (e.g., "cup," "pencil," "keys") and responding to yes-and-no questions. MQ demonstrated difficulty, however, matching written words to pictures, matching printed words to spoken words, and orally reading printed words. MQ's performance on the latter two tasks, however, improved when she was tested in Arabic. Her performance on the first was similar to that in English. Difficulty with the oral reading task in both languages is most likely due to MQ's speech apraxia difficulties.

The following verbal skills were also assessed in both English and Arabic: (1) answering simple questions, (2) counting to 20, and (3) naming the days of the week. MQ had difficulty initiating verbal responses to simple questions (e.g., "What do you do with a hammer?") in both languages, often responding by using hand gestures. MQ also had difficulty counting past the number 4 in English and the number 6 in Arabic, even when cued. In addition, she had difficulty naming days of the week beyond Monday in English and Thursday in Arabic without cues from the clinician. MQ performed better on all three tasks when they were administered in Arabic than when they were administered in English.

13B: Reporting of Test Administration and Scoring Modifications

Sample Report 1: African American Child With Suspected Articulation and Expressive Language Disorder (Chronologic Age = 6 Years, 4 Months)

The Preschool Language Scale-3 (PLS-3) was administered to obtain a general measure of expressive and receptive language skills. Test scores are not reported, since this test was standardized primarily on children from a different cultural background than C. In addition, testing was continued below the basal on the first subtest (auditory comprehension) to obtain a more comprehensive view of C's language strengths and weaknesses.

13C: Descriptive and Criterion-Referenced Analyses of Test Performance

Sample Report 1: African American Adolescent with Suspected Articulation and Expressive Language Problems (Chronologic Age = 12 Years, 3 Months)

Three subtests from the Test of Word Finding (TOWF) were administered to assess B's word-retrieval skills. On the first subtest, Picture Naming Nouns, B correctly named 21 of the 29 possible pictures (72%). She was unable to label four items and gave incorrect responses for the remaining four. In many cases, her error responses involved using a word that was at least indirectly related to the target in semantic reference. For example, she used the word "treasure box" to refer to the picture of a trunk. Slight delays in responding (approximately 2 seconds) were noted on five of the 21 items she labeled correctly. At this time, it is not clear how much of B's labeling difficulties can be attributed to language deficits and how much of the difficulties can be attributed to cultural bias resulting from limited exposure to and familiarity with pictured test stimuli.

Sample Report 2: African American Child with Suspected Articulation and Expressive Language Disorder (Chronologic Age = 6 Years, 4 Months)

On the Auditory Comprehension subtest of the PLS-3, C demonstrated strengths in grouping objects (e.g., "Show me all the things we eat"); identifying colors; making inferences; labeling objects; and understanding descriptive (e.g., heavy, same, empty), time (e.g., night, day), and quantity (e.g., five, three) concepts. C demonstrated difficulty, however, with comparisons (e.g., "Which one is heavier?"), labeling small body parts, spatial concepts (e.g., under, in back of, next to), following complex directions, understanding advanced morphosyntactic forms (e.g., *-er* endings as in "Find the skater") and negatives (e.g., "Show me who is not eating?"), and passive constructions (e.g., "Show me the dog was chased by the boy").

Stimuli from the Linguistic Concepts subtest of the Clinical Evaluation of Language Fundamentals-Preschool were also informally administered to evaluate C's auditory comprehension of basic concepts and verbal commands. Analysis of test results revealed that C was able to successfully follow one- and two-step commands with 70% and 80% accuracy, respectively. Three-step commands were more difficult, with C achieving only 50% accuracy. In addition, C performed best on commands involving spatial concepts (75% accuracy) but demonstrated difficulty with commands containing coordination (and), inclusion and exclusion (one, or, all, either, one), temporal relation and order (first, and then, after, before), and quantitative (all except, all, except) vocabulary terms.

13D: Alternative Methods for Reporting Scores

Sample Report 1: African American Child with Suspected Expressive Language Disorder (Chronologic Age = 3 Years, 11 Months)

Expressive language abilities, as measured by the PLS-3 Expressive Communication subtest, revealed a raw score of 26, which corresponds to a standard score of 83 and places T within 1.0–1.5 standard deviations of the norm for his age group. This score also places him at the thirteenth percentile (90% confidence interval of fifth to twenty-fifth percentile) and represents an age-equivalent score of 2 years, 10 months (90% confidence interval of 2 years, one month to 3 years, 10 months). Although these scores would normally indicate a mild language impairment, it is the examiner's impression that they reflect normal language abilities when cultural test bias influences are taken into consideration.

13E: Citing Potential Test Bias

Sample Report 1: Bilingual Spanish-English Child Speaker with Suspected Language Disorder (Chronologic Age = 5 Years, 6 Months)

All three subtests of the Test of Auditory Comprehension of Language-Revised (TACL-R) were administered to assess M's processing of English grammatic structures. Results from the first subtest (Word Classes and Relations) were as follows:

Raw score	26
Age-equivalent score	51–54 months

M's score places him approximately 1 year below his current chronologic age compared with monolingual English child speakers of the same age. He demonstrated difficulty with comprehension of the following grammatical forms: present progressive -*ing* (e.g., *jumping*), quantitative terms (e.g., *half*), comparative terms (e.g., *alike*), and adjectives (e.g., *soft*). These results, however, should be interpreted with caution given M's bilingual language background and the fact that this test was normed on monolingual English speakers. Many of his errors may be the result of his limited English language abilities.

13F: Differentiating Difference from Disorder

Sample Report 1: Bilingual Arabic-English Child Speaker with Suspected Articulation Disorder (Chronologic Age = 4 Years, 10 Months)

A whole-word transcription of G's English speech sound productions revealed persisting use of several phonologic processes, including (1) the deaffrication of /tʃ, dʒ/; (2) stopping of fricatives /v/, /z/, /θ/, and /ð/; (3) gliding of /r/ and /l/; (4) omission of final voiced and unvoiced sounds such as /b/, /z/, and /θ/; (5) deletion of unstressed syllables; and (6) consonant cluster reduction. It is important to note, however, that the majority of G's speech sound errors occurred on later developing English sounds such as /tʃ/, /dʒ/, /v/, /z/, /r/, /θ/, and /ð/, which generally do not stabilize in the speech of monolingual English speaking children until the age of 5–7 years. In addition, some of G's speech sound productions appear to be related to the fact that some of the previously mentioned sounds, such as /v/, do not exist in his dialect of Arabic.

Sample Report 2: African American Child with Suspected Articulation and Expressive Language Delay (Chronologic Age = 6 Years, 4 Months)

An informal analysis of A's language sample revealed several instances of missing grammatic forms, including (1) articles *a* and *the* (e.g., "Dog chase goat"), (2) possessive *-s* (e.g., "Caterpillar hair is black"), (3) personal pronouns (e.g., "Let do that"), (4) auxiliary *be* (e.g., "I gonna do three"), (5) plural *-s* (e.g., "Three caterpillar on it"), (6) third-person singular *-s* (e.g., "There it go"), (7) present progressive *-ing* (e.g., "He go right now"), and (8) infinitive *to* (e.g., "I want win"). Pronoun substitutions, such as *me* for *I* (e.g., "Me see"), were also noted. In addition, there were several instances of word-order errors (e.g., "Kitten three" and "a book, read it"). Although many of these productions, such as the absence of present progressive *-ing* and word-order differences, can be attributed to language disorder, it is still too early to determine whether others, such as A's grammatical omission of plural -s and third-person singular -s markers, are the result of language delay or emerging dialect differences.

Sample Report 3: Bilingual Spanish-English Child Speaker with Suspected but Unconfirmed Language Delay (Chronologic Age = 5 Years, 3 Months)

An informal analysis of R's language productions revealed occasional omissions of morphosyntactic forms, such as past-tense -ed ("And I was turn four"), copula am ("I not four"), and infinitive to ("They ask the mommy smell"). In addition, nonstandard productions of the following grammatic forms were noted: irregular past tense verbs (e.g., "see" for saw), third-person singular verbs (e.g., "don't" for doesn't), and pronouns (e.g., "them" for their). The majority of these omissions and nonstandard productions, however, are common in the speech of bilingual children acquiring English as a second language.

Sample Report 4: Bilingual German-English Aphasic Adult with Suspected Apraxia and Dysarthria

Results from administration of the Photo Articulation Test revealed several difficulties with the pronunciation of English sounds, with many of Ms. P's productions being inconsistent. Noted substitutions included /m/ for /w/ (initial), /k/ for /g/ (initial), /d/ for /g/ (final), /w/ for /r/ (initial, medial), /b/ for /v/ (initial), /ʃ/ for /s/ (initial, medial), /ts/ for /tʃ/ (initial, final), /k/for /dʒ/ (initial), /f/ for /v/ (medial), /ʃ/ for /tʃ/ (medial), /z/ for /dʒ/ (medial), /f/ for /θ/ (final), and /ts/for /z/ (final). Some of these substitutions, such as those occurring on the phonemes /r/, /dʒ/, /θ/, and /ð/, can most likely be attributed to first-language influences, since none of these sounds are part of the standard German phonetic inventory. It is important to also note, however, that at least one of these phonemes, /w/, appears in the phonetic inventory of some German dialects.

Sample Report 5: Adult Native Chinese Speaker Interested in Accent Modification Services

Ms. T exhibited difficulties with the pronunciation of several English sounds, including /ð/, /v/, /r/, /dʒ/, /ʒ/ and, /z/ in at least one word position; /r/ and /l/ blends; and vowels /ɪ/, /æ/, /ʊ/, /ɛ/, and /aɪ/. Frequent devoicing of final voiced sounds was also observed. No major differences were noted in the use of English stress and intonation patterns. Examination of English grammatic forms revealed occasional omission of articles, present progressive *-ing*, the contracted negative, prepositions, auxiliary verbs, plural *-s* markers, and past-tense *-ed*. These differences appear to have a moderate impact on Ms. T's overall speech intelligibility in English, but all represent normal differences common in the speech of native Chinese speakers learning English as a second language.

13G: Establishing Appropriate Intervention Goals and Targets

Sample Report 1: African American Child with Articulation and Expressive Language Delay (Chronologic Age = 6 Years, 4 Months)

Therapy using contrastive minimal word pair approaches should be considered for eliminating C's persisting use of inappropriate phonologic processes. Processes that should be targeted as a first priority include gliding, stopping of fricatives (with the exception of /θ/ and /ð/), fronting and backing of sounds due to assimilation, reduction of consonant blends, omission of final voiceless sounds, devoicing of initial voiced sounds, glottalization of final stops, and the insertion of intrusive medial /t/. Second priority should be given to omission of final voiced sounds and deletion of unstressed syllables, since the use of these two processes can vary between different dialects of English and A's current dialect status is not yet clear.

Therapy should also focus on increasing C's mean length of utterance and production of age-appropriate morphosyntactic forms through the use of naturalistic language activities conducted within a functional communication context. First priority should be given to the stabilization of forms that are non–dialect-specific (obligatory in all dialects of English), such as the articles *a* and *the*.

14

Clinical Practice Issues

Priscilla Nellum Davis,
Betholyn Gentry,
and Pamela Hubbard-Wiley

To provide more effective service to multicultural clients, speech-language pathologists and audiologists have recognized the need to become more knowledgeable about various cultural groups. According to Taylor (in press), the clinical practice setting should be perceived as a social setting. Taylor has voiced consistent and constant concern over the neglect of the multicultural issue in clinical training and service delivery. The cultural views of both client and clinician influence every aspect of the clinical setting. Clients engage in the therapy process based on their cultural beliefs and values. The activities, materials, and clinical procedures that professionals have been trained to use may be sources of cultural conflict for some clients from various cultural, ethnic, religious, and geographical backgrounds. As a result of these conflicts in the clinical setting, high absenteeism, tardiness, and termination of clinical services may occur. This chapter discusses cultural factors that affect the therapy process. It also provides a list of technological resources available to assist the speech-language pathologist in providing culturally appropriate clinical services.

Religious Practices and Clinical Practice

Ethnography is the study of culture, the work of describing culture (Spradley 1979). The main purpose of ethnography is to understand another person's way of living and how it is alike or different from their cultures. Ethnography makes it possible to learn from other cultures. The people clinicians seek to help have a way of life and a culture of their own.

Ethnography offers the educator a way of seeing a school through the eyes of the students; it offers health professionals the opportunity of seeing health and disease through the eyes of patients from a myriad of different backgrounds. Ethnography offers a pathway into understanding the cultural differences that make us what we are as human beings. Perhaps the most important force behind the quiet ethnographic revolution is the widespread realization that cultural diversity is one of the greatest resources of the human species.

Religious beliefs are cultural factors that have a great impact on the delivery of clinical services. They influence what clients eat, what they wear, and how they participate in the clinical program. Clinical practices are typically given from the religious point of view of the clinician, with little attention to the religious views of the client. This could be due to the American tenet of freedom of religion, which was a central belief of the founders of this country. Our educational and clinical practices are based on a European Christian model, which seemed appropriate when most of the people living in this country were Christian descendants of European countries. The demographic changes that have occurred, however, have made the United States a land of many peoples. The country is becoming more culturally diverse, with new immigrants coming from non-European countries. Cultural diversity means an increase in religious diversity. Clients are no longer exclusively white middle-class Christians.

Little has been written about the impact of religious practices on clinical practices. However, Davis (1992) obtained information about the religious practices and beliefs practices of various religious groups and how they affect the delivery of clinical services by using an ethnographic interview format. In this study, cultural informants were interviewed to obtain information about the impact of major recognized religions on clinical service delivery. All informants were familiar with speech-language hearing services and some of the activities used in the clinical setting. The informants stated that they were aware of some practices in mainstream America that were different from practices in their culture. The information that was given was based on experiences and opinions of the respondents to a hypothetical situation that showed the effect their culture would have on clinical services.

A questionnaire format adapted from Taylor (1986) called "Cultural Identities, Values, and Rules of Interaction" was used in each interview for uniformity. Questions were asked concerning family structure, interpersonal relationships, decorum and discipline, foods, holidays and customs, values, and beliefs about health care. Questions included the following: (1) Who is considered part of the "family"? (2) What are the rights, roles, and responsibilities of the members of the family? (3) How do people greet each other? (4) Who may disagree with whom? (5) How are insults expressed? (6) How do people behave at home and in public? (7) What means of discipline are used? (8) Who has authority over whom? (9) What is eaten? (10) What foods are taboo? (11) What holidays are observed? and (12) What are the concerns about medicine and health care? The interviews also addressed how these factors could influence clinical services.

Information from the interviews with religious groups indicated a wide range of beliefs and practices that directly affected the delivery of clinical services. The religious preferences of the groups interviewed were shown to influence scheduling, test and therapy materials, interpersonal communication, and nonverbal interactions. Some of the major practices for each of the groups interviewed and the implications for speech-language therapy are discussed in the following sections.

Hinduism and Buddhism

Hinduism and Buddhism are among the most prominent religious or moral systems among Southeast Asian cultures. Many of their basic beliefs and principles are in conflict with clinical practices.

Hinduism, or Brahmanism, is the major religion of India and is also found in Cambodia and Laos. It is the oldest religion still practiced in the world, with its roots dating to prehistoric times. Although most Hindus live in India, their literature and philosophy have influenced people throughout the world. Hinduism was not founded on the beliefs of one man but rather developed gradually over thousands of years and was shaped by many cultures, races, and other religions. It is associated with Indian philosophy, deities, and traditional worship of Brahma, the supreme being who is at once the Creator, the Preserver, and the Destroyer, with a different wife for each form he manifests. The views of Hinduism, or Brahmanism, are often combined with animism, in which it is believed that spiritual and supernatural powers are present throughout the universe and that all natural phenomena and things both animate and inanimate possess an innate soul.

Buddhism, one of the major religions of the world, was founded in India about 500 B.C. by a teacher called *Buddha*. The nearly 200 million followers of Buddhism live or have their roots in Southeast Asia and Japan. More than 780,000 followers of Buddhism live in the United States (World Almanac 1997).

At various times, Buddhism has been a dominant religious, cultural, and social force in most of Asia. There are two branches of Buddhism: (1) Mahayana, or Great Vehicle, is prominent in Vietnam, China, Japan, and

Korea, and (2) Hinayana, or Little Vehicle, flourishes in Cambodia, Laos, Burma, Thailand, and Sri Lanka. Buddhist doctrine is summarized in the four noble truths: (1) All life is suffering, (2) suffering is caused by desire or attachment to the world, (3) suffering can be extinguished and attachment to all things can be overcome by desire, and (4) to eliminate desire, one must live a virtuous life (Chan 1992). The Buddhist goal is to be released from the wheel of life, or circle of reincarnation, and reach nirvana. Nirvana is a state of complete redemption wherein all suffering is transcended, and one's soul is merged into the cosmic and only true reality.

Buddhism, together with the teachings of Confucius, Lao-tzu, and the tenet of ancestral worship, have a profound influence on the lives of Asians. Confucianism was founded by Confucius in 551 B.C. Its major beliefs involve individual virtue and the moral fabric of a society. Believers of the teaching of Confucius embody five virtues that are embodied in the duties owed to parents and ancestors and reverence for ancestors whose spirits must be appeased. Ancestral worship is characterized by three basic assumptions: (1) All living people owe their fortunes to their ancestors, (2) all departed ancestors have needs that are the same as the living, and (3) departed ancestors continue to assist their relatives in the world, just as their descendants can assist them. With such belief in the connection of all things living and dead, it is not surprising that there are many clinical practices that conflict with Buddhist beliefs.

The following are factors to be considered in the delivery of clinical services to those who are Confucianists, Buddhists, or the Hindus. They are not meant to be all inclusive nor are they meant to apply to all. They are intended as a guide to assist the clinician.

1. Meats are not included in the diet. Most Buddhists and Hindus are vegetarians and eat diets of vegetables and grains. Meat categories should be avoided in activities, especially beef because cows are thought to be sacred. Scenes and stories that depict the killing of animals should be avoided.
2. Knowledge of kinship terms is important. This relates to the belief in the importance of ancestors. The birth of a child and the death of an elder are significant events.
3. For some Hindus, no photographs or videotapes should be taken of female clients. Photographs of women are to be looked at only by male family members or other females. Care must be taken to obtain permission before audiotaping, videotaping, or photographing female clients. Male clinicians should exercise caution and ask for permission before photographing, videotaping, or both.

4. For both Buddhists and Hindus, strict rules govern the relationship between the sexes. Men and women are not permitted to work together and do not touch each other. Opposite-sex clinicians would not be permitted to work with some Hindus.

5. The head is the purest body part because it contains the human spirit. Patting a child's or adult's head is a great offense. Explanations should be given when touching the head is required in the therapy setting for audiologic testing and oral peripheral examinations. Permission should be granted before engaging in any activity that involves touching the head.

6. It is considered rude to blow one's nose, talk loudly, or show one's teeth in public. This can have an impact on the client's willingness to participate in an examination of the oral mechanism or to increase vocal intensity as part of an evaluation for voice disorder. In addition, the clinician can mistake decreased vocal intensity for a pathology rather than a cultural behavior.

7. Children respect their elders. They never address elders by their first names. Use Mr., Mrs., Miss, or other appropriate titles with the family name for Chinese and Koreans to establish the connection with the ancestors (e.g., Tien Chang-Lin would be addressed as Mrs. Tien). For Cambodians, Laotians, and Vietnamese use the first or given name. For example, Kamchong Laungpraseut would be addressed as Mr. Kamchong. Clinicians should refrain from addressing clients or their parents by their first name. This is especially important for elderly clients or new immigrants. Clinicians should also greet family members in order of age, beginning with the oldest man.

8. Conversations with clients and the family should begin with small talk before initiating the topic of the conversation or "getting to the point" for most Asian cultures.

9. Guests are welcomed warmly and invited to share in whatever meal the family has prepared. To decline the invitation to share the family meal or other food offerings is considered rude to the host or hostess.

10. Buddhists celebrate a special 3-day holiday in August. New Year's Day, the first day of the first month of the lunar calendar, is another holiday on which devout worshipers go to the shrine to pray.

11. The third, fifth, and seventh birthdays of children are important celebrations for Buddhists. Families travel to shrines on these birthdays to pray for the development of the young child.

12. Red is the color of good luck and represents life for most Asian cultures. White is the color of mourning and represents death. Wearing white medical smocks may be seen as a sign that the client is approaching death.

Islam

Islam was founded in the seventh century in the Empire of the Caliphs, which stretched from Spain and Morocco across the middle East to central Asia. People who practice the religion of Islam are called Muslims or Moslems. There are nearly 500 million Muslims in the world today. They form the majority of the population in the Middle East; North Africa; and Southeast Asian nations such as Pakistan, Malaysia, and Indonesia. Islam is the fastest growing religion in the United States, largely because of the increase of immigration of people from the Middle East and the conversion of many African Americans to Islam.

Followers of Islam believe that God gave his final revelation to the Prophet Mohammed, who they believe to be the last in a succession of prophets including Moses and Jesus. The Koran, the holy book containing Mohammed's revelations, is believed to be the full expression of the divine will for human life (Sharifzadeh 1992). Followers of Islam believe in the strength of the family and children. The Koran (Quar 18) says that "[w]ealth and children are the ornaments of this life."

Muslims follow the lunar calendar, which is based on the phases of the moon. Each new year begins on the second new moon after the winter solstice, or anytime between January and March.

Ramadan is a month-long observance of dedication and self-control. Since the time of Ramadan is determined by the lunar calendar, it begins on a different date each year on a solar or a Christian calendar. During Ramadan, no food or drink is consumed from sunrise to sunset. Children are required to participate for specified periods of time until they are 8 or 9 years of age. Children from the age of 8 or 9 years through adolescence are expected to participate from sunrise to sunset. Those who are ill or who have medical concerns are permitted to either not observe Ramadan at all or to participate on a limited basis. A large feast is held on Eid-al-Feter to mark the end of the month of Ramadan.

The following practices have been suggested for consideration by speech-language pathologists by Muslims from India, Kuwait, Saudi Arabia, Pakistan, and Africa currently living in the United States. Since many Muslims are from different cultural and geographical regions, some of the following information may be based on culture rather than on religion:

1.   No pork or food products containing pork should be used in clinical activities. This includes items such as bacon and sausage when discussing breakfast foods.

2.   Religious and secular activities related to Christian holidays, such as Easter and Christmas, should be avoided.

3.   Adult clients may observe Ramadan and may refuse food or water during the month-long observance. Although those with health problems are excused from the practice, many may wish to continue on a limited basis. Children may not participate in the observance, but some alteration in family patterns during the holiday period may still exist.

4.   Activities using violence or advocating hunting for sport should not be used. Animals are killed only for food, and religious teachings dictate how animals should be killed. Giving animals human-like characteristics and other forms of anthropomorphism is discouraged by some Muslims. For example, stories that use animals, such as a talking cat, may be taboo. Pigs should never be used.

5.   Activities about dressing and clothing should be used carefully. Devout Muslim women do not wear revealing clothes and often cover their faces. Activities involving dressing or bathing dolls should be avoided, unless previously discussed with parents and clients. Teaching body parts using anatomically correct dolls should be avoided. The use of cosmetics in language lessons is discouraged (i.e., lessons teaching face parts by using lipstick and eye shadow with female clients should be avoided).

6.   Friday is the Muslim Sabbath; it is called *Jum'a.* Some Muslims have restricted Jum'a celebrations to 1 PM on Friday afternoons. Others may celebrate *Jum'a* at a different time, depending on the time zone. Some Muslims agree to diagnostic and intervention sessions on Friday and others do not. Devout Muslims pray five times daily, with special prayers at sunrise, noon, and sunset. This can affect scheduling options.

7.   Islamic religions allow no physical contact between men and women in public. Women do not give orders or instructions to men. If services for a female client by a male clinician are accepted, strict rules would require that a parent or a family member be present at all times.

8.   Elders are considered authorities. Older clients may not comply when younger clinicians, especially female clinicians, give instructions or use direct requests with imperatives. Indirect requests and suggestions are more desirable methods.

9.   Extended families are common. Family members other than mother and father may be included in conferences. Fathers make the decisions regarding any member of the family. Their presence

is essential to the service-delivery process (i.e., at family conferences, individualized education program and individualized family service plan conferences, and whenever decisions are made about scheduling and treatment techniques).

10. Knowledge of kinship terms is important. For example, different names may be used for the maternal or the paternal grandparent. In addition, since polygamy is still practiced in some Muslim cultures, children may have more than one mother. Terms such as senior mother and natural mother may be used.

11. Touching, hugging, and gazing is considered overly familiar behavior, especially among members of the opposite sex. Men do not establish eye contact with women. To show respect for women, men avert their gaze. To show respect for adults, children do not look adults directly in the eyes. In conversational discourse and in the clinic setting, lack of eye contact from the client is considered respectful. In Ghana, when children are verbally reprimanded, the child is supposed to kneel at the feet of the elder. A child from Ghana would not look a teacher or clinician in the eye as he or she was being corrected.

12. Home visits are not encouraged. Because some Muslims view the home as private, business activities are not to be conducted in the home by outsiders. Some parents prefer to come to the clinic rather than have the clinician visit them at home. Friends, usually people of the same religion, may make unannounced visits. Outsiders, people who are not Muslims, are expected to wait for an invitation or to make an appointment.

13. Since it is thought that the Koran is carried in the head, touching, hitting, or patting the head should be avoided.

14. Devout Muslims believe that only Allah knows the future, and they therefore do not plan more than a few weeks ahead. Discussing long-term educational plans for infants may not seem important to parents and caregivers.

15. Use of the left hand to pass items is considered rude. When handing items to someone, place the item in the person's hand, not on the table or counter. To place materials, papers, and instrumentation on the counter is considered rude and offensive.

Judaism

Judaism is the religion of about 15 million people worldwide. There are more than 5 million Jews in the United States. Judaism is the oldest religion of the Western world and the first to teach monotheism. It is founded on the laws and teachings of the Hebrew Bible, or Old Testament, and of the Talmud. Christianity and Islam are both derived from Judaism, even though they both differ in many basic beliefs and practices. Because Jews do not recognize one single authority, they have found it possible to differ about their religion and still remain Jews. Today these differences are expressed through three major religious groups: Orthodox, Conservative, and Reformed.

Orthodox Jews represent a branch of Judaism that resists most change. They believe that they are observing the law as handed down to Moses on Mount Sinai. Orthodox Jews are the most devout. They observe all Jewish laws, including kosher dietary restrictions such as not eating pork or shellfish. They do not allow meat and dairy products to be served on the same dishes or to be served in the same meal. Many Orthodox Jews maintain two separate sets of dishes: one for meat meals and one for dairy meals.

Orthodox Jews observe all Jewish holy days. Jewish holidays are Rosh Hashanah, Yom Kippur, Succoth, Shemini Atzeret, Simchat Torah, Hanukkah, Passover, and Shavuoth. Each holiday begins at sunset of the day before the holiday. Orthodox Jews observe the Sabbath starting at sundown on Friday. Restrictions on the Sabbath include all forms of work, including riding in automobiles or pushing elevator buttons.

Conservative Jews accept Jewish law as the primary Jewish expression of all time. They observe many, but not all, Jewish holy days and may observe the dietary restrictions only during periods associated with the major holy days (e.g., Hanukkah, Yom Kippur, and Rosh Hashanah).

Reformed Jews are the largest and fastest-growing Jewish movement (Hoffman 1993). They are the most assimilated into American society. They believe that Jewish tradition constantly changes. They emphasize the need to interpret tradition from the perspective of individual conscious and informed choice. They may not follow all kosher dietary restrictions or strictly observe the rules of the Sabbath. They observe only the major Jewish holy days, such as Hanukkah, Rosh Hashanah, and Yom Kippur. The following information may not apply to all Jewish groups but should serve as a guide during clinical services.

1. Judaism has strict dietary rules. Foods that should not be discussed as a part of a therapy session are pork and shellfish. Food dishes requiring meat and dairy products to be mixed or served together are forbidden. Orthodox and Conservative Jews strictly observe all dietary rules. Reform Jews may or may not observe the dietary rules in accordance with their religious convictions. Activities and foods

used in the therapy setting should be selected with these considerations in mind.

2. Orthodox and Reform followers of Judaism observe Jewish holidays and nonsectarian American holidays.

Guidelines for Culturally Relevant Intervention

Furst (1971) identified teaching guidelines that helped increase student achievement and are applicable to clinicians as well. These guidelines can be adapted for the multicultural clinical setting. For successful intervention, the following guidelines should be observed:

1. Present clear explanations of objectives. The clinician should be clear about the objectives of the session and should make sure the client understands the objective of the assessment and treatment program.
2. Care should be taken to be certain the methods and procedures used in the sessions do not violate the beliefs of the client. A cultural informant could be used to assist the clinician in selecting culturally appropriate methods and materials.
3. Be flexible in selecting materials and activities. Clinicians should be willing to vary therapy content and teaching styles as needed. The learning environment should allow the client to be creative and motivated to take communication risks in the setting. Although an organized training program is desired, clinicians should be willing to change the content and activities as the situation dictates. Clinicians should adapt materials to the needs of the particular client.
4. Flexibility should be a major factor in scheduling. Avoid scheduling therapy on a Sabbath or on religious holidays when possible. Some absenteeism will be unavoidable when therapy falls on holidays. American Indians, African Americans, and some Hispanic groups have an elastic concept of time (e.g., they believe they have kept the appointment if they arrive 5–15 minutes after the scheduled appointment time or anytime within a flexible time period; they may consider it permissible to arrive between 2 PM and 3 PM for a 2:30 PM appointment).
5. Interact with clients according to their perception or expectation. In some cultures, the clinicians's showing enthusiasm, vigor, or confidence is a sign of competence. In other cultures, touching, showing

enthusiasm, using elevated pitch, and "gushing" over babies may be offensive. Some Native Americans do not permit hugging, kissing, and excessive handling of their babies by strangers.

6. Be businesslike and task oriented. Clients need to feel that the clinician has a purpose for activities and lessons. Examples from real-life situations could show the importance of the lesson and how to use the new information appropriately. Some individuals need to be shown how certain activities fit into their lifestyles and how they relate to the intervention process.

7. Use praise and encouragement. Criticism should be used wisely and sparingly. Too much negative criticism is not good. Some criticism, however, is desirable in that it reinforces and encourages the flow of communication. The clinician can never give too much praise and encouragement. In some groups, negative report of progress can result in punishment of the child.

8. Provide opportunities to learn. In the therapy setting the clinician should create a warm environment that enriches the social interaction and accepts the client's culture and communication style. The client should be given many opportunities to communicate. Activities should relate to the client's cultural patterns, customs, values, and holidays.

9. Preview and review lessons. Repetition and variety have been suggested as key factors to aid learning. Clients need to be told what the lesson is about and why it is important. The review reinforces any concepts that are not clear. Clients from some cultures are taught to review by repeating material themselves. Including the client as a participant in the review process can reinforce main points and give an opportunity for feedback where clarification is needed.

10. Use multiple levels of questions or cognitive discourse. Knowledge and use of different styles is important to increase the client's repertoire of useful language. Simplification of adult speech, repetition of phrases, expansions, and filling in omissions are ways that adults interact with young children. Knowledge of cultural activities and various speaking needs should be used to demonstrate different pragmatic aspects of language. The clinician should teach concepts in different settings and different ways.

The inclusion of multiculturalism into intervention is a concept that is gaining widespread support. Cultural competence is a goal for individuals as well as organizations. Therapy techniques, as well as environment, should create a feeling of inclusion that reflects the recognition and appreciation of diversity in America. By using a culturally competent approach to service provision, therapy becomes more relevant and interesting to clients (Lynch and Hanson 1992; Tiedt and Tiedt 1990). Additionally this approach promotes understanding of other groups and reduces potential racial conflicts. Addressing every possible source of cultural conflict that could occur in the therapy process is beyond the scope of this chapter. The following sections, however, provide additional suggestions that the clinician can refer to when encountering a client from a different culture.

Physical Environment

Waiting rooms and therapy rooms should be culturally inclusive. Signs and reading materials should be available in the languages of the clients served by the clinical program. Therapy rooms should be decorated with culturally relevant and appropriate pictures that reflect a multicultural society. Large pictures and posters are available that depict families of various racial and ethnic backgrounds living in varied communities and performing a variety of activities. These pictures should show nuclear families, extended families, multigenerational families, families with a person with disabilities, and families with mixed races. These pictures can be used to elicit language, as well as to make the therapy room appear inclusive.

Therapy Activities

Language and speech activities should focus on the various cultures represented in the caseload. Clients can be encouraged to share knowledge of their culture with the clinician and other clients.

Food

Culture can be incorporated into intervention programs by introducing food items likely to be found in the client's household while teaching basic vocabulary. For example, many Japanese families consume noodles as a staple for breakfast, lunch, and dinner. Likewise, many Hispanic families consume beans, *frijoles*, as a staple (Baedeker 1993). Additionally, an increasing number of families rely on fast food establishments for breakfast, lunch, and dinner. Actual food items can be tasted and experienced in the therapy setting. Permission should first be obtained from the parents, however, to determine if there are any types of foods that are not permitted.

Music

Music is integral to all groups and can be incorporated into therapy activities. Popular styles of music, such as rap, which many adults find offensive, have been found to be effective in teaching different language concepts. This is often the music listened to by many African American and non–African American children and young adults in the home. This style of music has been replicated by record makers who specialize in educational music for children. Use of these types of songs is an excellent way to promote language and include culture in therapy. The clinician could encourage children to write their own rap songs about assigned concepts or topics.

Literature

Culturally relevant children's literature can provide an excellent opportunity for introducing or reinforcing culture while teaching various aspects of language. There are many books available that teach and promote culture while providing interesting stories for all ages. Concepts taught include nouns, verbs, sequencing, retelling stories, predicting outcomes, discussing feelings, inferences, idiomatic expressions, and so on. Resources for this type of literature are presented in the chapter appendix.

Toys

Toys are an integral component of therapy when working with children. Animals and dolls are probably used more frequently than other types of toys. Today's market has many dolls that reflect various racial and cultural groups. Many African American dolls have braids and wear colorful clothing, whereas others are more mainstream in appearance. It is important for the therapist to be sensitive to the fact that many doll makers produce dolls that distort and magnify facial and physical characteristics of African Americans, which can be offensive at best. Time should be taken to select dolls that are appealing to children and create an accurate reflection of the racial group for which it is intended.

Play

All children play, but how children play can be affected by a child's culture; therefore, it should not be assumed that all children play the same way. One view of play involves adult-directed and structured play. In many cultures, however, children play alone, with little adult intervention. Also, not all children have the play space or toys commonly seen in middle-class American families. Schwartzman (1983) noted that children from poor, working-class environments use their imaginations and engage in very creative play using materials found in their environment (e.g., trash cans, junk cars, trees). In some countries and areas, such as Kenya, South Vietnam, England, Ghana, India, and East Africa, play is not encouraged (Ebbick 1971). In some rural American communities children may play while doing chores. For example, they may play a game of tag while milking cows. Blackburn (1992) reported, however, that after 3 or 4 years in the United States, Hispanic children adopted the toys, games and play habits of American children. The same may be true of children from other countries. Because play is often used as an assessment tool for young children, caution should be exercised when assessing the play of children from other cultures. Clinicians should not automatically place their values on the play of these children. For example, some children may be reluctant to engage in pretending activities. Pretend bahavior is not encouraged at home. In some homes pretend behaior is punished because it is perceived as lying. These children should not be penalized in this instance. For more information clinicians should see Lundsteen's (1997) extensive report on multicultural play.

Animals
Common animals that are typically assumed to be appropriate stimulators of language may be inappropriate when used with certain groups. Do not use a talking cow with children who hold the cow sacred. No pigs or hogs should be used with Jewish and Muslim clients. Some Indian tribes consider the owl to be a bad omen or evil force. Some groups do not have cats and dogs as pets: Asians and Arabic cultures are more likely to keep birds as pets. Therefore, animals and dolls should be selected based on one's knowledge of the cultural group to determine if the toys or images are acceptable and appropriate.

Events and Holidays
All cultural groups have holidays and events that are of great importance to them and often recognized or celebrated by the dominant culture. A discussion of these events in therapy provides a wealth of information relating to groups of people, as well as providing a therapist with a number of activities for therapy.

Significant cultural events, holidays, and festivals are excellent ways to incorporate a multicultural theme into therapy. Various ways of celebrating holidays such as Christmas, Hanukkah, and Cinco de Mayo can be incorporated into treatment sessions. However, although holidays can be beneficial to therapy, the use of some images should be carefully considered, and care should be taken not to incorporate into treatment sessions celebrations that may be offensive to the client and family. Halloween, for example, is celebrated by many in the United States. Although many cultural groups view this day as an innocent day of fun, many others take offense to some of the practices associated with the holiday. Some groups forbid the celebration of Halloween because of the frequency of "devil" themes. Many Native Americans link misfortune and etiology of disabilities to witchcraft, spirit loss, spells, and other supernatural causes. A witch poster or someone pretending to be a witch in the clinical setting may be perceived as offensive and frightening. In this case, the therapist should refrain from Halloween decorations, which could be offensive to others. Instead themes of fall could be used that include, for example, pumpkin pie instead of jack-o-lanterns.

Holidays with a connection to American history may not be understood by new immigrants. It should not be assumed that clients are familiar with the concepts of American history and historical figures. For example, discussions of Thanksgiving and the pilgrims can stimulate and elicit language from a cultural perspective. The therapist could ask clients with whom they will celebrate the holiday and what foods will be served. If therapy is being provided in a classroom setting, a Thanksgiving meal can be provided with foods representing the various cultures. A culturally-competent therapist would ensure that all cultural groups and their contributions to America are included.

The following are holidays and celebrations often overlooked by the mainstream culture:

- Kwanzaa is an African American cultural celebration started in 1966 by Dr. Ron Maulana Karenga. This celebration begins on December 26 and culminates on January 1. It celebrates cultural tradition, the strength of the family, and unity. It is not a religious holiday nor a substitution for Christmas.
- Cinco de Mayo (May 5), which may be considered a regionally specific celebration, is an event celebrated by many Mexican Americans in the Southwestern part of the United States. Mexican Americans, however, can be found in most parts of the United States. It is considered the independence day for Mexican Americans. Many schools and communities with large Hispanic populations have festivities, which include dancing, singing, and native dress.
- The principal holiday for many Asians is the Lunar New Year. Chinese usually celebrate this day in February, depending on the moon. Cambodians and Laotians celebrate their New Year's day in the fifth month of the lunar calendar, which usually occurs in mid-April, shortly after harvest time.

It is also important to note that some fundamental groups and Jehovah's Witnesses do not celebrate any holidays. Regardless of the holiday that the clinician emphasizes, he or she should keep in mind that new immigrants may not know many of the American holidays. The clinician should not assume, for example, that a new immigrant knows about Martin Luther King. An understanding of all American holidays and cultural events can be incorporated into activities designed to stimulate language development.

There are many cultures in the United States, and different beliefs and values are shared by each group. Students should be given ongoing opportunities to celebrate their culture and to learn about another's. Thematic units can be developed that incorporate multiculturalism in everyday activities. The clinician should be careful not to become an "expert" on another's culture but to consider himself or herself a "student," always learning and evolving to another level.

Learning Styles

Not all people learn in the same way. There are many styles of learning. Dunn and Griggs (1988) described learning styles in terms of how the individual's ability to learn new or difficult material is affected by the following variables: (1) the immediate environment (noise level, temperature, amount of light, and furniture design), (2) emotionality (degree of motivation, persistence, responsibility, and need for structure), (3) sociological needs (learning alone or with peers, learning with adults present, learning in groups), (4) physical characteristics (auditory, visual, tactile, and kinesthetic strengths; best time of day for learning; need for food and drink while learning; and mobility requirements), and (5) psychological inclinations (global and analytical strengths).

Most Americans have been educated using one teaching style. There is no one teaching style that is best for all people. It is important to determine what teaching style works best for a particular individual. Carbo and Hodges (1988) determined that many disabled children, behaviorally disordered children, and at-risk children have been trained using teaching styles that are at odds with their learning styles. In the clinical setting, a communication gap can exist between the teaching style of the clinician and the learning style of the client.

Anderson (1988) determined that there are different learning styles for multicultural groups. White children do best on analytic tasks—that is, they learn material that is inanimate and impersonal more easily, and their performance is not greatly affected by the opinions of others. Many Mexican American, Puerto Rican, and African American children are thought to be more global in their learning styles.

In the clinical setting, cultural and cognitive conflicts occur when a client is asked to perform in a manner and setting that is different from the style that he or she prefers. Using therapy techniques based on an analytical learning style in the clinical setting can place the multicultural client at a disadvantage. Anderson (1988) summarized his findings by stating that "what is a valuable and valid communication process under one cognitive style becomes a deformed example of cognitive/linguistic deficits under another."

In the effective delivery of services, clinicians should be aware of cultural differences in learning styles. Carbo and Hodges (1988) suggested that instruction should be based on learning styles. For example, for the global learner the following approaches should be used: (1) listening to and reading good literature, (2) acting in plays, (3) creating models, (4) drawing pictures and writing about them, and (5) using puppets as characters in storytelling activities.

The following strategies, adapted from Carbo and Hodges (1988), are suggestions for considering the preferred learning styles of clients in clinical intervention:

1. During an informal assessment or in the diagnostic setting, the clinician should determine what learning style the client uses most often. Most information available on the different ethnic groups, with the exception of the Asian group, suggests that analytic styles are not preferred.

2. The clinician should explain to the client what he or she is trying to determine. He should also share with the client the results of findings. If an ethnographic interview is performed, the clinician should discuss how cultural views differ and make every effort to include the cultural views of the client in decisions about therapy and materials. Objectives should be structured, flexible, and clearly stated.

3. Therapy materials should appeal to the emotions. Action and active involvement in therapy with clear objectives that relate to real life are prerequisites for good therapy sessions. Acting out situations, modeling, using pantomime, and using songs and chants can help the client relate therapy to real life. Demonstrations and motor and kinesthetic approaches that involve the hands and the whole body should be used rather than drills, work sheets, and some board games. Variety and action are the key words for successful intervention sessions.

4. The clinician should allow clients to work in a cooperative style with peers, friends, or adults. School-age clients often want a friend or buddy to come with them. If the environment is conducive to this arrangement, friends should be allowed. Most individuals from

non-Western groups prefer activities in which they work with others and help others in a cooperative style. Competitive activities should be excluded.

5. Language stories, story boards, and picture stories rooted in the client's culture should be used whenever possible.

6. Structured real-life situations are imperative for teaching pragmatic skills. These situations can be set up, for example, in group settings, special field trip assignments, role playing, films and videotapes, and storytelling.

Conclusion

This chapter outlines differences in religious beliefs and learning styles that affect clinical service delivery. Continual research is needed, as well as more innovative strategies and methods of effective service delivery to those from various religious groups. Knowledge of culture groups and their beliefs, customs, attitudes, and values is essential to overcome barriers to successful intervention programs.

References

Anderson, J. (1988). Cognitive styles and multicultural populations. In L. Cole (Ed.), *Communication sciences and disorders: Marketing careers to minority students*. Rockville, MD: American Speech-Language-Hearing Association.

Baedeker, K. (1993). *Baedeker's Mexico*. Englewood Cliffs, NJ: Prentice Hall.

Blackburn, J. (1992). *Hispanic play*. Minisession within the session, "Multicultural Play," at the American Association for the Child's Right to Play. Denton, TX.

Carbo, M., & Hodges, H. (1988). Learning styles and strategies can help students at risk. *Teaching Exceptional Children, 55*, 55–56.

Chan, S. (1992). Families with Asian roots. In E.W. Lynch, & M.J. Hanson (Eds.), *Developing cross-cultural competence: A guide for working with young children and their families* (pp. 181–257). Baltimore: Brookes.

Davis, P. (1992). Clinical practice issues. In D. Battle (Ed.), *Communication disorders in multicultural populations* (pp. 306–316). Boston: Andover Medical Publishers.

Dunn, R., & Griggs, S.A. (1988). The learning styles of multicultural groups and counseling implications. *Journal of Multi-Cultural Counseling and Development, 17*, 146–153.

Ebbeck, F.N. (1971). Learning from play in other cultures. *Childhood Education, 48(2)*, 69–74.

Furst, N. (1971). *International analysis in teacher education: A review of studies*. Washington, DC: Washington Association of Teacher Education in Collaboration with ERIC Clearinghouse of Teacher Education.

Hoffman, L. (1993). *What's a Jew?* New York: Macmillan.

Lundsteen, S. (1997). *Multicultural play awareness*. http://www.earlychildhood.com/articles/multplay.html

Lynch, E., & Hanson, M.J. (1992). *Developing cross-cultural competence: A guide for working with young children and their families*. Baltimore: Brookes.

Sharifzadeh, V. (1992). Families with Asian roots. In E.W. Lynch, & M.J. Hanson (Eds.), *Developing cross-cultural competence: A guide for working with young children and their families* (pp. 319–352). Baltimore: Brookes.

Schwartzman, H.B. (1983). Child-structured play: A cross-cultural perspective. In F. Manning (Ed.), *The world of play* (pp. 25–33). West Point, NY: Leisure Press.

Spradley, J.P. (1979). *The bilingual child*. New York: Academic.

Taylor, O. (1986). *Treatment of communication disorders in culturally and linguistically diverse populations*. San Diego: College Hill.

Taylor, O. (in press). Communication as a social process. In G. Cole & V. Deal (Eds.), *Communication disorders in multicultural populations*. Rockville, MD: American Speech-Language-Hearing Association.

Teidt, P.L., & Tiedt, L.M. (1990). *Multicultural teachings: A handbook of activities, information and resources (3rd ed.)*. Boston: Allyn & Bacon.

The world almanac and book of facts. (1997). New York: Press Publishing (The New York World).

Appendix

Resources for Information on Cultural Awareness

In addition to the therapy activities listed in this chapter, there are many resources available to the clinician that provide information, instruction, and education about cultural awareness. With the availability of information on the Internet, clinicians have a wealth of information at their disposal. The following list of resources includes books and website addresses for more information.

Books

Buchman D. Family Fill-In Book: Discovering Your Roots. New York: Scholastic, 1994. *A book that provides an opportunity for children to engage in discussions with parents about family history and roots.*

Hudson W. I Love My Family. New York: Scholastic, 1993. *A book for primary-age children that talks about family pride.*

Lynch E, Hanson M. Developing Cross-Cultural Competence: A Guide for Working with Young Children and Their Families. Baltimore: Brookes, 1992. *A landmark resource that provides strategies for effective cross-cultural interactions with families of young children who may be at risk for speech-language and hearing problems. Each of eight chapters describes a particular cultural group, including Anglo-European, Native American, African American, Latino, Asian, Filipino, Native Hawaiian and Pacific island, and Middle Eastern. Chapters describe geographic and historical origins, values, beliefs, and language and provide recommendations for effective cross-cultural interaction.*

Randall-David E. Strategies for Working with Culturally Diverse Communities and Clients. Baltimore: Association for the Care of Children's Health, 1989. *A guide to train project participants in learning principles applicable to working with families caring for children from diverse cultures. Exercises are provided that are designed to increase cultural awareness of the importance cultures play in shaping attitudes, values, and practices. Cultural awareness should lead to more culturally appropriate community outreach and culturally sensitive health care.*

Spector R. Cultural Diversity in Health and Illness. New Haven, CT: Appleton & Lange, 1993. *A book that discusses North American societies and describes beliefs about illness, health beliefs, and practices. It focuses on the trend toward home health care and why it is important for service providers to understand cultural backgrounds of clients and families that they serve.*

Multicultural Websites

The following is a list of websites providing information about more than 20 languages and cultures. The information provided in these websites may be of interest to people learning a language or looking for more information about a specific country or culture. *Please keep in mind that many websites change, move, or are down or discontinued; however, at the time of this writing, the websites listed in this appendix are accurate.*

Languages

http://www.writingco.com/10/PH343.html
Multicultural Art Activities Kit: Ready-to-Use Lessons and Projects with 194 Drawings, Photos, and Color Prints.

http://www.udel.edu/sine/educ/multcult.htm
Multicultural Education Resources. "Presents resources available on the Internet to support Multicultural Education."

http://www.bluepearl.com/latinlnks/index.html
Blue Pearl Latin Links.

http://www.lib.umich.edu/libhome/rrs/classes/multicul-as-lat-nat.html
Multicultural Studies—Selected Asian, Latino, and Native American Resources on the Web.

http://humanitas.ucsb.edu/shuttle/minority.html
Voice of the Shuttle: Minority Studies Page. Provides links to general resources websites and to African American, Asian American, Chicano,

Latino, Hispanic, immigrant/refugee, Jewish, Native American and Native Alaskan (also includes world indigenous and aboriginal cultures), Pacific, and other (minority cultures in Europe) websites.

http://www.echo-on.net/~sharpe/main.htm
Honouring Diversity—A Cross-Cultural Approach to Infant Development for Babies with Special Needs: A Handbook.

http://www.echo-on.net/~sharpe/nav.htm
Centennial Infant and Child Center.

http://curry.edschool.virginia.edu/go/multicultural/initial.html
Multicultural Pavilion. Provides resources on multiculturalism to educators.

http://www.cc.swarthmore.edu/Library/Interdisc/area.html
Resources in Area & Ethnic Studies. Provides links to World Wide Web, gopher, and Telnet resources of ethnic interest (African American, Asian, Latino, Native American, multicultural).

http://www.tcm.org/resources/clubhouse/thecc.html
The Computer Clubhouse. "An after-school learning environment where young people explore their own interests and become confident learners through the use of technology." Contains games and activities for children for a variety of cultures.

Bilingualism

http://www.edb.utexas.edu/coe/depts/ci/bilingue/resources.html
Bilingual Education Resources on the Internet.

http://www.estrellita.com/bil.html
Estrellita: Accelerated Beginning Spanish Reading: Bilingual Education Resources on the Net. Links readers to other Web pages that have information on bilingual education.

http://www.csusm.edu/campus_centers/csb/index.htm
Center for the Study of Books in Spanish for Children and Adolescents. Provides information on literacy materials available in Spanish for preschool through high-school children.

http://www.nvg.unit.no/~cindy/biling-fam.html
Bilingual Families Web Page. Provides parents who are raising their children bilingually with information and resources concerning bilingual language development.

http://www.ncbe.gwu.edu/
National Clearinghouse for Bilingual Education. Highlights the purpose of the organization: to collect, analyze, and disseminate information concerning the education of linguistically and culturally diverse individuals in the United States.

http://205.218.11.254/overlode/net1.html
Teacher Training for ESL Students—Multicultural Classrooms.

Hispanic Culture

gopher://latino.sscnet.ucla.edu:70/77/.index/index
Gopher search of Latino websites.

gopher://latino.sscnet.ucla.edu/diversity1.html
Latino website.

http://latino.sscnet.ucla.edu/
Building Chicana/o Latina/o Communities Through Networking.

http://latino.sscnet.ucla.edu/women/womenHP.html
Chicana Studies Web Page.

http://www.library.vanderbilt.edu/central/span.html
Resources for Spanish and Latin American languages, literature, and culture.

African American Culture

http://nuinfo.nwu.edu/registrar/nucatalog/catalog9597/cascourses/afrasilanguage.html
African and Asian Languages Program. "Offers an opportunity to explore through language study some of the fascinating cultures that are most vital for Americans to understand: those of Africa, China, Japan, Korea, and the Middle East."

http://www.rain.org/~kmw/aa.html
African American information.

http://www.gatech.edu/bgsa/blackpages/essential.html
The Universal Black Pages.

http://www.melanet.com/watoto/watoto.html
Melanet's Watoto World. Website for Children, Parents, and Educators of African Descent.

http://www.sas.upenn.edu/~africa
The African Studies Center Online.

http://www.sas.upenn.edu/African_Studies/AS.html
African Studies WWW (University of Pennsylvania).

Asian American Culture

http://latino.sscnet.ucla.edu/Asian.links.html
Asian-American Internet Sites. Provides links to listservs, websites, and newsgroups.

http://www.mit.edu:8001/afs/athena.mit.edu/user/i/r/irie/www/aar.html
Asian-American Resources.

asiarain@iss.nus.sg (e-mail)

http://www.iss.nus.sg/RND/MLP/Projects/MT/mt.html
AsiaRain Automated Translators. "Specializes in large-scale translation for technical documents and software messages from English to Chinese and other Asian Languages."

http://nuinfo.nwu.edu/registrar/nucatalog/catalog9597/cascourses/afrasilanguage.html
African and Asian Languages Program. "Offers an opportunity to explore through language study some of the fascinating cultures that are most vital for Americans to understand: those of Africa, China, Japan, Korea, and the Middle East."

Native American Culture

http://wbs.net/webchat3.so?cmd=cmd_doorway:Native_American_Chat
American Indian Chat.

http://users.aol.com/Donh523/navapage/index.html
The Flags of the Native American People of the United States.

http://www.best.com/~jantypas/aicap/visiting_artist1.html
American Indian arts page.

http://www.indians.org/
The Native American Adventure. ·